The ABC of CBC
Interpretation of Complete Blood Count and Histograms

The ABC of CBC
Interpretation of Complete Blood Count and Histograms

Second Edition

DP Lokwani MD
Former Founder Vice-Chancellor
Madhya Pradesh Medical Sciences University
Jabalpur, Madhya Pradesh, India

Professor and Head
Department of Pathology
Netaji Subhash Chandra Bose (NSCB) Medical College
Jabalpur, Madhya Pradesh, India

Former Honorary Dean (Academics)
Diplomate National Board Courses
Jabalpur Hospital and Research Center
Jabalpur, Madhya Pradesh, India

Sunit Lokwani MD DM
Consultant Hematologist and Medical Oncologist
Shalby Group of Hospitals
Jabalpur, Madhya Pradesh, India

Foreword
MB Agarwal

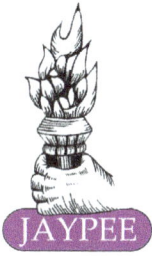

JAYPEE BROTHERS MEDICAL PUBLISHERS
The Health Sciences Publisher
New Delhi | London

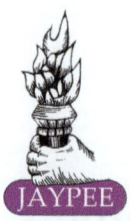 **Jaypee Brothers Medical Publishers (P) Ltd**

Headquarters
Jaypee Brothers Medical Publishers (P) Ltd
EMCA House, 23/23-B
Ansari Road, Daryaganj
New Delhi 110 002, India
Landline: +91-11-23272143, +91-11-23272703
+91-11-23282021, +91-11-23245672
Email: jaypee@jaypeebrothers.com

Corporate Office
Jaypee Brothers Medical Publishers (P) Ltd
4838/24, Ansari Road, Daryaganj
New Delhi 110 002, India
Phone: +91-11-43574357
Fax: +91-11-43574314
Email: jaypee@jaypeebrothers.com

Overseas Office
J.P. Medical Ltd
83 Victoria Street, London
SW1H 0HW (UK)
Phone: +44 20 3170 8910
Fax: +44 (0)20 3008 6180
Email: info@jpmedpub.com

Website: www.jaypeebrothers.com
Website: www.jaypeedigital.com

© 2022, Jaypee Brothers Medical Publishers

The views and opinions expressed in this book are solely those of the original contributor(s)/author(s) and do not necessarily represent those of editor(s) of the book.

All rights reserved. No part of this publication may be reproduced, stored or transmitted in any form or by any means, electronic, mechanical, photocopying, recording or otherwise, without the prior permission in writing of the publishers.

All brand names and product names used in this book are trade names, service marks, trademarks or registered trademarks of their respective owners. The publisher is not associated with any product or vendor mentioned in this book.

Medical knowledge and practice change constantly. This book is designed to provide accurate, authoritative information about the subject matter in question. However, readers are advised to check the most current information available on procedures included and check information from the manufacturer of each product to be administered, to verify the recommended dose, formula, method and duration of administration, adverse effects and contraindications. It is the responsibility of the practitioner to take all appropriate safety precautions. Neither the publisher nor the author(s)/editor(s) assume any liability for any injury and/or damage to persons or property arising from or related to use of material in this book.

This book is sold on the understanding that the publisher is not engaged in providing professional medical services. If such advice or services are required, the services of a competent medical professional should be sought.

Every effort has been made where necessary to contact holders of copyright to obtain permission to reproduce copyright material. If any have been inadvertently overlooked, the publisher will be pleased to make the necessary arrangements at the first opportunity.

Inquiries for bulk sales may be solicited at: jaypee@jaypeebrothers.com

The ABC of CBC: Interpretation of Complete Blood Count and Histograms

First Edition: 2013

Second Edition: **2022**

ISBN: 978-93-90595-98-3

Dedicated to

Babaji—*My Spiritual Master*

My Parents—*My Blessings*

My Teachers—*My Strength*

My Students—*My Treasure*

My Patients—*My Experience*

Foreword

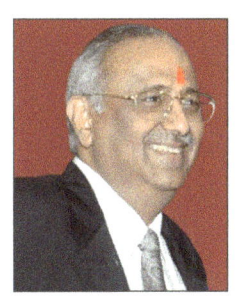

Hematology has advanced by leaps and bounds during the last two decades. Sophisticated laboratory investigations have moved from research to clinical laboratories. This is an era of polymerase chain reaction (PCR), fluorescence in situ hybridization (FISH), flow cytometry, etc. One may feel that trying to read a book dedicated to complete blood count (CBC), may not be worth the time spent. However, we teach our students that in clinical practice, history and examination of the patient are of more importance than various investigations ordered costing thousands of rupees. Similarly, a well-executed "CBC" followed by its proper interpretation has its worth in gold and a shrewd clinician can make tremendous use of this simple and cheap test for diagnosing hematological or even non-hematological disorders.

All of us order CBC as the first and unavoidable test in our clinical practice. A student also talks of CBC as a routine test without giving it any importance. To write a book on such a test is bringing back some respect to the test that it deserves.

DP Lokwani has done a laudable job in writing this book on "CBC" and histograms in the era of sophisticated laboratory techniques. I have been told that he has utilized data collected over thousands of CBCs and histograms to prepare this book and that makes the book even more important. There is no match to the knowledge generated out of the experience and this is what he has done. The book has been written based on material collected over seven long years of his huge practice and hence the information provided is useful not only to students but also to the practicing clinicians and teachers in the field of hematology, pathology, and allied branches.

I had the opportunity of going through the book which also has 30 case illustrations. This makes the discussion even more lively and practical. I have no hesitation in recommending the book to be on the shelf of everyone even remotely connected with CBC.

MB Agarwal MD MNAMS
Head
Department of Hematology
Bombay Hospital Institute of Medical Sciences
Mumbai, Maharashtra, India

Book Review

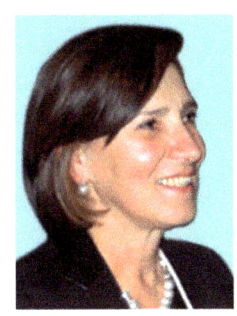

Despite the enormous advances made in immunophenotyping and cytogenetics and molecular aspects of hematology, the analysis of the composition of peripheral blood and the observation of the peripheral blood smear at the microscope remains fundamental in the diagnosis of hematological disorders, as well as in many other areas of clinical medicine. The complete blood count (CBC), in effect, has evolved during the last decades from a short-list of numerical results to a real-time representation of the functional status of hematopoiesis. New automated instruments have immensely improved the speed and reproducibility of quantitative measurement of the EDTA-anticoagulated blood. Original cellular parameters, in addition to the classical CBC and WBC differential count, have been devised and made available to the laboratory operators, such as RDW, IRF, CHr, Ret-He. Flags for abnormal cells are important to identify samples that need a microscope review, and their sensitivity and specificity are continuously improving with a reduction in the rates of false-positive and false-negative results. Such instruments, including the morphology of cell distribution in histograms and scattergrams, must be interpreted by the trained and skilled human eye and brain so that the full spectrum of diagnostic information present in such a simple analytical report is fully exploited. Thus, the study of the new methods is a necessary complement to practice for those who are approaching the laboratory hematology of the year 2000. Similarly, the knowledge of hematological pathologies and cellular aberrations in the different diseases remains a cornerstone for the interpretation.

The ABC of CBC, wisely conceived, scientifically devised, and skillfully written by DP Lokwani, represents an excellent and authoritative reference tool to answer the need for knowledge in the area of laboratory hematology.

Besides a clear and comprehensive text, the book is full of microscope cell images, diagrams, histograms, and scattergrams. It indicates to the reader the best approach to fully appreciate and exploit all the new information and the advanced diagnostic features of the current automated technologies for CBC. Throughout the pages, it is easy to appreciate the value of the wide spectrum of clinical information present in an instrumental report. In the different chapters, we find technical descriptions of diagnostic methods, often in a historical perspective (for instance, see page 7 and chapter 6), as well as a description of both the basic and the new hematological measurements. These include some valuable time-honored practical information, such as the "rule of 3" (page 12). The pages are also rich in colorful drawings, visually illustrating some otherwise abstract concepts so that the rigorous scientific approach does not impede the Author's lively creativity and artistic talent. the use of images is very important to catch the imagination, the interest, and the concentration of students and readers; a representative and vivid figure will never be forgotten. Updated scientific information also covers very specific areas, with significant practical impacts, such as the possibility of detection of malaria parasites using automated blood cell count (page 31) or the importance of osmotic changes in red cells due to hyperglycemia (page 105). Chapter 6 describes the interwoven roles of automated and manual methods, while chapter 7 gives detailed and original clues for the interpretation of cell distribution in the instrument histograms. Cell distributions in a large number of disorders are also shown and explained, from aplastic anemia to HBH disease, from iron deficiency to myelofibrosis. Chapter 10, in which the author presents 30 well-documented clinical cases selected to represent a wide range of clinical conditions is among the most valuable features of this textbook. Finally, the author does not forget that perfect technical quality of testing represents an unavoidable premise to any diagnostic observation; the last chapter thus reminds the important rules of quality control, that all laboratory operators must know and use with great attention.

"The ABC of CBC" indicates to us how correct and informed use of the automated blood cell count can represent a bridge between the traditional laboratory diagnosis of blood disorders and the latest diagnostic technologies. Discoveries and capabilities have not canceled or replaced the classical methods, but have increased their value. Even in the era of molecular medicine textbooks like this still play a central and unique role in the training of the new generation of blood professionals in laboratory hematology.

Prof. Gina Zini
Director of Blood Bank
Director of UNICATT Cord Blood Bank
Fondazione Policlinico Universitario A. Gemelli IRCCS - Roma
Università Cattolica del Sacro Cuore, Rome

Preface to the Second Edition

The second edition, a step forward from the first edition, has been derived from the marked increase in documented innovations over the last few years and their applicability in diagnostic improvisation.

Increasingly enough, medical practitioners have recognized the use of these improved techniques and equipment. I have kept the essential backbone of the informatics; the story is the same as in the previous edition.

All the old chapters have been overhauled, most of them significantly restructured, updated, and extended. There are many new sections within the updates chapter covering relevant recent advances and applications in clinical practice.

As the test menu in the clinical laboratory is complex and as computer's increasing ability to generate and interpret newer and newer parameters within the same sample of CBC is getting incorporated in the cell counter technology, it becomes a call of the times to update the commonly referred elaborate document *ABC of CBC* for the better understanding of this very basic and most demanded investigation.

Updates in this ever-evolving subject have been happening by leaps and bounds. It seemed a foolhardy mission for me to cope up with the ever-changing dynamism of the subject of CBC, with the diversity of philosophies and their products of cell counters of various brands, this homogenous take would not have been possible without the help of Dr. Sunit Lokwani, who made this exercise more workable in the available time as well as in the scientific frame.

Apart from many relevant changes and additions made to each chapter, the most liked chapter of this book "Interpretation of Histograms" has been enriched with RBC cytograms and WBC scatterograms in various disease conditions with their interpretation and practical application in diagnostic medicine.

DP Lokwani

Preface to the First Edition

Diagnosis is not the end but the beginning of practice—Martin H Fischer

The complete blood count (CBC) is one of the most frequently ordered and routinely done investigations in the hematology laboratory. It is a Pandora's Box of information, which aids in the diagnosis of a multitude of diseases and disorders in the human body. This simple investigation, aptly labeled as the "meat and potatoes of hematology", is economical, the time-honoring, minimally invasive, and exorbitantly informative.

This book is a navigation guide for students and practitioners alike related to pathology and clinical subjects, as nearly all body ailments have a direct or indirect influence on the blood picture. Hematology is all about relationships, like the relationships of the bone marrow to the systemic circulation, the plasma environment to the red cell lifespan, and hemoglobin to the red cell, so the book and you, the students and practitioners, are a vital part of this relationship.

With the changing dynamics of technology, the last decade has brought forth a radical change in hematology. The wheels of hematology have moved from predominantly manual practice to highly advanced automation. The Coulter principle and Coulter counter was a landmark in the field of hematology, and the prolific Coulter's revolutionized laboratory procedures changed the face of medicine by turning hematology guesswork into accuracy. What is needed for the novice practitioner is a way to approach interpreting the visual automated data. This skill is neither necessarily practiced at university programs, nor much of the literature is available in the racks of medical libraries dedicated to the subject of CBC in this era of automation.

The book aims to help the student bridge the gap between the classroom and clinical practice; introducing the automation principles in hematology along with interpretation and deciphering of various parameters like red cell distribution width (RDW) and histograms which carry a lot of encrypted diagnostic information because eyes can see only those things which brain knows. Although the data of the automated blood count alone will not guarantee specific diagnosis in every case, yet does every disease have a single pattern of abnormality. Rather these values should be used to narrow the differential diagnosis as much as possible, so that more expensive and time requiring, a confirmatory battery of expensive investigations like vitamin B_{12}, folic acid, serum iron, total iron-binding capacity (TIBC) estimations, or Hb electrophoresis, etc., is done only selectively and invasive procedures like bone marrow aspiration and biopsy can be avoided, by proper evaluation of CBC.

The approach of the book is as simple, straightforward, and user-friendly as possible. I hope that clinical residents and consultants will find the book useful and also the text will travel with you, as you continue your career in the laboratory profession and the information will motivate you arousing your intellectual curiosity.

Attempt is virgin, mistakes are mandatory, corrections and suggestions are solicited.

DP Lokwani

Acknowledgments

A long time back, I had this dream, a vision of presenting a book on Hematology to the members of my fraternity.

And here I am with my pristine venture, 2nd edition of *The ABC of CBC*.

First and foremost, I thank Babaji (My Spiritual Master), for giving me the ability, skill, and courage to complete this arduous task and fulfill this long-awaited dream.

Most humbly I am indebted and grateful to my mother, Mrs Heerdevi, for her incessant prayers and blessings and to my father, Mr Kishinchand Lokwani, for making me what I am today and instilling in me his virtues.

I am immensely grateful to my siblings, Shobha, Roopa, Vasu, Chandar and Pushpa, for having staunch faith in me and my capabilities.

I acknowledge my gratitude to all my teachers, both formal and informal, who have influenced my professional standing the most with a special mention to Dr PL Tandon and Dr BC Chhaparwal.

It is gratifying to be able to acknowledge at this platform my immeasurable gratitude and admiration for Dr MB Agarwal, who has been my role model and a perpetual source of inspiration.

I will fail in my duty if I don't especially mention the hardwork put in by beloved Shweta to shape the 2nd edition.

My professional growth has been nurtured by my supportive wife, Dr Lakshmi Lokwani, who made it possible for me to spend endless uninterrupted evenings at my desk, and encouraging me all the way.

I am immensely grateful to my beloved friend and my source of inspiration Dr Rajesh B Dhirawani, an eminent maxillofacial surgeon, who has guided the sails of my life towards a prosperous shore.

A very special mention to Dr Pushpraj Singh Baghel, my student, for his untiring efforts and dedication; without his support, this mammoth task would not have been completed in time. He has spent with me endless strenuous hours in the shaping and framing of the book. He has been a cardinal buttress in the foundation of the book. I consider myself extremely fortunate to have such a prized student and also thank my student Dr Apoorva.

I sincerely acknowledge the efforts and elementary research on this subject by Dr Bessman, who systematically addressed the use of histograms and dedicate to him, with deference, humility, and respect.

A special thanks to my workplace, Jabalpur Hospital and Research Center, Jabalpur, Madhya Pradesh, India, and all its consultants and patients and my colleagues at Netaji Subhash Chandra Bose (NSCB) Medical College, Jabalpur, Madhya Pradesh, India, and Mahatma Gandhi Memorial (MGM) Medical College, Indore, Madhya Pradesh, India.

Most importantly, my beloved children, Anita, Manisha, Hitesh, Kavneet, and my dearest granddaughter Kavya, for being my source of energy. I will fail in my duty if I don't especially mention the hard work and skilled efforts put in by my daughter-in-law Dr Shweta Lokwani to shape the 2nd edition.

It will be lapse on my part if I don't appreciate the cooperation and contribution of cell counter research and manufacturing giants Siemens, Mindray, Abbott, Sysmex, and others.

Gratitude towards all the students, practicing doctors, and all readers who have taught me so much about laboratory medicine and inspired me to bring forward this second edition.

Sincere thanks to Prof Gina Zini of Rome for her very sincere review with expert guidance.

I am extremely grateful to M/s Jaypee Brothers Medical Publishers (P) Ltd, New Delhi, India, for giving me this opportunity to dissipate my work to the people of my fraternity.

Contents

1. **Introduction and Significance of CBC** 1

2. **Red Blood Cells** 5
   Red Blood Cells *5*
   - Erythrocyte (RBC) *5*

   Hemoglobin *7*
   Reticulocyte *9*
   Hematocrit—Packed Cell Volume (PCV) *11*
   Mean Corpuscular Volume *13*
   Mean Corpuscular Hemoglobin *14*
   Mean Corpuscular Hemoglobin Concentration (MCHC) *14*
   Red Cell Distribution Width *15*

3. **RBCs on Peripheral Smear** 18
   - Peripheral Blood Smear Preparation *18*
   - Peripheral Blood Smear Examination *18*

   RBCs on Peripheral Smear *19*
   - Clinical Importance of RBC Morphology *19*

   Hemoparasites *27*
   - Malaria Parasite *27*
   - Diagnosis of Malaria *27*
   - Filariasis *33*

4. **White Blood Cells** 35
   White Blood Cell Count *35*
   - Leukocytosis—High WBC Count *35*
   - Stages of Leukocyte Maturation *36*

   Polymorphs *38*
   - Leukemoid Reaction *42*

   Eosinophils *44*
   Basophils *44*
   - Monocytes *45*
   - Lymphocytes *46*

5. **Platelets** 50
   Platelet Count *50*
   - Causes of Thrombocytopenia *51*

   Disorders of Platelets *54*
   Mean Platelet Volume *55*
   Platelet Distribution Width *56*
   Plateletcrit *56*
   Immature Platelet Fraction (IPF) *56*

6. **Manual versus Automation in Hematology** 60
   - Sample Collection for Complete Blood Cell *61*
   - Collection of Blood Smear Direct from Finger *61*
   - Manual Cell Counting (WBC, RBC and Platelet) *62*
   - Hematology Automation *63*
   - Role of Flow Cytometry in Laboratory Medicine *66*

- Application of Laser Light to Identify Cell Types 66
- Fluorescent Dyes Augmentation of Flow Cytometry 67
- Hydrodynamic Focusing 69

7. General Principle of Histogram Generation and Interpretation 71
- General Principle of Histogram Generation 71

Statistical Definitions 72

Histogram In Hematology 73
- Histogram Characteristics 73

8. RBC Histogram and Cytogram 75

The Volume Histogram for Erythrocytes 76
- Abnormal RBC Histograms and Red Cell Flags 77
- RBC Cytogram 80

9. WBC and Platelet Histogram and Scatterogram 107

The Volume Histogram for WBCs 107
- Flagging and Abnormal WBC Histogram 108
- Various Types of WBC Histograms 111
- The Volume Histogram for Platelets 113
- Scatter Plots (Scattergram) 115

Dual WBC - Perox and Basolobularity Methods 117
- Peroxidase Staining 117
- Perox Method 117
- Baso Method 118

Platelet Scatter Cytogram 122

10. Case Studies 123
Case 1: Improper Collection: Spurious Results 124
Case 2: Iron Deficiency Anemia 125
Case 3: Beta Thalassemia Major 126
Case 4: Beta Thalassemia Minor 127
Case 5: Heterozygous Alpha Thalassemia 128
Case 6: Sickle Cell Anemia 129
Case 7: Megaloblastic Anemia–Vitamin B_{12} Deficiency 130
Case 8: Megaloblastic Anemia–Vitamin B_{12} Deficiency (Post-Therapy) 131
Case 9: Chronic Macrocytic Anemia—Drug Induced 132
Case 10: Red Cell Fragmentations 133
Case 11: Hemolytic Disease of Newborn 134
Case 12: Cold Agglutinins 135
Case 13: Aplastic Anemia 136
Case 14: Recovery from Aplastic Anemia 137
Case 15: Bimodal RBC Curve-Transfusion Related 138
Case 16: Acute Lymphocytic Leukemia 139
Case 17: Septicemia 140
Case 18: Multiple Myeloma 141
Case 19: Acute Myeloid Leukemia (FAB – M1) 142
Case 20: Chronic Lymphocytic Leukemia 143
Case 21: Acute Myeloid Leukemia (FAB – M4) 144
Case 22: CML in Blast Crisis 145
Case 23: Infectious Mononucleosis 146
Case 24: Myelodysplasia 147
Case 25: Cytotoxic Chemotherapy 148

Case 26: Eosinophilia *149*
Case 27: EDTA-induced Platelet Agglutination (EIPA) *150*
Case 28: Essential (Primary) Thrombocythemia *151*
Case 29: Thrombocytopenic Purpura *152*
Case 30: Coagulopathy (DIC) *153*

11. Quality Control 154
- Quality Assurance in the Hematology Laboratory *154*
- Purpose of Quality Control (QC) *154*
- Indirect Quality Control *154*
- Direct Quality Control *155*
- Standards or Calibrators *158*
- Controls *158*
- Analysis of QC Data *159*
- Specimen-related Problems *160*
- Instrument Problems and Troubleshooting *160*
- Sources of Error in Cell Counts *161*
- Quality Control—Review of Histograms *162*
- Variations Observed in WBC Histogram *162*
- Variations Observed in Platelet Histogram *162*

Suggested Reading 165

Index 167

Glossary of Terms Employed in Automation and Hematology

- **Anisochromia:** Variation of hemoglobinization of cells.
- **Anisopoikilocytosis:** Anisocytosis is variation of cell size more than normal. Poikilocytosis is variation of cell shape. In practice, the two terms are used as a single phrase "anisopoikilocytosis" means variation of cell size and shape.
- **Aperture:** A small opening in a device by which blood cells may be drawn into an analyzer for counting.
- **Backlighting:** An alert mechanism to visualize a potential problem or an error. The instrument can highlight a parameter that falls outside the reference interval.
- **Cluster Analysis:** A type of analysis that is based upon the instrument's ability to cluster different cell populations together based upon size, staining characteristics, absorption characteristics and other parameters. The analysis of abnormal cell populations is accomplished.
- **Coincidence:** When two or more cells pass through an aperture at the same time and are counted as a single cell.
- **Continuous Flow Analysis:** Analysis of cells that flow past a laser beam and is based upon the cellular characteristics.
- **Contour Grating:** A means of analysis where information is plotted on an x-, y-, and z-axis. The result is a three-dimensional plot that can separate subpopulations of cells.
- **Coulter Principle:** Sizing and counting cells by detecting and measuring changes in electrical resistance when a cell passes through a small aperture.
- **Cytometry:** Measurement of the cell can be visual or automated.
- **Diffraction:** The ability of a light beam to break up into its component parts as it bends across the surface of a cell. Light is bent to project at a new angle.
- **Dimorphic:** Two populations of cells in a single sample of blood.
- **EDTA:** Anticoagulant commonly used for hematologic studies.
- **Electrical Impedance:** Cell counting principle is dependent upon the detection and measurement of changes in the electrical resistance produced by cells in a conduction solution as they move through an aperture.
- **Erythropoiesis:** The process of RBC production in the bone marrow.
- **Flow Cell:** A structure made of quartz. Quartz is transparent and does not bend the light that passes through it. It also allows ultraviolet light to pass through. Glass does not have these two properties. The counting of the cells and their evaluation occurs in the flow cell.
- **Forward Angle Light Scatter:** Light from a laser source is scattered in a forward direction (at a zero degree angle) when it strikes a cell or particle. The larger the object, then there is more forward light scatter.
- **Forward High Angle Light Scatter:** Similar to forward angle light scatter, except the forward direction is with a 5 to15° variation.
- **Forward Low Angle Light Scatter:** Similar to forward angle light scatter, except the forward direction is with a 2 to 3 degree variation.
- **Hemoglobinopathy:** Amino acid abnormality of the globin component of the hemoglobin molecule.
- **Hemolysis:** Accelerated destruction of the "short-lived" RBCs. It may be due to intrinsic (defect of the red cell itself) or extrinsic (destructive environment) causes.
- **Histogram:** A visualization graph that can be created based upon cell size and/or cell number and can indicate frequency of distribution.
- **Hydrodynamic Focusing:** The ability of an analyzer to create a gradient differential and cause cells and/or particles to flow in a single column in which a central column of the sample fluid flows inside a column of sheath fluid. The laminar flow physics principles cause the sample stream to flow in a narrow lumen and at a rate faster than the sheath fluid. This narrowing phenomenon allows the cells to separate and align into a single file for passage through the sensory zone of the flow cell.
- **Hypoproliferative:** Quantitative decreased blood cell formation, also known as hypoplastic, the extreme of which is aplastic.
- **Isovolumetric Sphering:** A technique in which cells are placed in a buffered diluent that results in each cell becoming spherical, without altering the volume of the cell.
- **Laminar Flow:** A mathematical and physical term that describes the flow properties of fluids as they move through a tubular system. In laminar flow, particles will flow in parallel lines and are dependent of flow velocity, channel diameter, and fluid density.

- **Laser Light:** Monochromatic light or light of a single wavelength or frequency that is intense and small with the tendency to radiate as an almost non-divergent beam.
- **Light Scatter:** A light phenomenon that is composed of three independent processes that include diffraction, reflection, and refraction. The light scatter is actually in all directions. Diffraction is light that is bent at small angles relative to the light source. Refraction is that light bent at large angles to the light source.
- **Linearity Limits:** The instrument will be accurate as long as the results fall within a certain range known as the linearity range. Linearity ranges vary by instrument.
- **Morphology:** Description of cell size, shape, color, contour, etc., by light or electron microscopy or flow cytometry.
- **Myelophthisic:** Literal meaning consumption of marrow. It is the replacement of marrow by granuloma, tumor, or fibrous tissue (myelofibrosis), resulting in hypoproliferative marrow with presence of premature cells in peripheral blood.
- **Myeloproliferative:** Increased abnormal marrow production, it includes polycythemia vera, CML, essential thrombocythemia, etc., but not the acute leukemias.
- **Optical Scatter:** A cell counting principle that employs both laser and nonlaser light. The cell is identified and differentiated on the basis of light scatter and effects when it strikes the cell.
- **Parameter:** A statistical term that refers to any numerical value that describes an entire population.
- **Random Access:** Technological capability of an analyzer to process patient specimens independent of each other or to perform individual runs or panel of tests.
- **Reagent Blank:** The reagents and diluents (minus the patient specimen) that measure the degree of absorbance to eliminate false increases (due to reagent color) in the actual patient sample.
- **Reflection:** Forward light rays are bent or turned backward as the result of striking an obstruction.
- **Refraction:** The light beam or rays bend because of a change in speed and move in an oblique direction when passing from one medium into another because of changes in density.
- **Scatter Plots:** A two dimensional dot-plot histogram that allows definition of subpopulations of cells, in particular leukocytes.
- **Sheath Fluid:** Usually a 0.85% saline solution, it is the fluid that fills the flow cell and surrounds the sample stream as it passes through the flow cell. The sheath fluid keeps the flow cell clean, preventing the accumulation of reagents, cell debris, and any other substance onto the surface of the flow cell that would interfere with the laser light analysis. The sheath fluid also facilitates hydrodynamic focusing.
- **Side Light Scatter:** Also called "orthogonal light scatter", this is laser light that is scattered away from the cell at a 90°degree angle. This is caused due to internal granularity of the cell. The more numerous the granules, the more there is side scatter.
- **Threshold Limit:** A limit imposed that will selectively eliminate or include cells of certain sizes to be counted. For the cell counter, it is the minimal electrical signal that will produce a pulse that will include a cell in the total count.

CHAPTER 1

Introduction and Significance of CBC

INTRODUCTION

The subject of Hematology (the Greek word "haima" meaning "blood") has grown by leaps and bounds ever since the invention of the microscope. Hematology is a unique super-specialty in Medicine that encompasses the fields of Pathology, Physiology, Molecular Biology, Biochemistry, Obstetrics and Gynecology, Medicine, and Pediatrics.

The era of diagnosis has changed from simple microscopy and manual methodologies to complex automated counters, application of cytogenetics, flow cytometry, and molecular technology.

The basic test performed on the peripheral blood – "Complete Blood Count" (CBC) is one of the most informative single investigations, expressing the health and disease status of the body, in the whole menu of laboratory medicine. A long journey is travelled by this single investigation from the era of only hematocrit/hemoglobin as a diagnostic tool to the most sophisticated multi-parts multi-parameters automation.

Automation, because of its accuracy, has changed the principles and methodologies, approaches, and conclusions of various disciplines of medicine. Few branches are modified to the extent that their entire philosophy is so much reoriented that it needs to be rewritten and hematology is one of them. Although the fact remains that, automation is no replacement for the study of a peripheral smear, it just compliments manual microscopy, just like ECG and X-ray chest compliments manual auscultation in clinical medicine.

Over the past 5 decades, hematology analyzers have evolved from semiautomated to fully automated ones. Many additional parameters have become available now. From the earlier instruments that used electrical impedance as the sole counting principle for blood cells, modern-day analyzers, also, use conductivity differences, cytochemical staining, light scatter, and flow cytometric principles. While enhancing the speed, accuracy, and precision of test results, these have also added a new dimension to hematology reporting. However, even in the wake of much technological advancement, the attention to numerical data with regards to the interpretation of test results has not changed.

As the automated analyzers become more advanced, their precision has shown enormous improvement and manual blood smear review rates have been on a steady decline. Still, many hematologists and trainee residents in laboratories have been performing a validation function rather than an interpretative one. An experienced reviewer can weigh the relative significance of observed findings and assess their importance within the context of other clinical data. A trained eye will also appreciate other morphological abnormalities that may be undetected by automated review.

Hematology analyzers are marketed by multiple instrument manufacturers with varying levels of sophistication and technical complexity. These analyzers are equipped to produce, not only the traditional RBC, WBC, Platelet parameters but also many research and clinically important reportable parameters, along with three part, five-part, or six-part differential leukocyte count in less than one minute with a micro-volume of whole blood. Leucocyte positional parameters, which may diagnose specific diseases (e.g. differentiate between abnormal lymphocytes in leukemia and viral conditions and may also detect malarial infection) are now available.

Automated analyzer principles of operation, vary technologically. Electronic impedance and optical scatter are used by most of the analyzers. Sometimes Radiofrequency (RF) is used in conjunction with other methods. RF signals are proportionate to cell interior density or conductivity. Impedance and conductivity plotted against two-dimensional distribution cytogram or scatterplot, to evaluate cell populations with cluster analysis technology.

Flow cytometers with optical scatter system detect interference in a laser beam or light source to differentiate and evaluate cell types. The use of peroxidase (PEROX) and basophil - lobularity (BASO) channels, further improvises the generated results. Most of the sophisticated cell counters perform reticulocyte analysis using either fluorescent or other dyes. Limitations of the instruments result in specific flagging, which warrants evaluation with an alternative methodology.

There is a need for hematologists to give more clinically useful diagnostic opinions and further evaluation guidelines on blood samples run on automated analyzers instead of signing out a parameter-littered automated report printout.

In automation generated CBC reports, graphical representation of results in the form of histograms or scatter plots, red cell distribution width (RDW), hemoglobin distribution width (HDW), and reticulocyte hemoglobin, immature platelet fraction, etc., have been largely ignored in favor of traditional numerical parameters over the years. These CBC parameters are very important as they provide useful information for the precise diagnosis and management of the patient.

What is CBC?

A complete blood count (CBC) is a series of tests used to evaluate the composition and concentration of the various cellular components of blood. It consists of the following tests:
- Red blood cell (RBC) count, white blood cell (WBC) count, and platelet count.
- Measurement of hemoglobin and calculation of hematocrit and red blood cell indices.
- White blood cells (WBC) total and differential count.
- Platelet count, mean platelet volume, plateletcrit, PDW, etc.
- Histograms, cytograms, scatterplots of RBC, WBC and platelets, etc.

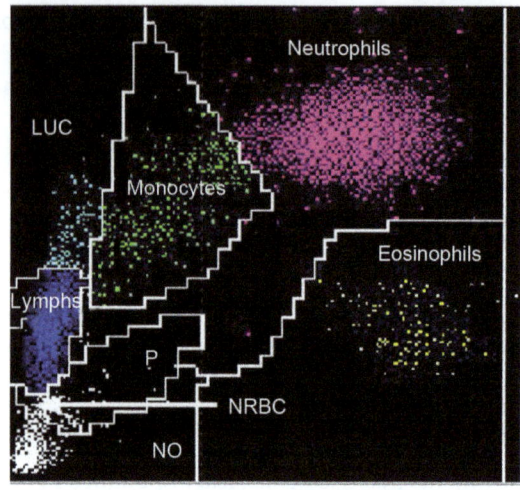

Courtesy: © Siemens Healthcare GmbH 2020

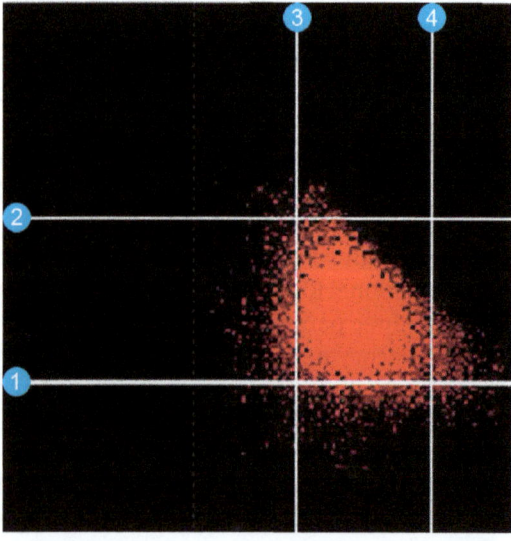

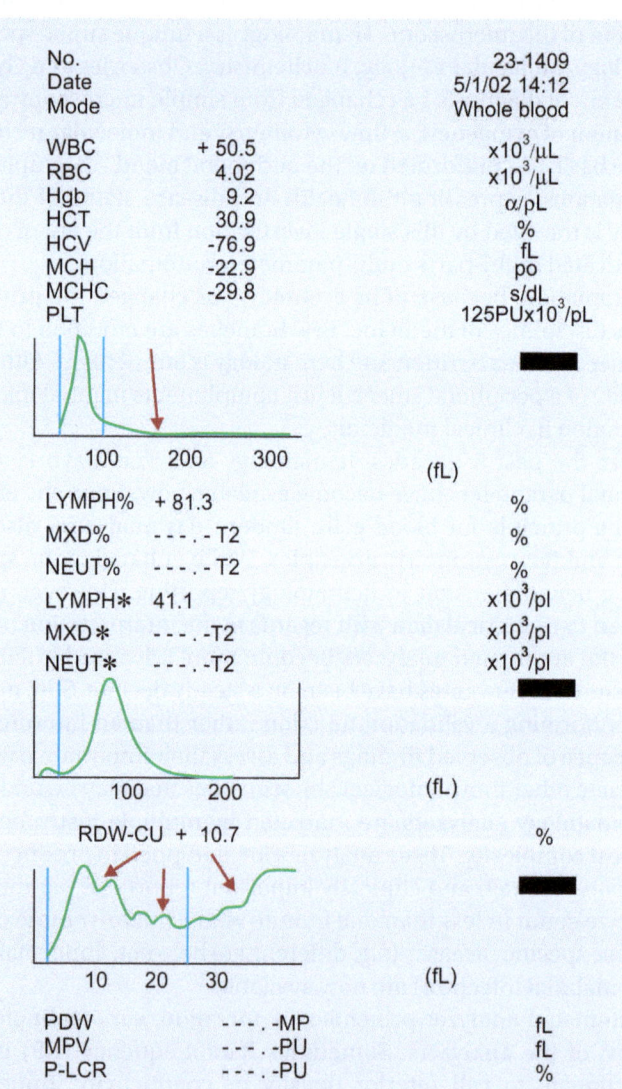

How Important is CBC?
To know the importance of CBC we need to know: • What is CBC? • What are the variations in CBC parameters? • Why CBC? • What these variations can tell us? • What are the various parameters of CBC? • How these variations affect the assessment and care of patients?

Why CBC?

CBC is a comparatively inexpensive but powerful diagnostic tool in a variety of hematological and non-hematological conditions. It provides a myriad of valuable information about blood and to some extent the bone marrow, and also some direct or indirect shreds of evidence of health and disease status of various systems of the body. CBC is a window into the functional status of the bone marrow, the factory producing all blood elements. It is easily obtained, easily performed, relatively cheap, and serial measurements can evaluate response to therapy. The CBC may be used as informative tool for various sets of situations like:

- Diagnosis of anemia (Etiological and morphological types)
- Hemoglobinopathies (Thalassemia, sickle cell anemia, and hemolytic anemia)
- Bone marrow aplasia (Single lineage and multilineage)
- Nutritional deficiencies (Iron, vitamin B_{12}, folic acid)
- Parasitemia (Malaria, filaria, leishmania)
- Thrombocytopenia [Primary (due to nonproduction), secondary (due to peripheral destruction) and bleeding disorders]
- Various viral fevers, and autoimmune conditions
- To diagnose infections, leukocytosis, leukopenia, eosinophilia, monocytosis, lymphocytosis, etc.
- Various hematopoietic malignancies like leukemias, various dysplasias like myelodysplastic syndrome, spillage of lymphoproliferative solid tumors, metastatic malignancies
- To diagnose the effect of various drugs including chemotherapy and radiation therapy and effects of various toxins and chemicals
- To diagnose effect of various types of stresses like traumatic, metabolic, neoplastic, and surgical stresses.

To conclude, it may be emphasized that not all hematological and nonhematological disorders can be diagnosed after an automated analysis of CBC but some direct or indirect, indicative, or diagnostic feature may be picked up by the instrument or on a peripheral smear. Along with numerical data, the histograms and scattergrams from automated hematology analyzers provide valuable information regarding common hematological conditions. It is important that operators and the end-users must have a basic understanding of the graphical output while interpreting their numerical data. This can enhance the diagnostic utility of automated data, ultimately benefiting the patient with better diagnosis and outcome.

Various Parameters of CBC

About 33 parameters can be obtained by most sophisticated counters (observed and calculated), which include:

RBC parameters	WBC parameters	Platelet parameters
• rBC count	• WBC count	• PLATELET count
• Hgb	• NEUT%	• MPV
• Hct	• LYMPH%	• Pct
• MCV	• MONO%	• PDW
• MCH	• EO%	• IPF-Immature platelet fraction (measurement of reticulated platelets) to monitor thrombopoietic activity of the marrow
• MCHC	• BASO%	
• RDW-SD	• NEUT#	
• RDW-CV	• LYMPH #	
• NRBC	• MONO#	• HPC-Quantitative hematopoietic progenitor cell count as a screen for the optimal presence of hematopoietic progenitor cells in peripheral blood and cord blood samples
• NRBC#	• EO#	
• RET%	• BASO#	
• RET#	• Immature Granulocyte Count (IG)%	
• IRF (Immature Reticulocyte Fraction)	• Immature Granulocyte Count (IG)#	
• RET-He	• Neutrophil volume (NV)	• Mean platelet component (MPC).
• Fragmented Red Cells	• Neutrophil granularity index.	• Platelet larger cell ratio (P-LCR).
• Reticulocyte hemoglobin content (CHr)	• Neutrophil reactivity intensity (Neut-Ri)	• Platelet component distribution width (PCDW)
• RBC Hemoglobin Content (RBC He)	• Neutrophil granularity intensity (Neut-Gi)	
• Mean Reticulocyte Volume (MCVr)	• Reactive lymphocytes (Re-lymp)	• Mean platelet component (MPC)
• %MACRO	• Antibody-synthesizing lymphocytes (As-lymp)	
• %MICRO		
• %HYPER	• Large Immature Cells	
• %HYPO	• Large Undifferentiated Cells (LUC)	
• Low Fluorescence Reticulocytes (LFR)		
• Medium Fluorescence Reticulocytes (MFR)		
• High Fluorescence Reticulocytes (HFR)		
(# = absolute count, % = percent count)		

Chapter 1: Introduction and Significance of CBC

Normal Values of Various Parameters of CBC

CBC values vary by age, sex, race, and demography. Normal values (reference range) are ultimately determined by the laboratory performing the test in the particular population. As a guide, the normal values for men and women are as follows:

RBC parameters

- RBC count: 4.2–5.0 × 10^6/mm^3 for women, 4.6–6 × 10^6/mm^3 for men
- Hemoglobin: 12.0–15.8 g/dL for women, 13.3–16.2 g/dL for men
- Hematocrit: 35.4–44.4% for women, 38.8–46.4% for men
- Mean corpuscular volume (MCV): 79–98 fL
- Mean corpuscular hemoglobin (MCH): 26.7–31.9 pg
- Mean corpuscular hemoglobin concentration (MCHC): 32–36%
- Red cell distribution width (RDW-CV): 11.5–14.5%
- Red cell distribution width (RDW-SD): 35–45 fL
- Reticulocyte count: 0.8–2.3%

WBC parameters

- Total WBCs: 4,500–11,000/mm^3 for women and men
- Neutrophils: 50–70%
- Lymphocytes: 25–35%
- Monocytes: 4–6%
- Eosinophils: 1–3%
- Basophils: 0.4–1%
- Bands: 0–5%

Platelet parameters

- Platelets: 150000–450000/mm^3
- Mean platelet volume: 7.4–10.4 fL
- Platelet distribution width: 9–13 fL
- Plateletcrit: 0.108–0.282

Various Indices by Age Group and Conditions

Newborn		
	Normal range	*SI unit*
Hematocrit	42–68%	0.42–0.68%
Hemoglobin	15.4–24.5 g/dL	9.6–15.3 mmol/L
RBC count	4.1–6.2 million/µL	4.1–6.2 × 10^{12}/L
MCV	103–106 µ^3	103–106 fL
MCH	36–38 pg	2.24–2.37 fmol
MCHC	34–36 %	21.10–22.34 mmol/L
Platelets	100000–300000/µL or mm^3	100–300 × 10^9/L

Up to one year of age		
	Normal range	*SI unit*
Hematocrit	29–41%	0.29–0.42%
Hemoglobin	9.0–14.5 g/dL	5.6–9.1 mmol/L
RBC count	3.6–5.5 million/µL	3.6–5.5 10^{12}/L
MCV	78 µ^3	78 fL
MCH	25 pg	1.55 fmol
MCHC	32%	19.86 mmol/L

Pregnancy		
	Normal range	*SI unit*
Hematocrit		
Trimester 1	35–46 %	0.35–0.46%
Trimester 2	30–42 %	0.30–0.42%
Trimester 3	34–44 %	0.34–0.44%
RBC count		
Trimester 1	4.0–5.0 million/µL	4.0–5.0 × 10^{12}/L
Trimester 2	3.2–4.5 million/µL	3.2–4.5 × 10^{12}/L
Trimester 3	3.0–4.9 million/µL	3.0–4.9 × 10^{12}/L

CHAPTER 2

Red Blood Cells

RED BLOOD CELLS

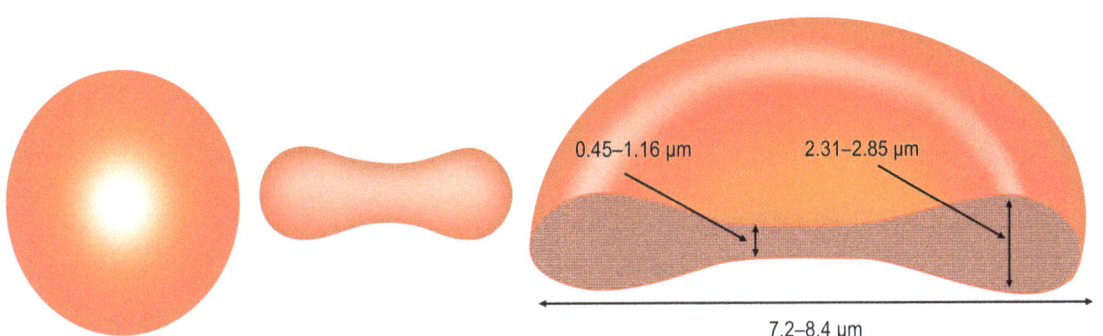

The diagram of red blood cell including cross section.

ERYTHROCYTE (RBC)

- RBCs are produced in the bone marrow with the help of metals (iron, cobalt, manganese), vitamins (B_{12}, B_6, C, E, folate, riboflavin, pantothenic acid, thiamine), and amino acids.
- Erythropoiesis is regulated by erythropoietin, thyroid hormone, and androgens.
- The biconcave erythrocyte is thinner in the middle, creating a central pallor on blood smears that is ordinarily less than 1/3rd of the cell's diameter. Such a cell, possessing the normal amount of hemoglobin, is called normochromic.
- The mature red blood cell (also known as an erythrocyte) carries oxygen attached to the iron present in hemoglobin.
- The mature red blood cell is an anucleate structure with no capacity to synthesize protein, yet it is capable of a limited metabolism, which enables it to survive for 120 days.
- Assessment of the RBC is to check for anemia and to evaluate normal erythropoiesis (the production of red blood cells).
- The number of red blood cells is determined by age, sex, altitude, exercise, diet, pollution, drug use, tobacco/nicotine use, kidney function, health and disease status, etc.
- The clinical importance of the test is that it is a measure of the oxygen carrying capacity of the blood.

Normal Red Blood Cells Values at Various Ages	
♦ Newborn	: 4.1–6.1 million/mm³
♦ Children	: 3.6–5.5 million/mm³
♦ Adult	: (Males): 4.6–6.0 million/mm³
	: (Females): 4.2–5.0 million/mm³
♦ Pregnancy	: Slightly lower than normal adult values

Broadly, the causes of decreased RBC count may be classified as:
- Impaired red blood cell (RBC) production
- Increased RBC destruction (hemolytic anemias)
- Blood loss
- Fluid overload (hemodilution).

(I) Decreased RBC Count Due to Impaired Production

- **Disturbance of proliferation and differentiation of stem cells:**
  - Pure red cell aplasia
  - Aplastic anemia (affecting all kinds of blood cells)
  - Fanconi anemia (a hereditary disorder featuring aplastic anemia and other abnormalities)
  - Anemia of renal failure (insufficient erythropoietin production)
  - Anemia of endocrine disorders
- **Disturbance of proliferation and maturation of erythroblasts:**
  - Pernicious anemia (macrocytic anemia due to impaired absorption of vitamin B_{12})
  - Anemia of folic acid and vitamin B_{12} deficiency (megaloblastic anemia)
  - Anemia of prematurity (diminished erythropoietin response in premature infants)
  - Iron deficiency anemia (resulting in deficient heme synthesis)
  - Thalassemias (causing deficient globin synthesis)
  - Anemia of renal failure (erythropoietin deficiency)
- **Other mechanisms of impaired RBC production:**
  - Myelodysplastic syndrome
  - Anemia of chronic inflammation
  - Myelophthisic anemia or Myelophthisis (a severe type of anemia resulting from the replacement of bone marrow by malignant tumors or granulomas)

(II) Decreased RBC Count Due to Increased Destruction: Hemolytic Disorders

- **Intrinsic (intracorpuscular) abnormalities**
  (Where the red blood cells have defects that cause premature destruction)
  - Hereditary spherocytosis (a hereditary membrane defect, causing RBC to be sequestered by the spleen)
  - Hereditary elliptocytosis(defect in membrane skeleton proteins)
  - Abetalipoproteinemia (causing defects in membrane lipids)
  - Enzyme deficiencies
    - Pyruvate kinase and hexokinase deficiencies (causing defective glycolysis)
    - Glucose-6-phosphate dehydrogenase deficiency (causing increased oxidative stress)
  - Hemoglobinopathies
    - Sickle cell anemia
    - Hemoglobinopathies causing unstable hemoglobins
  - Paroxysmal nocturnal hemoglobinuria
- **Extrinsic (extracorpuscular) abnormalities**
  - Antibody-mediated
    - Warm autoimmune hemolytic anemia is an anemia caused by autoimmune attack against red blood cells, primarily by IgG
    - It is the most common of the autoimmune hemolytic diseases. It can be idiopathic, drug-associated or secondary to systemic lupus erythematosus, or a malignancy, such as chronic lymphocytic leukemia (CLL)
    - Cold agglutinin hemolytic anemia (IgM mediated,can be idiopathic or secondary)
    - Hemolytic disease of the newborn
    - Mismatch transfusion reactions
  - Mechanical trauma to red cells
    - Microangiopathic hemolytic anemias including TTP, HUS
    - Disseminated intravascular coagulation (DIC)
    - Infections, including malaria
    - Prosthetic valve/heart surgery

(III) Decreased RBC Count Due to Blood Loss

- Trauma or surgery, causing acute blood loss
- Gastrointestinal tract lesions (causing chronic blood loss)
- Gynecologic disturbances (also generally causing chronic blood loss)
- Hypervolemia causes spurious low RBC count (due to hemodilution)

(IV) Causes of High Red Blood Cell Count

- Polycythemia vera (often a hereditary problem)
- Excessive smoking
- High altitudes
- Renal neoplasia (the kidneys are producing too much erythropoietin)
- Heart failure or some heart diseases
- Lung diseases like emphysema, pulmonary fibrosis, etc.
- Dehydration
- Erythropoietin doping by athletes to boost their performance
- Hemoglobinopathies
- Adrenal cortical hyperfunction
- Anabolic metabolism

HEMOGLOBIN

- Hemoglobin is the oxygen-carrying component of the red cell. Each organ in the human body depends on oxygenation for growth and function.
- By measuring the hemoglobin concentration of the blood, the oxygen-carrying capacity of the blood is evaluated.
- Both high and low hemoglobin counts indicate defects in the balance of red blood cells, and may indicate disease.
- Hemoglobin is synthesized at the polychromatic normoblast stage of red cell development.
- This synthesis is visualized by the change in cytoplasmic color from a deep blue to a lavender-tinged cytoplasmic color.
  - The hemoglobin molecule consists of two primary structures:
  - Heme portion and globin portion.
  - Each heme molecule consists of four heme structures with iron at the center and two pairs of globin chains.
- The normal range for hemoglobin is highly age and sex-dependent with men having higher values than women and adults having higher values than children except neonates which have the highest value of all.
  - Hemoglobin, bound to O_2 gives RBCs their "chrom" color; therefore variations in hemoglobin are referred to as "chromic" changes.

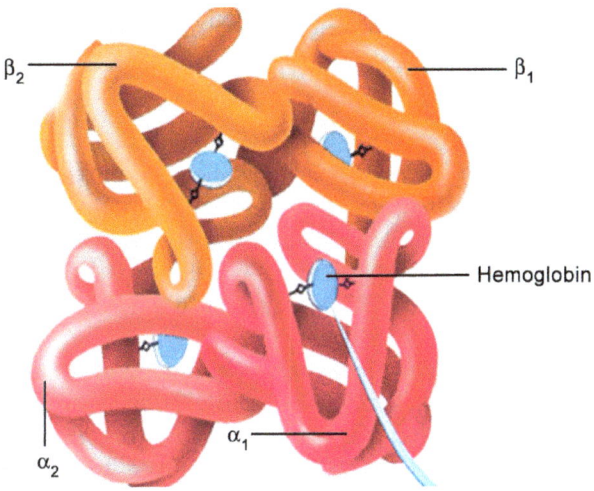

| Hemoglobin normal range | Male 13.3–16.2 g/L | Female 12.0–15.8 g/L |

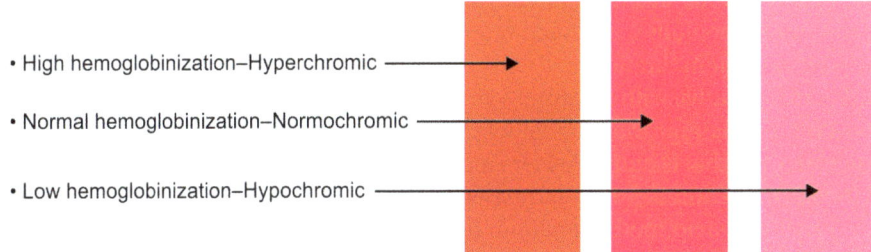

- High hemoglobinization–Hyperchromic
- Normal hemoglobinization–Normochromic
- Low hemoglobinization–Hypochromic

Hemoglobin Concentration Measurement

To measure hemoglobin concentration (Hb), a known volume of well-mixed whole blood is added to a diluent which lyses red cells to produce a hemoglobin solution. Lysis occurs because of the hypotonicity of the diluent, but may be accelerated by the inclusion in the diluent of a nonionic detergent to act as a lytic agent. The Hb is determined from the light absorbance (optical density) of the solution of hemoglobin or its derivative at a selected wavelength.

Cyanmethemoglobin Method

The International Council for Standardization in Hematology (ICSH) has recommended a reference method in which hemoglobin is converted to cyanmethemoglobin.

Method

The basis of the method is the dilution of blood in the solution of potassium cyanide and potassium ferricyanide.

A volume of 20 μL of blood is added to 5.0 mL of diluents (1:250), mixed well, and allowed to stand at room temperature for at least 5 minutes the absorbance is measured, against the reagent blank, in the photocalorimeter at 540 nm and compared against the absorbance of HiCN standard. Calculate the Hb concentration by

Hb (g/dL) = (Test sample abs./Standard abs) × Concentration of standard × Dilution factor.

Advantages

- Hemoglobin, methemoglobin, and carboxyhemoglobin are all converted to cyanmethemoglobin and are therefore included in the measurement.

- Cyanmethemoglobin has an absorbance band at 540 nm, which is broad and relatively flat and thus measurements can be made either on a narrow-band spectrophotometer or on a filter photometer or colorimeter that reads over a wide band of wavelengths.
- (Stable secondary) International Standard are readily available for calibration.

Disadvantages

- The presence of sulfhemoglobin will lead to a slight underestimation of total hemoglobin.
- The slow conversion of carboxyhemoglobin to methemoglobin.
- The maximum possible error that could be caused if 20% of the hemoglobin were in the form of carboxyhemoglobin, a degree of abnormality that may be found in heavy smokers, would be 6%.
- Increased turbidity causes a factitiously elevated estimate of Hb.....
  - **When the WBC is high**, turbidity effects are circumvented by centrifugation or filtration of the solution prior to reading the absorbance.
  - **When turbidity is due to a high level of plasma protein** (either when a paraprotein is present or when there is polyclonal hypergammaglobulinemia resulting from severe chronic infection or inflammation), it can be cleared by the addition of either potassium carbonate or a drop of 25% ammonia solution.
  - **When turbidity is due to hyperlipidemia**, the lipid can be removed by diethyl ether extraction and centrifugation.
  - **When turbidity is due to red cells containing hemoglobin S or C**, which may fail to lyse in the diluent and, produces a factitiously high reading of Hb making a 1:1 dilution in distilled water ensures complete lysis of osmotically resistant cells.

Other Methods

Alternative methods of measuring Hb are not widely used except when they have been incorporated into hemoglobinometers. Such methods usually require standardization by reference back to a cyanmethemoglobin standard.

- Hb can be measured as hematin produced under alkaline conditions. The alkaline–hematin method measures carboxyhemoglobin, sulfhemoglobin and methemoglobin, although it does not adequately measure hemoglobin F or hemoglobin Bart's, which are resistant to alkaline denaturation.
- Hemoglobin can be converted into a sulfated derivative with maximum absorbance at 534 nm by the addition of sodium lauryl sulfate. Conversion is almost instantaneous and methemoglobin, but not sulfhemoglobin, is converted. This method correlates well with the reference method that is employed for calibration. This method is suitable for use with a spectrophotometer and has also been incorporated into several automated instruments.
- Hb can also be measured following conversion to acid methemoglobin by the addition of sodium nitrate and sodium azide. This is the method permit compensation for turbidity.
- Hb can be measured as oxyhemoglobin; in this case concentration of carboxyhemoglobin, sulfhemoglobin and methemoglobin will not be measured accurately.
- Acid hematin method (Sahli's hemoglobinometer) is commonly used but less reliable.

Hemoglobin Measurement by Sahli Acid Hematin Method

Materials required for Hb measurement:
- Distilled water.
- Sahli-Hellige hemoglobinometer kit containing:
  - Small bottle of dilute (approx. 0.1N) hydrochloric acid.
  - Graduated tube, with a scale on two sides. On one side is the percentage scale, and on the opposite side is the Gram scale. The percentage scale reads from 0 to 170. The Gram scale reads from 0 to 24.
  - Pipette, marked at the 20 mm level.
  - Stirring rod.
  - Color comparator, with a window on the side. On the right and left sides of this opening is the color standard for comparison. The center has an open slot to hold the graduated tube.

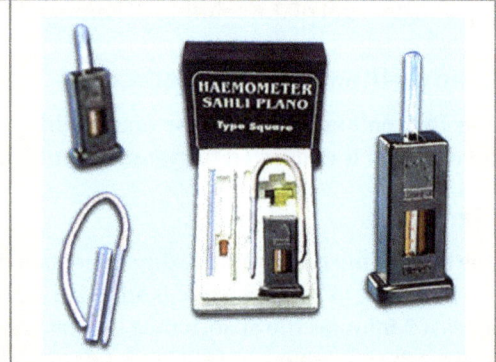

Procedure

- With a dropper, place 5 drops of the 0.1 NHCl in the bottom of the graduated tube. Place the tube in the color comparator.
- Using well-mixed venous blood or fingertip blood, fill the pipette to the 20 mm mark.
- Wipe the blood from the outside of the pipette. Transfer blood to the Sahli tube.

- Aspirate distilled water into the pipette two or three times and transfer these washings to the tube.
- Shake until the blood is well-mixed and the tube is a uniform color.
- Add distilled water, drop by drop, each time mixing the solution with the stirring rod. Keep adding water and mixing until the color of the solution matches the standards on either side. Remove the stirring rod from the tube each time before comparing. Natural light makes more accurate readings possible.
- Five minutes after the time noted, read the result from the scale on the tube by noting the graduation mark at the lower edge of the meniscus.

Hemoglobin is decreased in:
Area of central pallor takes up more than 1/3rd of the area of the RBC (hypochromia)
- Blood loss (lung, gastrointestinal, hemorrhoids, ulcers, colitis, uterine, menses, in urine via kidneys, hemorrhage)
- Deficiency (protein malnutrition, iron, copper, vitamin C, vitamin B_1, folic acid, B_{12}), chronic disease (liver, kidney, rheumatoid arthritis, carcinoid, etc.)
- Bone marrow insufficiency (infiltration with tumor or tuberculosis, toxic, immune or drug-induced hypoplasia)
- Digestive inflammation (with occult or obvious blood loss) as might occur with parasites, colitis, hemorrhoids, etc.
- Free radical pathology
- Adrenal cortical hypofunction
- Hereditary anemia(s)
- Hemodilution (pregnancy, edema)

Hemoglobin is increased in:
Area of central pallor takes up less than 1/3rd of the area of RBC (hyperchromia)
- Polycythemia vera
- High altitude adaptation
- Pulmonary pathology
- Splenic hypofunction
- Testosterone supplementation
- Dehydration as might occur with prolonged or severe diarrhea
- Emphysema, severe asthma, and other long-standing respiratory distress
- Macrocytosis (deficiency of B6, B12, folic acid, or hypothyroid)
- Adrenal cortex overactivity

RETICULOCYTE

In the journey of erythropoiesis, a reticulocyte is a cell just one stage prior to the mature erythrocyte.

Normal range of reticulocyte count is - 0.5% to 1.5%

An increased number of reticulocytes is seen when the marrow is churning out RBCs at excessive speed (presumably to make up for those lost to hemolysis or hemorrhage).

The reticulocyte count is usually performed when patients are evaluated for anemia and response to its treatment.

The lifespan of erythrocytes is approximately 120 days, and about 0.8% of the red cells need to be replaced daily by young cells released from the bone marrow.

Manual reticulocyte count
- These immature cells (reticulocytes) contain ribosomal RNA that can be precipitated and stained by supravital dyes, such as new methylene blue or brilliant cresyl blue.
- The blood and stain are mixed and allowed to stand for about 15 minutes before the films are prepared and air-dried.
- The cells containing blue granules or reticulum are counted as a percentage of total red cells or as an absolute number per volume.

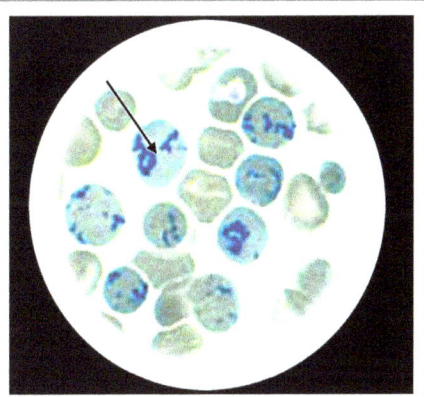

Automated Reticulocyte Count by Fluorescent Method

Automated methods employ a substance, such as thiazole orange, that binds to RNA and fluoresces.
With the use of fluorescent technology, the retic channel provides:
- Accurate reticulocyte counting in both % and absolute count
- Improved immature reticulocyte information (IRF-Immature Reticulocyte Fraction) for earlier diagnosis and treatment by clinicians.
- Elimination of common interferences such as Howell-Jolly bodies, Pappenheimer bodies, and immature reticulocytes to avoid manual count errors.

Reticulocyte Production Index or Corrected Reticulocyte Count

- Reticulocyte count must be adjusted for the level of anemia to obtain the reticulocyte index, a more accurate reflection of erythropoiesis.
- Reticulocyte index = Reticulocyte count × Patient's hematocrit/Normal hematocrit.
  For example: Reticulocyte count 6%, hematocrit 15, then Reticulocyte index = (6 × 15)/45 = 2%.

Reticulocyte Proliferation Index and Shift Correction Factor

Normally reticulocytes survive 3.5 days in the marrow and one day in peripheral circulation at normal PCV. In case of anemia and reduced hematocrit, the survival time in circulation is increased and this may cause a poor correlation of retic count with marrow response. This situation can be dealt with the calculation of corrected retic count or reticulocyte proliferation index.

Reticulocyte proliferation index =
Corrected retic count/shift correction factor
For example, Corrected retic count 7%, PCV—25, RPI = 7/2 = 3.5

Reticulocyte proliferation index	
PCV %	**Maturation time in days**
45	1
35	1.5
25	2
15	2.5

Increased Retic Count

- Hemolytic anemias
- Response to treatment of iron and Vit B_{12} and folic acid in anemia
- Recent hemorrhage
- Thalassemia
- Pregnancy
- Erythroblastosis fetalis
- HbC disease
- Leukemias
- Hypoxia

An increased count indicates active erythropoiesis

Retic Count is Decreased in:

- Decreased adrenocortical and anterior pituitary activity
- Aplastic anemia
- Cirrhosis
- Megaloblastic anemia
- Exposure to radiation
- Anemia of chronic diseases
- MDS

Reticulocyte Hemoglobin Measurement (RET-He)

RET-H*e* is a parameter measured in the reticulocyte channel and is used to measure the incorporation of iron into erythrocyte hemoglobin beyond traditional biochemical tests (e.g. iron, ferritin, TIBC, % Sat).

The RET-H*e* parameter supports:
- Assessment of anemia and is an established parameter used in KDOQI (Kidney Disease Outcomes Quality Initiative) guidelines for assessing the initial iron status of patients.
- Rapid, direct analysis of an earlier stage of RBC development for prompt clinical follow-up.
- Accuracy and sensitivity in measurement of red cell production that supports effective monitoring of costly drug protocols for cell stimulation.
- Screening of infants for iron deficiency,
- Evaluation of iron deficiency in end stage renal disease (ESRD)/chronic dialysis patients
- In other chronic diseases associated with inflammation in which traditional biochemical tests may be misleading.
- Ret-He is a Sysmex instrument parameter and CHr is a Siemens instrument parameter
- While not identical, these parameters essentially measure the same thing in reticulocytes
- Reticulocyte Hemoglobin content provides an idea regarding the amount of iron available for RBC production in the bone marrow. It is a newer parameter that is being used in the research area to check the utility in diagnosing iron deficiency.

Low, Medium and High Fluorescence Reticulocytes

The newer fluorescence flow cytometry technique now allows us to categorize the reticulocytes based on their degree of maturation.
This is done by measuring the RNA content of the reticulocyte as fluorescence intensity. The higher the RNA content, the less mature the cells are:
- Low fluorescence reticulocyte: Mature
- Medium fluorescence reticulocyte: Medium maturity
- High fluorescence reticulocyte: Most immature

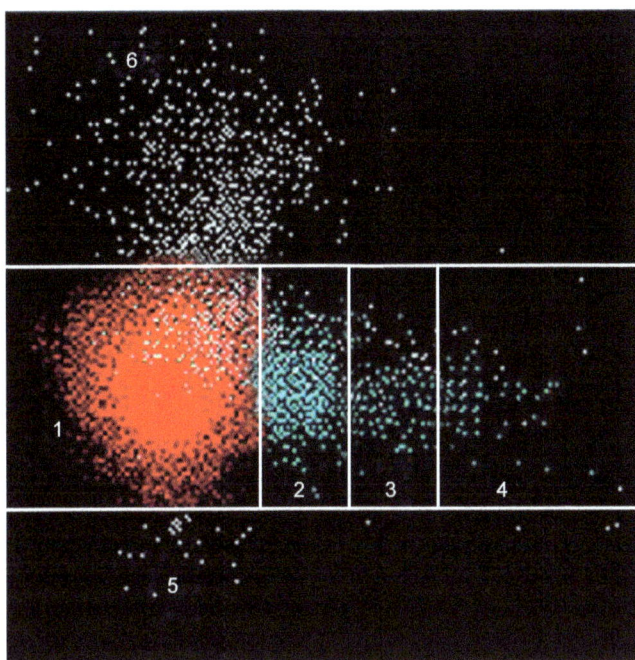

Retic scatter absorption
Courtesy: © Siemens Healthcare GmbH 2020.

1. Mature RBCs
2. Low absorption retics
3. Medium absorption retics
4. High absorption retics
5. Platelets
6. Coincidence events

Immature Reticulocyte Fraction (IRF)

- IRF is a marker to show the effectiveness of erythropoiesis in a patient.
- IRF is a calculated ratio of newly released reticulocytes to total reticulocytes.
- It is a very sensitive measure of marrow erythropoietic activity.
- Evaluate patients after bone marrow transplantation to indicate early engraftment
- In patients treated with EPO to measure the response to EPO therapy
- Red cell inclusions (e.g. Howell-Jolly bodies, Pappenheimer bodies, basophilic stippling) may cause interference with this parameter
- For most practical purposes, evaluation of the combination of IRF along with reticulocyte count (RET) may be used to define the etiology of anemia in a particular patient.

For example:

- **Low RET + Low IRF** would suggest *aplastic anemia or renal failure.*
- **High RET + High IRF** would suggest *hemolytic anemia or blood loss.*
- **Low/normal RET + High IRF** would suggest *iron, folate, or B-12 deficiency.*
- **Low/normal RET + Normal IRF** would suggest *anemia of chronic disease.*

To summarize in terms of practical diagnosis,

The reticulocyte count is a very valuable measure of assessment of the rate of production of the red cells, and efficacy of the marrow in terms of responding to anemia.

To oversimplify,

- *If the disease-causing the anemia is inside the marrow, the reticulocyte count is decreased.*
- *If the disease-causing the anemia is outside the marrow, the reticulocyte count is increased.*

HEMATOCRIT—PACKED CELL VOLUME (PCV)

- The hematocrit (Hct) or packed cell volume (PCV) or erythrocyte volume fraction (EVF) is the ratio of the volume of erythrocytes to that of the whole blood and is reported as a percentage.
- This is the earliest RBC parameter identified and is used for red cell disorders differentiation.
- The hematocrit is one of the most precise methods of determining the degree of anemia or polycythemia, i.e. increase or decrease in RBC concentration.

Hematocrit normal range	Male	Female
	38.8–46.4%	35.4–44.4%

- The manual method of measuring Hct has proved to be a simple and accurate method of assessing red cell status.
- It is easily performed with little specialized equipment – The spun.
- However, several sources of error are inherent in the technique.
- The spun Hct measures the red cell concentration, not red cell mass.
- Therefore, patients in shock or with volume depletion may have normal or high Hct measurements due to hemoconcentration despite a decreased red cell mass.
- Technical sources of error in manual Hct determinations usually arise from inappropriate concentrations of anticoagulants, poor mixing of samples, or insufficient centrifugation.

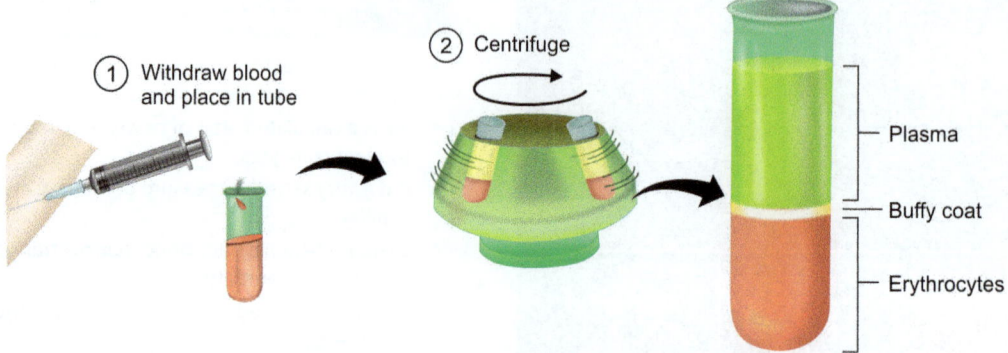

Another inherent error in manual Hct determinations arises from the trapping of plasma in the red cell column. This may account for 1-3% of the volume in microcapillary tube methods, and more trapping of plasma is noted in the macrotube methods.
- Abnormal red cells (e.g. sickle cells, microcytic cells, macrocytic cells, or spherocytes) often trap higher volumes of plasma due to increased cellular rigidity, possibly accounting for up to 6% of the red cell volume.
- Very high Hct, as in polycythemia, may also have excess plasma trapping. Manual Hct methods typically have a precision [coefficient of variation (CV)] of approximately 2%.

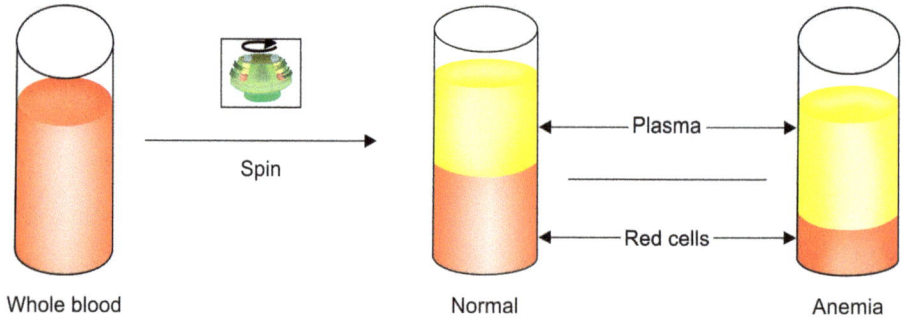

- Automated analyzers do not depend on centrifugation techniques to determine Hct, but instead calculate Hct by direct measurements of red cell number and red cell volume (Hct = Red cell number × red cell volume).
- Errors of automated Hct calculation are more common in patients with polycythemia or abnormal plasma osmotic pressures. Manual methods of Hct determination may be preferable in these cases.
- The precision of most automated Hct is less than 1% (CV).

High Hematocrit is due to:	Low Hematocrit is due to:
♦ Dehydration (such as from severe diarrhea) ♦ Kidney disease with high erythropoietin production ♦ Low oxygen level in the blood ♦ Congenital heart disease ♦ Cor pulmonale ♦ Pulmonary fibrosis ♦ High altitude ♦ Dengue hemorrhagic fever ♦ Polycythemia vera ♦ Smoking	♦ Blood loss (hemorrhage) ♦ Bone marrow failure (for example, aplasia or hypoplasia due to radiation, infections, drugs, neoplasia, autoimmune, etc.). ♦ Erythropoietin deficiency (usually secondary to kidney disease) ♦ Hemolysis (RBC destruction due to varied etiologies) ♦ Leukemia ♦ Malnutrition (nutritional deficiencies of iron, folate, vit. B_{12}, or vit. B_6) ♦ Multiple myeloma ♦ Autoimmune/collagen-vascular diseases, such as lupus erythematosus or rheumatoid arthritis

An elevated hematocrit may be due to spleen hyperfunction, and a reduced hematocrit may indicate low thymus function.

Rule of three
Correlation checks between the Hgb and Hct are a significant part of quality assurance for the CBC and are known as the "rule of three." The formulas for correlation checks/rule of three are as follows:

$$Hgb \times 3 = Hct \pm 3, \text{ and } RBC \times 3 = Hgb.$$

Example: 14.8 (*Hgb*) × 3 = 44 (patients actual hematocrit result is 45%)
11.0 (*Hgb*) × 3 = 33 (patients actual hematocrit result is 32%)

The exception to this rule is in patients with hypochromic red cells. These patients will have hematocrits that are more than three times the hemoglobin

MEAN CORPUSCULAR VOLUME

Mean corpuscular volume (MCV) is the average volume of the red blood cell
- MCV = (hematocrit/red cell count) × 100.
- Can be directly measured by automated cell counters.
- With impedance analyzers, the MCV is measured by averaging the amplitude of the pulses created as the cells pass through the aperture of the counter.
- Mean corpuscular volume (MCV), mean corpuscular hemoglobin (MCH), and mean corpuscular hemoglobin concentration (MCHC) were first introduced by Wintrobe to define the size (MCV) and hemoglobin content (MCH, MCHC) of red blood cells.

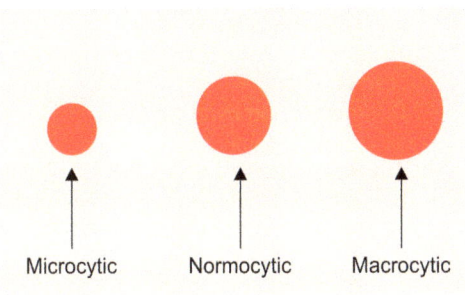

MCV normal range	Men and Women
	79–98 fL (femtoliters)

Cells are classified as microcytic if MCV < 79 fL and macrocytic when > 98 fL and normocytic when indices are within normal limits.
- MCV is higher at birth, decreases rapidly during first 6 months of life.
- The blood analyzer gives us a superior determination of the red cell size whereas the microscopic observation gives us a crude impression of the same.
- Anemias in which red cells are normal in both size and hemoglobin content are called "normocytic normochromic".

- *Presence of microcytic and macrocytic cells in the same sample may result in a normal MCV.*
- *MCV <72 fL without heterogeneity, i.e., with normal RDW, has sensitivity and specificity (S/S) of 88% and 84% respectively as a predictor of thalassemia trait.*

Normal MCV (Normocytic Anemia)

- Following acute hemorrhage
- Dimorphic anemia
- Hemoglobinopathies
- Anemias due to inadequate blood cell formation
  - Myelophthisic
  - Hypoplastic
  - Aplastic.
- Endocrinopathies—(hypopituitarism, hypothyroidism, hypoadrenalism, hypogonadism)
- Anemia of chronic disease (chronic infections, neoplasms, uremia).

Increased MCV (Macrocytic Anemia - MCV >98 fL)

- Megaloblastic anemia
- Pernicious anemia (vitamin B_{12} or folate deficiency)
- Sprue (e.g., steatorrhea, celiac disease, intestinal resection or fistula)
- Macrocytic anemia of pregnancy
- Megaloblastic anemia of infancy
- Di Guglielmo disease
- Myelodysplastic syndromes (aplastic anemia, sideroblastic anemia)
- Myelophthisic anemia
- Post splenectomy
- Infants and newborns
- Nonmegaloblastic macrocytic anemias
- Alcoholism
- Liver disease
- Anemia of hypothyroidism
- Drugs:
  - Oral contraceptives
  - Anticonvulsants (e.g., phenytoin, primidone, phenobarbital)
  - Antitumor agents (e.g., methotrexate, hydroxyurea, cyclophosphamide)
  - Antimicrobials (e.g., sulfamethoxazole, sulfasalazine, trimethoprim, zidovudine, pyrimethamine).

Decreased MCV (Microcytic Anemia – MCV <79 fL)	Interferences in MCV

• Usually hypochromic
  – Iron deficiency anemia
  – Thalassemia (major or combined with hemoglobinopathy)
  – Lead poisoning
  – Disorders of porphyrin synthesis
• Usually normochromic
  – Anemia of chronic diseases (<1/3rd of patients)
  – Heterozygous thalassemia and hemoglobinopathies
	• Cold agglutinins (increased values)
	• Warm autoantibodies
	• Marked hyperglycemia (>600 mg/dL) (increases MCV)
	• Marked leukocytosis (>50,000/μL) (increased values)
	• In vitro hemolysis or fragmentation of RBCs (decreased values)
	• Methanol poisoning (increased values)
	• Marked reticulocytosis (>50%) from any cause (increases MCV)

MEAN CORPUSCULAR HEMOGLOBIN

Mean corpuscular hemoglobin (MCH) is the amount of hemoglobin in a single red blood cell.

$$MCH = (hemoglobin/red\ cell\ count) \times 100$$

MCH normal range	Men and women
	26.7–31.9 pg/cell

- MCH if low—Hypochromasia
- MCH if high—Hyperchromasia.

MCH decreases in:	Interferences in MCH
• Microcytic and normocytic anemias	• Lipemia • Marked leukocytosis (>50,000/μL) • Cold agglutinins • In vivo hemolysis • Monoclonal proteins in blood • High heparin concentration
MCH increases in:	
• Macrocytic anemias • Infants and newborns	

MEAN CORPUSCULAR HEMOGLOBIN CONCENTRATION (MCHC)

- The average hemoglobin concentration per unit volume (100 mL) of packed red cells is indicated by MCHC.
- In contrast to MCH, MCHC correlates the hemoglobin content with the volume of the cell.
- It is expressed as g/dL of red blood cells.

$$MCHC = (Hemoglobin/Hematocrit) \times 10$$

MCHC normal value	Male and female
	32–36 g/dL

MCHC decreased in (decrease is defined as ≤ 30.1 g/dL):	Interferences: MCHC decreased in:
• Hypochromic microcytic anemia. Normal value does not rule out any of these anemias. • Low MCHC may not occur in IDA when performed with automated instruments.	• Marked leukocytosis (>50,000/μL)
MCHC increased in:	**MCHC increased in:**
• Hereditary spherocytosis • In spherocytosis, the MCHC is increased due to loss of membrane and the consequent spherical shape assumed by the cell • Infants and newborns • Autoagglutination • Artifactual (abnormal MCHC may be most valuable clue to artefact)	• Hemolysis (e.g., sickle cell anemia, hereditary spherocytosis, autoimmune hemolytic anemia) with shrinkage of RBCs making them hyperdense • Conditions with cold agglutinins or severe lipemia of serum • Rouleaux or RBC agglutinates • High heparin concentration

The microcytic-to-hypochromic ratio
(Siemens %HYPO, Sysmex %HYPO-He)

- To distinguish thalassemia from iron deficiency anemia (IDA), as the former tends to show more prominent microcytosis, while severe hypochromasia is more characteristic of the latter.
- Iron deficiency superimposed on certain thalassemia variants can result in marked hypochromia, yielding a ratio similar to that of a non-thalassemic patient with IDA.

- $\text{\% Macro} = 100 \times \dfrac{\text{Cell count in RBC volume histogram} > 120 \text{ fL}}{\text{Total cell count in RBC volume histogram}}$

- $\text{\% Micro} = 100 \times \dfrac{\text{Cell count in RBC volume histogram} < 60 \text{ fL}}{\text{Total cell count in RBC volume histogram}}$

- $\text{\% Hyper} = 100 \times \dfrac{\text{Cell count in RBC HC histogram} > 41 \text{ g/dL (*HC = Hemoglobin conc.)}}{\text{Total cell count in RBC HC histogram}}$

- $\text{\% Hypo} = 100 \times \dfrac{\text{Cell count in RBC HC histogram} < 28 \text{ g/dL}}{\text{Total cell count in RBC HC histogram}}$

RED CELL DISTRIBUTION WIDTH

Red cell distribution width (RDW) is a quantitative measure or numerical expression of anisocytosis. It is a coefficient of variation of the distribution of individual RBC volume, as determined by an automated blood cell counting instrument.

- The RDW value reflects size variability in red cells.
- High RDW values mirror a large range in red cell size.
- The RDW can provide insight into the basis of anemia because some processes increase their value while others do not.
- Microcytosis, for instance, exists with either iron deficiency or thalassemia minor. The former condition increases the RDW while the latter does not. Therefore, marked microcytosis with a normal RDW suggests thalassemia minor early in the work-up.
- Anisocytosis of RBCs is a variation of cell size in a given population of cells or excessive heterogeneity on smear or the visual equivalent of increased CV (coefficient of variation).
- The coefficient of variation (CV) means how reproducible repetitive measurement is.
- The reproducibility of values among a cell population reflects not only variability in the measurement but also the biological heterogeneity of the cells.
- Cells excessively heterogeneous in size would not present a reliable amount of oxygen-diffusion surface to the capillary endothelium. On the other hand, the more rigidly the red cell size is controlled, the large number of cells would be quickly destroyed by the spleen.
- The heterogeneity of a red cell property, therefore, is a result of a balance of acceptable function versus the cost of quality control.
- The coefficient of variation (CV) of red cell size is reported as "red cell distribution width" or RDW.
- The index of red cell heterogeneity should not be simply the width of the histogram, because this measures only the SD.
- The CV is the ratio of the standard deviation–SD (width of the histogram) to the "mean corpuscular volume" (MCV).

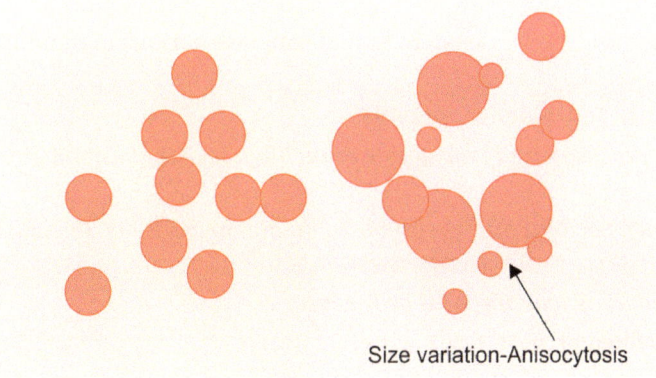

Size variation-Anisocytosis

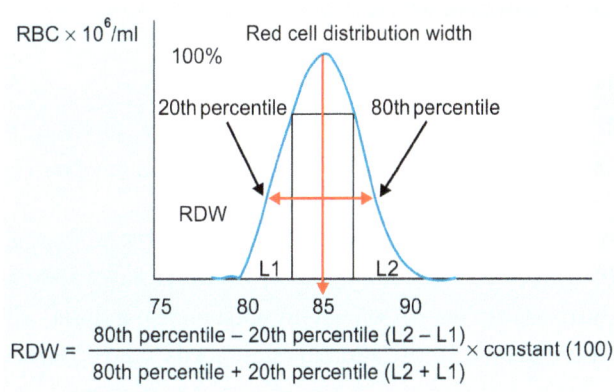

$$\text{RDW} = \dfrac{\text{80th percentile} - \text{20th percentile (L2} - \text{L1)}}{\text{80th percentile} + \text{20th percentile (L2} + \text{L1)}} \times \text{constant (100)}$$

RDW-CV:
The RDW-CV is calculated from the formula:
RDW-CV = (Standard deviation of RBC volume/mean MCV) × 100
1SD reflects the size variation of the erythrocytes round the mean. As the 1SD is divided by the MCV, the RDW-CV also depends on the mean size (MCV) of the erythrocytes.
Reference values: 11.5–14.5%

The RDW is markedly elevated in newborns, ranging from 14.5% to 19.5%, gradually decreases, and reaches adult levels by the age of 6 months.

RDW-SD:

The determination of the RDW-SD is an actual measurement of the width of the erythrocyte distribution curve. This measurement is performed at a relative height of 20% above the baseline. The wider the curve is spread by erythrocytes of different sizes, the higher the RDW-SD value will be.
Reference values: 35–45 fL.

Thus, a given SD may be normal or abnormal depending on MCV, therefore, more important is the calculation of RDW-CV.

Unlike most variables, in which, these are abnormally high and abnormally low values – No disorder is known to have abnormally low RDW.

Role of RDW in Modern Classification of RBC disorder

Anemia has been classified by two main methods.
1. **Morphologic**: In which classification is based on RBC size and is classified into:
   – Normocytic, (normal MCV)
   – Microcytic (low MCV)
   – Macrocytic (higher MCV).

   Usually, MCV is the classifier in this classification but this parameter can be deceptive in conditions like mixed nutritional deficiency, where microcytic and macrocytic RBCs, average the MCV to the normocytic range.
2. **Physiologic**: Usually bone marrow studies, biochemical markers and reticulocyte count are used as a classifier in this classification and is classified as:
   – Hypoproliferative or bone marrow production defect
     • Marrow aplasia
     • Chronic disease
     • Myeloproliferative disorder
     • Organ failure, (e.g. renal failure)
     • Blood dyscrasias.
   – RBC maturation defect or ineffective erythropoiesis
     • Cytoplasmic: Hypochromic
     • Nuclear: Megaloblastic
     • Combined: Myelodysplastic syndrome
   – Decreased RBC survival (hypoproliferative)
     • Hemorrhagic: Acute blood loss
     • Hemolytic: Primary, immune, hemoglobinopathies, enzymopathies, and parasites, etc.
     • Dilutional : Pregnancy, splenomegaly

Bone marrow studies help to differentiate hypoproliferative anemia (no erythroid hyperplasia) from maturation disorder (erythroid hyperplasia).

Biochemical markers such as serum iron, ferritin, TIBC, folate and vit. B_{12} assay help to distinguish various maturation disorders.

Reticulocyte production distinguishes between hypoproliferative and hemolytic anemia.

But bone marrow studies are invasive, biochemical markers are expensive and reticulocyte count has a high duplication error without automation.

Older parameters like MCHC, MCH, and HCT have always shown variable disproportionate findings towards the diagnosis. Therefore, the discussion of red cell disorders focuses primarily on directly measured parameters of RBC.

The modern time classification based on two indices – *MCV and RDW was proposed by Bessman.*
Although this classification method needs to be prospectively validated.

RDW is mathematically derived from the RBC histogram with a portion of each of the extreme ends of the histogram curve excluded. This allows for a computation to exclude platelets, platelet clumps, and electrical interference from left side of the curve.
The exclusion of the right side of the curve eliminates clumped RBCs (from Rouleaux or agglutination) or overly large RBCs.
The MCV is calculated using the entire RBC histogram.
The RDW independent of the MCV may be normal when the MCV is normal, low, or high.

The six possible combinations classify almost all major possible causes of anemia.
- Low MCV   with   Normal RDW   or   High RDW
- Normal MCV   with   Normal RDW   or   High RDW
- High MCV   with   Normal RDW   or   High RDW

	MCV Normal (Normocytic)	MCV High (Macrocytic)	MCV Low (Microcytic)
Normal RDW (Nonheterogeneous)	<ul><li>Anemia of chronic disease</li><li>Acute blood loss</li><li>Hemolysis</li><li>Chronic lymphocytic Leukemia (CLL)</li><li>Chronic myelogenous leukemia (CML)</li><li>Hemoglobinopathy</li><li>Normal variant</li></ul>	<ul><li>Aplastic anemia</li><li>Preleukemia</li><li>Myelodysplastic syndrome</li></ul>	<ul><li>Anemia of chronic disease</li><li>Thalassemia (heterozygous)</li></ul>

High RDW (Heterogeneous)	1. RDW increases before MCV becomes abnormal
	  – Early iron deficiency anemia
	  – Early vitamin B_{12} deficiency
	  – Early folate deficiency
	2. Anemic globinopathy like Sickle cell anemia
		<ul><li>Vitamin B_{12} deficiency</li><li>Folate deficiency</li><li>Immune hemolytic anemia</li><li>Liver disease</li><li>Cold agglutinins</li><li>Alcoholism</li></ul>	<ul><li>Iron deficiency anemia</li><li>RBC fragmentation</li><li>HbH</li><li>Thalassemia intermedia</li><li>G6PD deficiency</li></ul>

Low RDW	Low RDW is not observed normally but theoretically, it is possible only at the marrow level when RBC produced by marrow has less heterogeneity than the accepted normal. Some observers quote low RDW low MCV in thalassemia minor and low RDW with high MCV in aplastic anemia but the author includes both these under normal RDW		

The classification may be grossly summarized as:
- Hypoproliferative disorders—Independent of MCV have normal heterogeneity.
- Nutritional disorders—Independent of MCV have increased heterogeneity.
- Hemolytic disorders—Independent of MCV have heterogeneity that is increased in direct proportion to the degree of anemia caused by the disorder.

Hemoglobin distribution width (HDW)

- HDW is a measurement of anisochromia, or variation in hemoglobin concentration, similar to the red cell distribution width (RDW) which is an automated measurement of anisocytosis (variation in red cell size),
- The HDW is useful to differentiate between causes of microcytosis and macrocytosis and is only available on haematology analysers that use optical red cell technology.
- The normal range for HDW is 22 to 32 g/L.
- Cases of microcytosis caused by iron deficiency anaemia often have a raised HDW (and RDW), whereas microcytosis caused by thalassaemia trait usually has a normal HDW (and RDW).
- In cases of macrocytosis, the HDW is typically below the reference range in alcoholic liver disease (ALD), normal (or borderline raised) in megaloblastic anemia and raised in hemolytic anemia.
- Different HDW values for different causes of microcytosis and macrocytosis, as well as different cytogram appearances are helping parameter in diagnosis.

CHAPTER 3

RBCs on Peripheral Smear

In this era of automation in hematology, despite the availability of the most sophisticated multiparameter cell counters, the significance of the skilled peripheral smear examination cannot be underestimated.

Peripheral smear examination is the gold standard investigation in the study of hematology. It is the true window of bone marrow, the home of all hematopoietic cell production.

PERIPHERAL BLOOD SMEAR PREPARATION

- The wedge slide (push slide) technique developed by Maxwell Wintrobe remains the standard method for the preparation of peripheral blood smears (films).
- Place a 1 × 3 glass microscope slide with a frosted end on a flat surface (usually the counter top of a laboratory bench).
- Attach a label on the slide or write the specimen identification number, on the frosted surface.
- Place a 2–3 mm drop of blood approximately ¼" from the frosted slide, using a glass capillary tube.
- Hold the slide by the narrow side between the thumb and forefinger of one hand at the end farthest from the frosted end.
- Grasp a second slide (spreader slide) between the thumb and forefinger of the other hand at the frosted end.
- Place the edge of the spreader slide on the lower slide in front of the drop of blood (side farthest from the frosted end).
- Pull the spreader slide toward the frosted end until it touches the drop of blood. Permit the blood to spread by capillary motion until it almost reaches the edges of the spreader slide.
- Push the spreader slide forward at a 30° angle with a rapid, even motion. Let the weight of the slide do the work.

A well-made peripheral smear is thick at the frosted end and becomes progressively thinner toward the opposite end. The "zone of morphology" (area of optimal thickness for light microscopic examination) should be at least 2 cm in length. The smear should occupy the central area of the slide and be margin-free at the edges.

PERIPHERAL BLOOD SMEAR EXAMINATION

Peripheral smear examination requires a systematic approach in order to gather all possible information. The following approach is recommended:

An examination at low power (10X ocular, 10X objectives) is first performed to evaluate the quality of the smear, ascertain the approximate number of white blood cells and platelets, and detect rouleaux formation, platelet clumps, and leukocyte clumps and other abnormalities visible at low magnification. An optimal area for evaluation at higher magnification is also chosen. This should be an intact portion of the smear-free of preparation artifact where the red blood cells are separated by 1/3rd to 1/2nd of cell diameter. Optimal preparation and staining of the peripheral blood smear are critical for morphologic examination; an inadequate smear should not be examined.

Following low power examination of a peripheral blood smear, the 40X or 100X objective of the microscope is selected (400X or 1000X total magnification when using a 10X ocular) and the area of morphology is examined in a consistent scanning pattern to avoid counting the same cell(s) twice. A differential count of at least 100 white blood cells (200, 500, or 1000 is even better) is performed, and any abnormal morphology of RBCs, WBCs, and platelets observed during the differential count is recorded. Each morphologic abnormality observed should be quantitated (graded) separately as to severity (slight to marked or 1+ to 4+). A fairly accurate estimate of the white blood cell count (cells/mL) can be obtained by counting the total number of leukocytes in ten 40X microscopic fields, dividing the total by 10, and multiplying by 3000.

A peripheral smear must be interpreted in the context of the clinical situation. The age and sex of the patient must be known since absolute cell numbers and the significance of some findings vary with age. For example, relative lymphocytosis with nucleated RBCs and atypical lymphocytes would be unusual and pathologic in an adult but appear in any infant under stress.

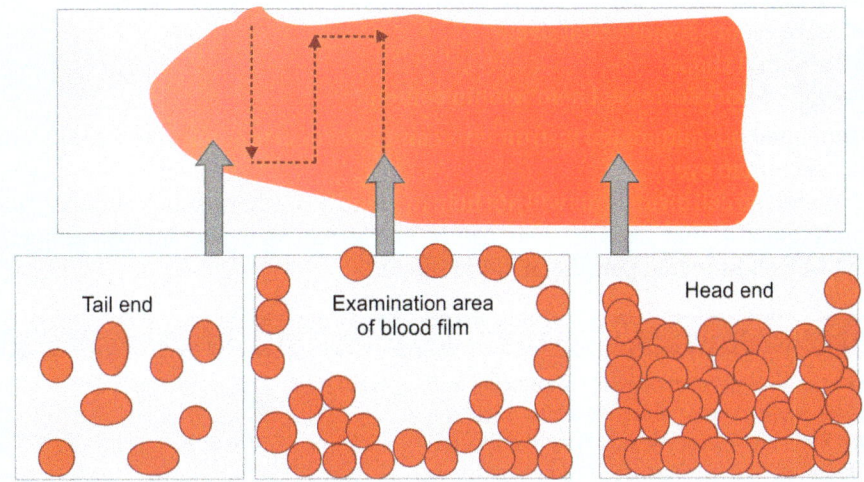

RBCs ON PERIPHERAL SMEAR

CLINICAL IMPORTANCE OF RBC MORPHOLOGY

Normal RBCs on smear are:
- Normocytic with normal cell size and shape.
- Normochromic, with normal hemoglobin content and color.
- Abnormal morphologic variations in red blood cells arise from different etiological processes, hence the proper interpretation of red blood cell morphology in conjunction with CBC data and other clinical information can help in the diagnosis of diseases.
- Red cell morphology is assessed according to size, shape, color (hemoglobin content), and the presence or absence of inclusions. Red cell morphology must be scanned in a good counting area.

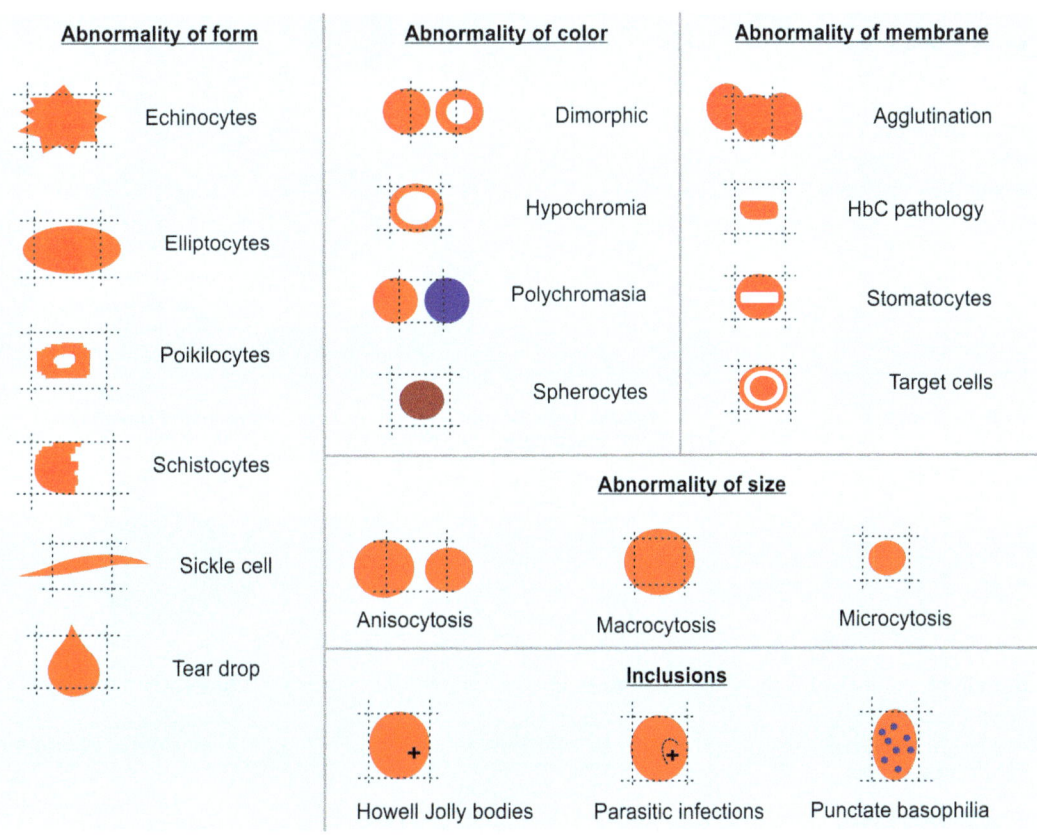

Morphological abnormalities of RBCs can be:
- Anisocytosis "Aniso" unequal or asymmetrical size
- Poikilocytosis "Poikilo" varied shape
- Hypochromic ("chromic"- color) decreased hemoglobin content.

Precession of data generated but automated instruments cannot recognize some of the significant abnormalities, which can be observed only by the human eye.

Red cell indices, RDW, and red cell histograms will not help to identify conditions such as red cell inclusions or membrane abnormalities such as spherocytosis that might be responsible for anemia. An evaluation of anemia is not complete without the careful examination of a well-prepared peripheral blood smear.

MICROCYTIC, HYPOCHROMIC RED CELLS

The RBCs are smaller than the nucleus of the small lymphocyte and have markedly increased central pallor, which exceeds 1/3rd the diameter of the RBC. Such RBCs are microcytic (<7.0 μm in diameter) and hypochromic. Both features, i.e., microcytosis, and hypochromia usually coexist and indicate abnormal hemoglobin synthesis.

The major causes are:
- Iron deficiency anemia
- Thalassemia minor
- Sideroblastic anemia
- Anemia of chronic disease
- Hemoglobinopathies.

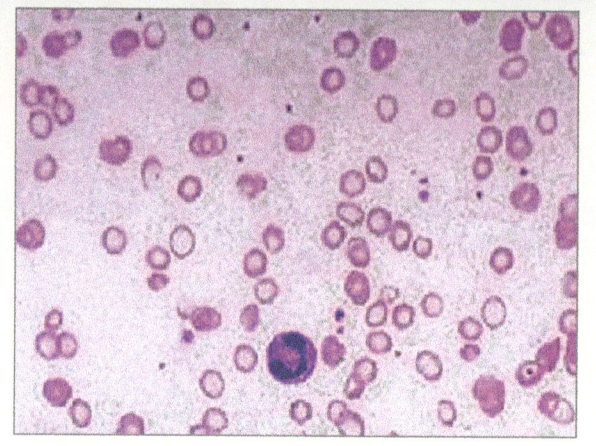

MACROCYTIC RED CELLS

Most of the red cells are larger than the nucleus of the small lymphocyte (size > 8.5 μm in diameter).

The major causes of macrocytic red cells are:
- Vitamin B_{12} or folate deficiency
- Alcoholism
- Liver disease
- Myelodysplastic syndrome (MDS)
- Hypothyroidism
- Drugs that impair DNA synthesis.

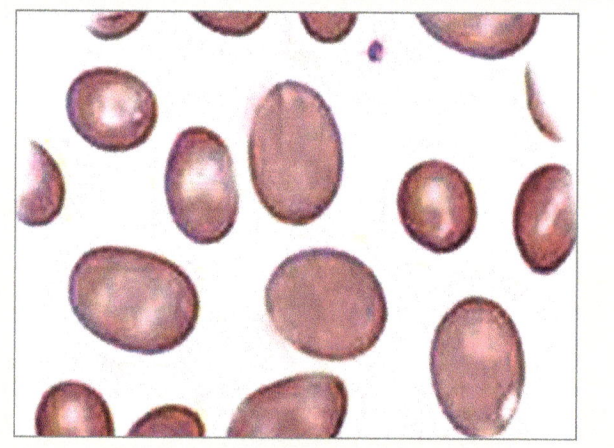

Oval macrocyte

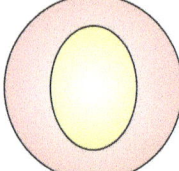

Seen in:
- Folic acid deficiency
- Vitamin-B_{12} deficiency
- Pernicious anemia
- MDS
- Postchemotherapy

Round hypochromic macrocyte

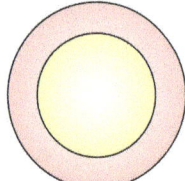

Seen in:
- Alcoholism
- Hypothyroidism
- Liver disease
- Postsplenectomy

Blue-tinged macrocyte

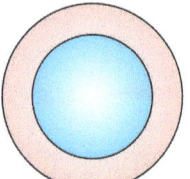

Seen in:
- Neonates
- Response to anemic stress

TARGET OR BELL CELLS

They have a characteristic ringed appearance. This configuration occurs because of the "increased surface area to volume ratio", i.e., there is an increase in the red cell membrane compared to the hemoglobin content, so the excess membrane pools in the middle of the cells.

Causes of target cells are:
- *Thalassemia* (most common cause)
- Hemoglobinopathies
  - Hb AC or CC
  - Hb SS, SC
- Liver disease
- Post-splenectomy or hyposplenic states
- Severe iron deficiency
- HbE (heterozygote and homozygote)
- Abetalipoproteinemia.

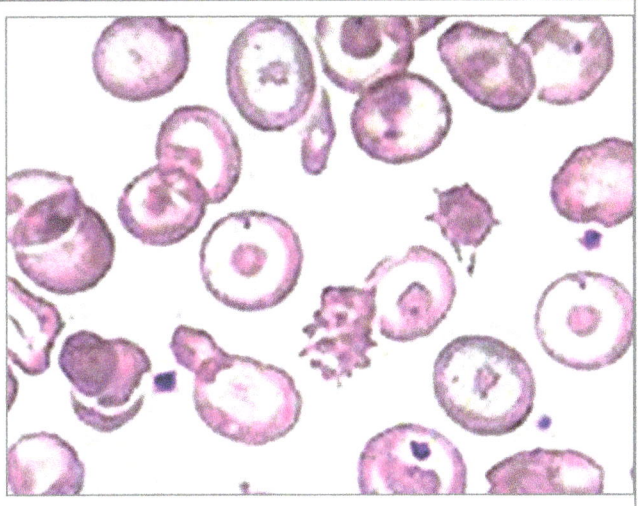

SCHISTOCYTES: "SCHISTO"—SPLIT OR CLEFT
(From GREEK schistos for "divided" and kytos for "cell")

Physical assault to erythrocytes within the bloodstream can create fragments called schistocytes, which include such strange forms as helmet cells, triangles, crescents, and microspherocytes. Such cells are seen when intravascular destruction of RBCs occurs, like in:
- Disseminated intravascular coagulation (DIC)
- Severe hemolytic anemia (e.g., G6PD deficiency)
- Microangiopathic hemolytic anemia
- Hemolytic uremic syndrome
- Prosthetic cardiac valve, abnormal cardiac valve, cardiac patch, coarctation of the aorta
- Connective tissue disorder [e.g., systemic lupus erythematosus (SLE)]
- Burns (spheroschistocytes as a result of heat)
- Thrombotic thrombocytopenic purpura
- Uremia, acute tubular necrosis, glomerulonephritis
- Malignant hypertension, Systemic amyloidosis
- Liver cirrhosis
- Disseminated carcinomatosis
- Chronic relapsing schistocytic hemolytic anemia.

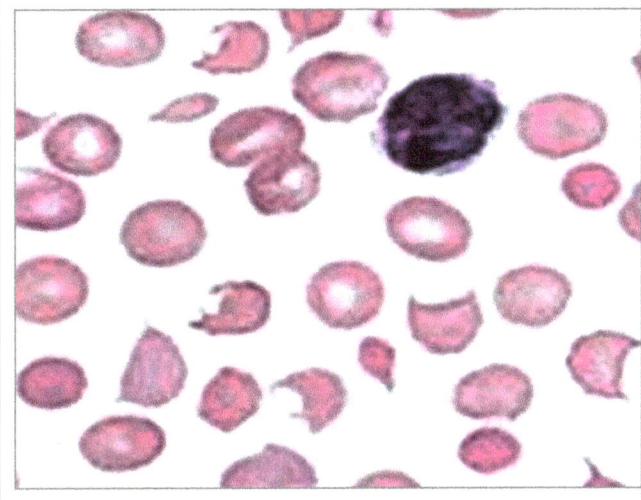

TEAR DROP CELLS (DACRYOCYTE)

Pear-shaped cells, usually microcytic, hypochromic.
Seen most prominently in:
- Newborn
- Thalassemia major
- Leukoerythroblastic reaction
- Myeloproliferative disorders.

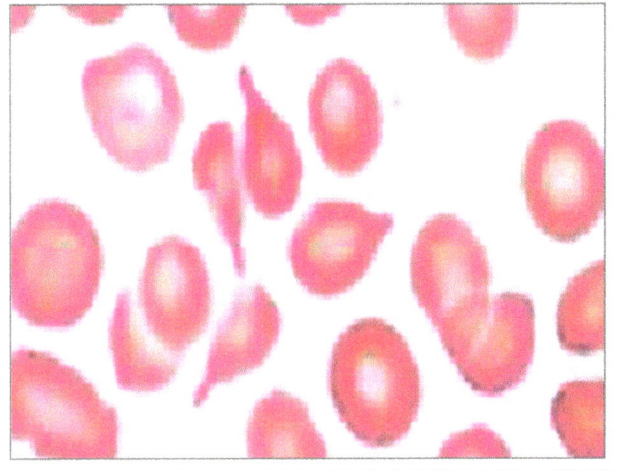

SPHEROCYTES

Ball-shaped red cells, decreased surface/volume ratio, hyperdense (increased MCHC)

Causes of spherocytosis are:
- Hereditary spherocytosis
- ABO incompatibility
- Autoimmune hemolytic anemia
- Microangiopathic hemolytic anemia (MAHA)
- SS disease
- Hypersplenism
- Burns
- Post-transfusion
- Pyruvate kinase deficiency
- Water-dilution hemolysis

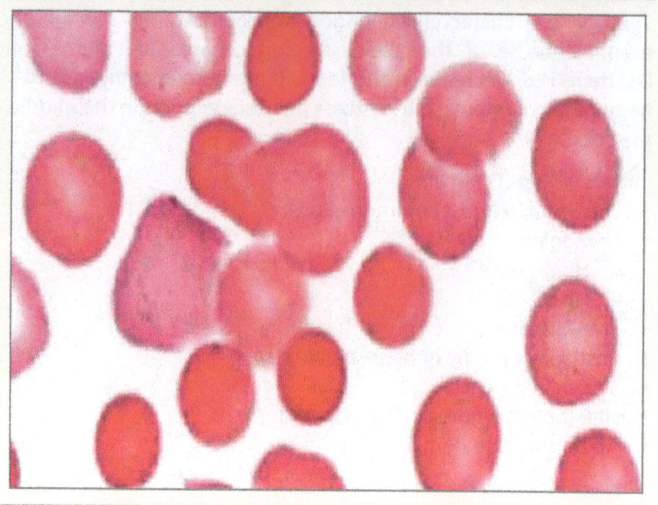

ELLIPTOCYTE

Elliptical and normochromic cells, seen normally in less than 1% of RBC's.

Causes of elliptocytes are:
- Hereditary elliptocytosis
- Iron deficiency anemia (increased with severity)
- SS disease and SA trait
- Thalassemia major
- Leukoerythroblastic reaction
- Malaria
- Megaloblastic anemia
- Any anemia may occasionally present with 5 to 10% elliptocytes.

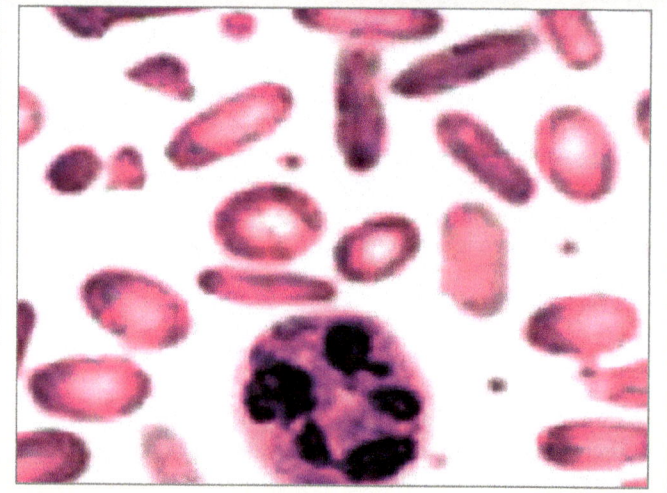

BURR CELLS (ECHINOCYTES)

10-30 spicules equal in size and evenly distributed over RBC surface; caused by alteration in extracellular environment.

Burr cells are seen in:
- Renal failure from any cause
- Liver diseases, especially when uremia coexists
- Storage artefact—if blood is kept in a tube for several hours before preparation of the smear
- Stomach cancer or bleeding peptic ulcer
- Dehydration
- Pyruvate kinase deficiency
- Immediately after red cell transfusion.

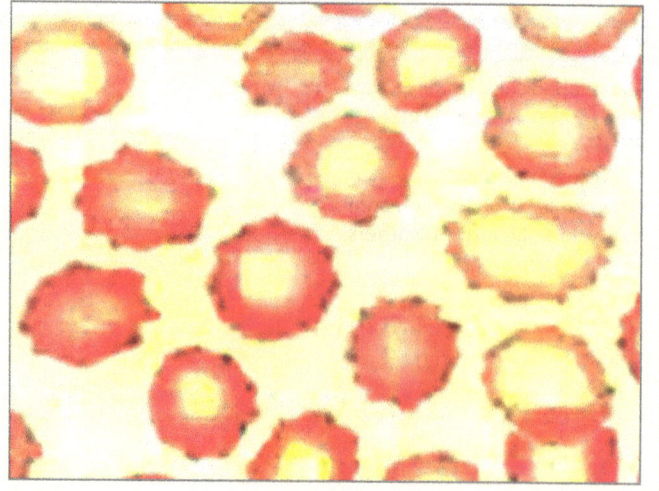

BITE CELL (DEGMACYTE)

Appears like a cookie with a bite taken out.
- These defects occur when certain drugs cause oxidative damage of hemoglobin, often in patients with glucose-6-phosphate dehydrogenase (G6PD) enzyme deficiency.
- Bite cells apparently occur when the spleen removes the Heinz bodies from the RBCs.

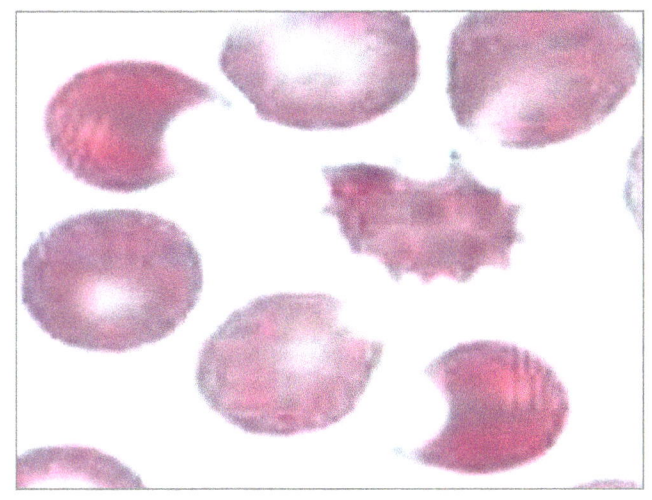

STOMATOCYTE

When examined on dry smears, it has a central slit or stoma (mouth). Seen in:
- Few stomatocytes may be present in normal people
- Various cardiovascular and pulmonary disorders
- Hereditary
- Alcoholism, liver disease, malignancies
- Drug induced.

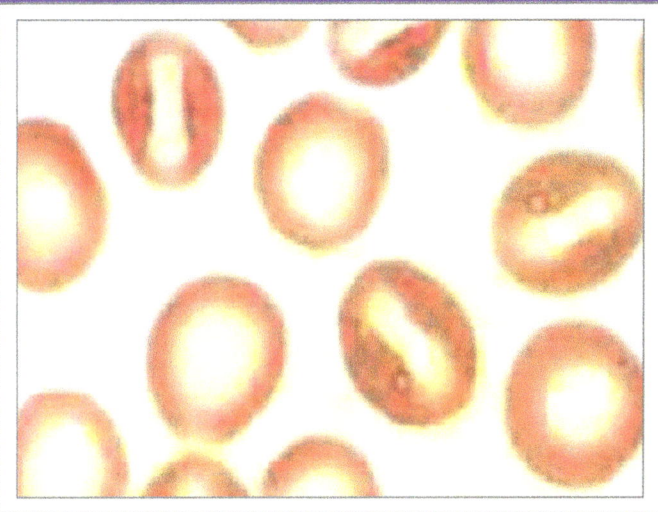

HOWELL-JOLLY BODIES

Small, well-defined, round, densely stained inclusions; 1 µm in diameter, eccentric in location that represent DNA fragments which were once part of the nucleus of immature red cells. Associated with rapid or abnormal RBC formation.

Howell-Jolly bodies are seen in:
- Post-splenectomy or hyposplenia (a normally functioning spleen usually removes all intraerythrocytic inclusions including nuclear remnants very efficiently)
- Newborn
- Megaloblastic anemias
- Dyserythropoietic anemias
- Rarely iron-deficiency anemia
- Hereditary spherocytosis.

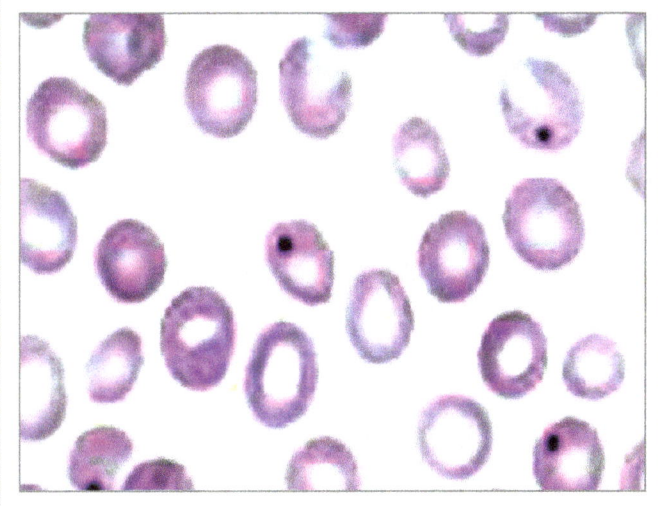

SPUR CELL (ACANTHOCYTES) – "ACANTHO"-THORN

Cells with 5-10 spicules of varying length; spicules irregular in space and thickness, with wide bases; appear smaller than normal cells because they assume a spheroid shape.
Results from changes in membrane lipid content.

Spur cell is seen in:
- Spur cell anemia, usually alcoholic cirrhosis, causes an increase in the cholesterol: phospholipid ratio in the red cell membrane, leading to hemolysis.
- Post-splenectomy or hyposplenic state
- Hypothyroidism
- Abetalipoproteinemia: 50–100% of cell acanthocytes
- Associated abnormalities (fat malabsorption, retinitis pigmentosa, neurologic abnormalities)
- Malabsorption
- Vitamin E deficiency.

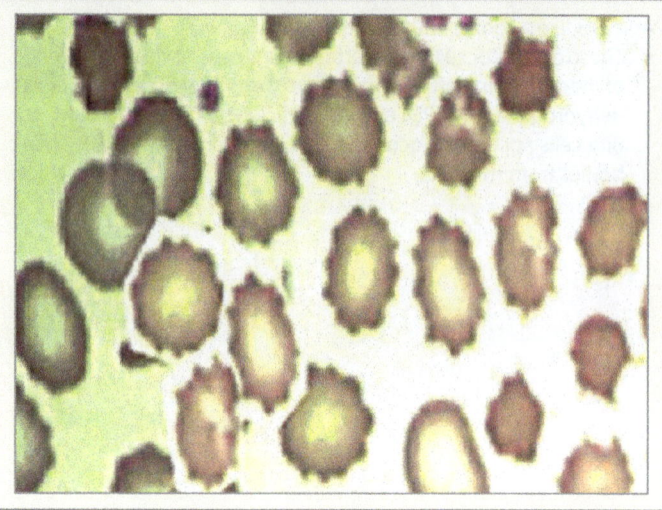

HEINZ BODIES

Heinz bodies are erythrocyte inclusions of denatured hemoglobin caused by oxidation of globin portion of hemoglobin molecule. Removal of Heinz bodies may lead to formation of bite cells.
- Trigger is drugs or certain foods like fava beans and onions.

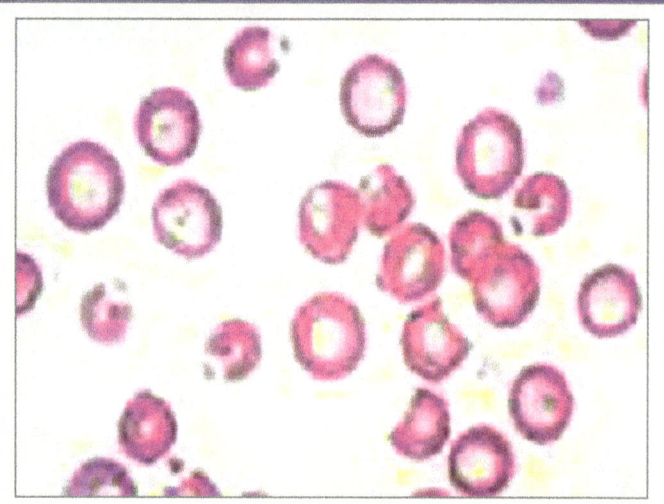

SIDEROTIC GRANULES/PAPPENHEIMER BODIES

They are irregular dark blue iron containing granules occurring in small clusters, predominantly in the cell periphery. Erythrocytes with Pappenheimer bodies are called siderocytes. These are iron-containing inclusions which can be demonstrated by Perl's or Prussian blue stains. Siderotic granules are seen in:
- Splenectomy
- Hemolytic anemia
- Myelodysplastic syndromes
- Lead poisoning
- Sideroblastic anemia
- Subsequent to transfusion therapy.

In their presence iron deficiency can be ruled out.

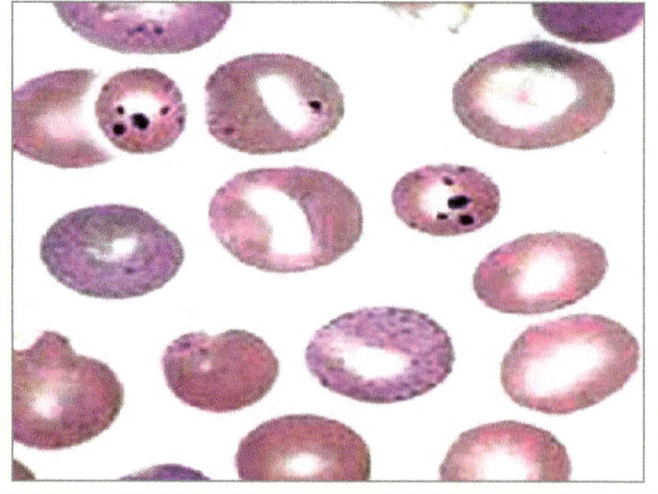

SICKLE CELLS

Crescent-shaped sickle cells develop in people homozygous for the hemoglobin S (HbS) gene and in those heterozygous for HbS and either thalassemia or another abnormal hemoglobin such as HbC. There is a substitution of valine for glutamic acid at the sixth residue of the beta chain, establishing sickle cell anemia as a disease of molecular structure, "a molecular disease" based on one point mutation.

Individuals with the sickle cell trait—Heterozygous for HbS and HbA—do not have sickle cells.

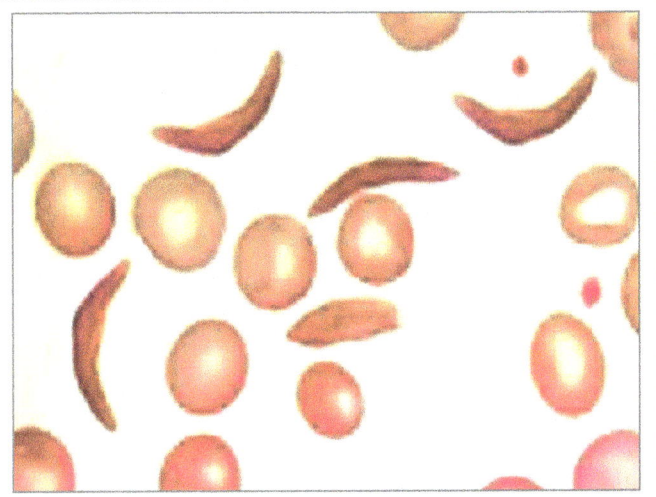

POLYCHROMATOPHILIA (POLYCHROMASIA) (more than one color)

- Primitive reticulocytes are larger than mature erythrocytes.
- They stain on Romanowsky preparations as bluish-gray or purple because of the substantial RNA remnants.
- This phenomenon is called polychromatophilia because the cells derive their hue from the combination of the blue from the RNA and red from the hemoglobin.
- Mostly they are present when a high level of erythropoietin circulates in a response to anemia.

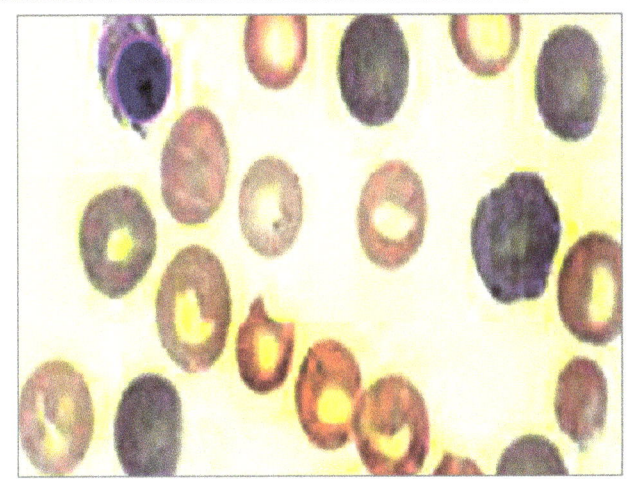

NUCLEATED RED BLOOD CELLS (nRBC)

These cells have a dark, dense nucleus in the center of a bluish (polychromatophilic) or red (orthochromatic) cell periphery.

They may result in response to marked stimulation of the bone marrow by erythropoietin in patients with severe anemia and the causes are:

- Newborn (first 3–4 days)
- Intense bone marrow stimulation
- Acute bleeding severe hemolytic anemia (e.g., thalassemia, SS hemoglobinopathy)
- Megaloblastic anemia
- Congenital infections (e.g., congenital syphilis, CMV, rubella)
- Post-splenectomy or hyposplenic states: Spleen normally removes nucleated RBCs
- Leukoerythroblastic reaction, seen with extramedullary hematopoiesis and bone marrow replacement
- Fungal and mycobacterial infection
- High WBC count with left shift
- Dyserythropoietic anemias
- Hypoxia, uremia, sepsis, liver disease

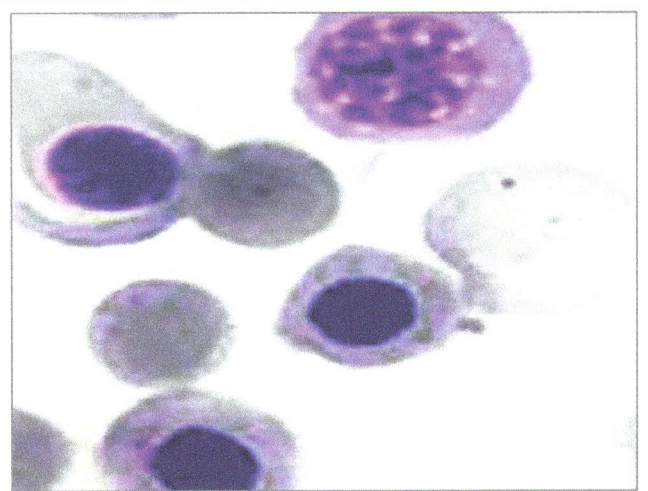

Except the newborns, presence of nucleated red cells is abnormal in the peripheral blood

BASOPHILIC STIPPLING

Numerous small, purplish inclusions, which result from RNA and mitochondrial remnants.

Seen in:
- Lead toxicity
- Thalassemias
- Hemoglobinopathies
- Macrocytic anemias

In their presence iron deficiency can be ruled out.

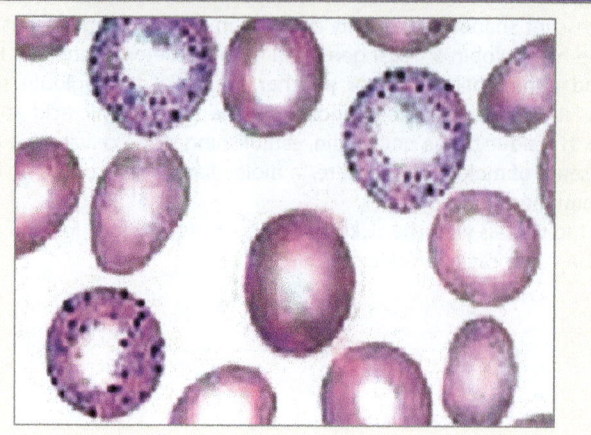

CABOT RINGS

Cabot rings are delicate thread-like inclusions, remnants of the nuclear membranes, in the RBC.
   They can take on a variety of shapes and sizes, such as basophilic.
   Purplish ring, figure-of-eight, incomplete rings appearing in the center or near the periphery of erythrocytes.

Significance: Cabot's rings are seen in:
- Pernicious anemia
- Lead poisoning
- Alcoholic jaundice
- Severe anemia
- Leukemia.

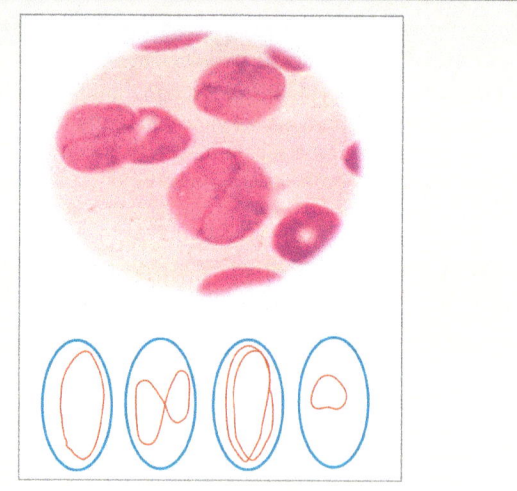

ROULEAUX FORMATION

A stack-like arrangement of red blood cells where the biconcave surfaces of RBCs are next to each other, a phenomenon that may be seen on a peripheral smear. The appearance of rouleaux may be artificially caused by poor preparation of the smear or by viewing the slide in a thickened area. Rouleaux formation may be seen in:
- An increase in cathodal proteins, such as immunoglobulins and fibrinogen
- Multiple myeloma
- Macroglobulinemias
- Acute and chronic infections
- Connective tissue diseases
- Chronic liver disease
- Diabetes mellitus
- Malignancies.

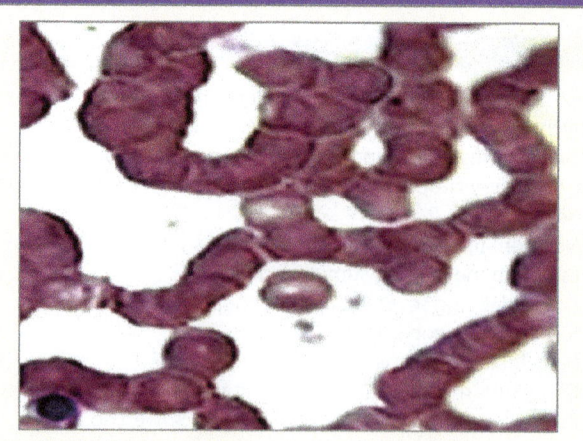

Grading of inclusions	
Rare	0 to 1/hpf
Few	1 to 2/hpf
Mod	2 to 4 /hpf
Many	> 5/hpf

Qualitative grading of abnormal RBC morphology

Grade	Degree of abnormalities
1 to 5 cells/10 fields	Slight
6 to 15 cells/10 fields	Moderate
> 15 cells/10 fields	Marked

HEMOPARASITES

MALARIA PARASITE

Malaria is a mosquito-borne infectious disease caused by Plasmodium. It is widespread in tropical and subtropical regions, including Sub-Saharan Africa, Asia, and America. The disease results from the multiplication of malaria parasites within red blood cells, causing symptoms that typically include fever with chills and headache, in severe cases progressing to coma, and death.

Four species of *Plasmodium* can infect and be transmitted by humans. Severe disease is largely caused by *Plasmodium falciparum*. Malaria caused by *Plasmodium vivax*, *Plasmodium ovale* and *Plasmodium malariae* is generally a milder disease that is rarely fatal. A fifth species, *Plasmodium knowlesi*, is a zoonosis that causes malaria in macaques but can also infect humans.

DIAGNOSIS OF MALARIA

A. Peripheral Blood Smear Examination

- Remains the gold standard for diagnosis
  - Giemsa stain distinguishes between species and life cycle stages
  - Parasitemia is quantifiable.
- Threshold of detection thin film: 100 parasites/l, thick film: 5–20 parasites/l.
- Accuracy depends on the laboratorian skill.
- Prepare smears as soon as possible after collecting venous blood to avoid changes in parasite morphology.

Interpreting Thick and Thin Film

Thick film
- Lysed RBCs
- Larger volume
- 0.25 μl blood/100 fields
- Blood elements more concentrated
- Good screening test for positive or negative parasitemia and parasite density-difficult to diagnose species

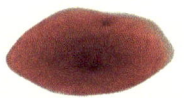

Thin film
Fixed RBCs
- Single layer
- Smaller volume
- 0.005 μl blood/100 fields
- Good species differentiation
- Requires more time to read-low density infections can be missed

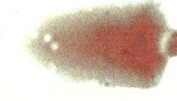

Appearance of *P. falciparum* in the Blood Films

Ring Forms or Trophozoites
• Many red cells infected – some with more than one parasite • Red cell size is unaltered • Ring size is 1.25–1.5 μm in diameter, nucleus often projecting beyond the ring • Parasite often attaches itself to the margin of the host cell; this is known as appliqué or Accole form (arrow).

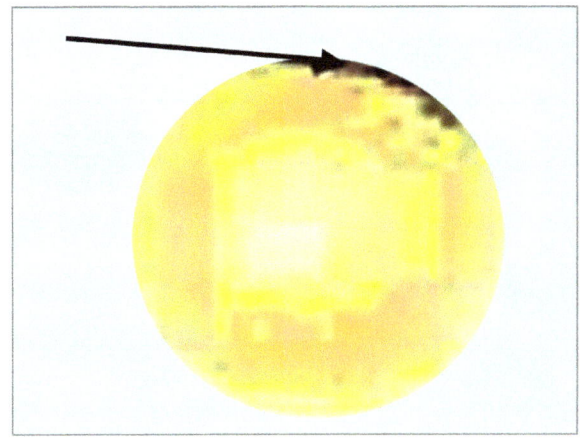
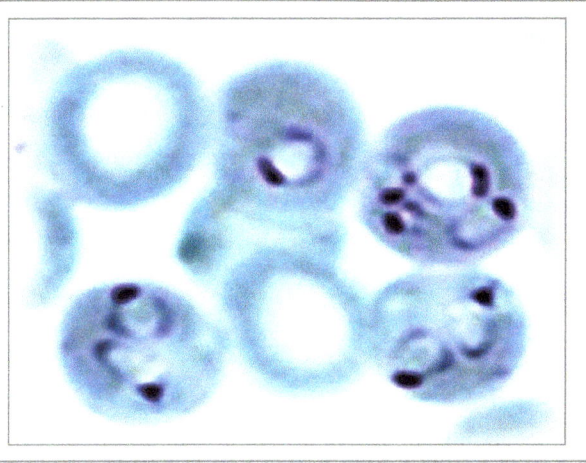

Schizont of *P. falciparum*
- Very rarely seen except in cerebral malaria. - A single brown pigment dot along with 18–32 merozoites. 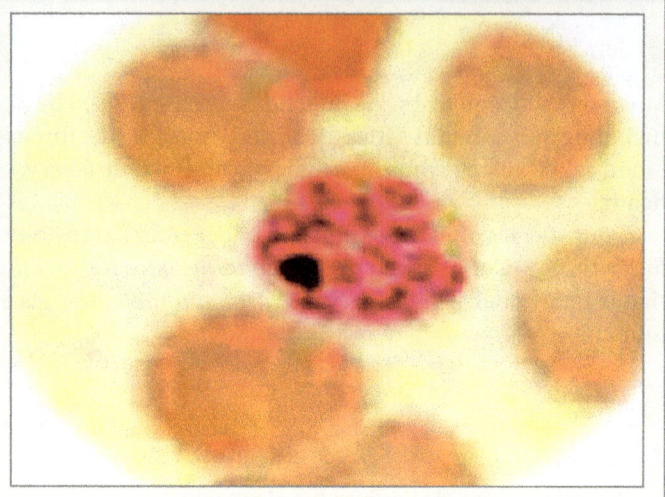

Gametocytes (Sexual Stages)

- These are sickle-shaped "crescents".
  The size of mature gametocyte is about 1½ times larger than RBC harbouring it.
- Microgametocyte–Broader, shorter, blunt ends. Cytoplasm stains light blue. The nucleus is scattered in fine granules over a wide area. Pigment is scattered throughout the cytoplasm.
- Macrogametocyte–Longer, narrower, pointed ends. The cytoplasm stains deep blue. The nucleus is condensed into a small compact mass at the center. The pigment aggregate like a wreath around nucleus.

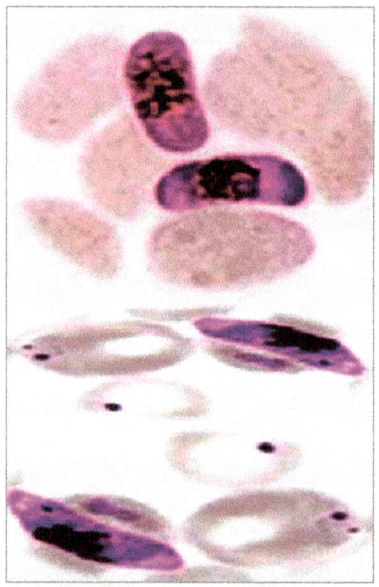

Appearance of *P. vivax* in the Blood Films

Ring Form or Trophozoite

- Red cell enlarged and distorted
- Unoccupied portion by parasite shows a dotted or stippled appearance called Schuffner's dot
- Trophozoite consists of a blue cytoplasmic ring, a red nuclear mass and an unstained area called the nutrient vacuole
- Diameter is about 2.5–3 μm
- One side of the ring is thicker and red chromatin at the thinner part.

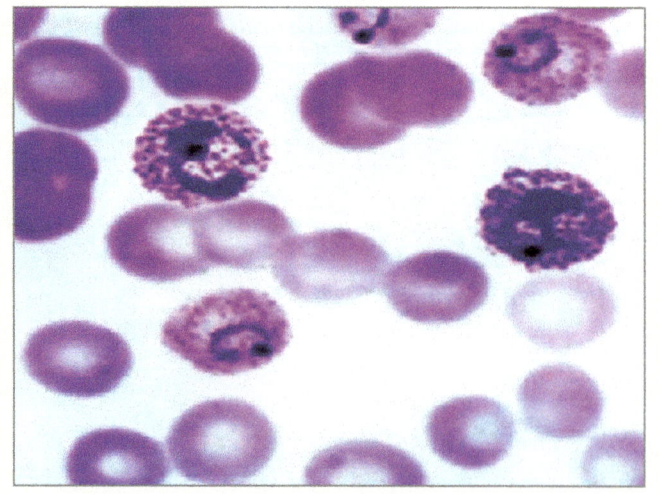

Schizont	
<ul><li>Represents the full grown trophozoite.</li><li>Measures 9–10 µm</li><li>Contains 12–24 merozoites</li><li>Arranged in form of a "rosette" with yellow-brown pigment at the center.</li></ul>	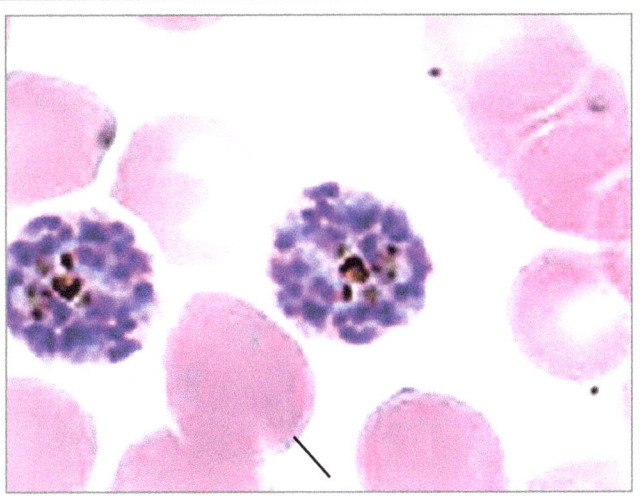

Gametocyte	
<ul><li>Certain schizonts become biologically modified and resultant merozoites are differentiated into sexual forms. Merozoites arising out of a single schizont are either all males (microgametes) or all females (macrogametes).</li><li>*Microgametes*–Spherical, 9–10 µm. Cytoplasm stains light blue with a large diffuse nucleus.</li><li>*Macrogametes*–Spherical, 10–12 µm. The cytoplasm stains deep blue and the nucleus is small compact.</li></ul>	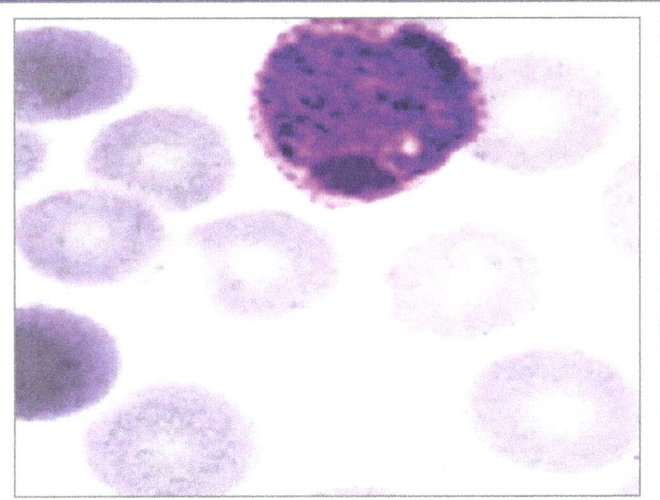

B. Fluorescent Microscopy

- Modification of light microscopy
  - Requires special equipment–fluorescent microscope.
- Dyes detect RNA and DNA contents of parasites.
- Nucleic material not seen normally in mature RBCs without parasitemia.
  - Stain thin film with acridine orange (AO).
  - Staining itself is cheap.
  - Sensitivities up to 90%.

C. Quantitative Buffy Coat (QBC) (Becton Dickinson)

- Fluorescent microscopy after centrifugation.
- Acridine orange—Coated capillary is filled with 50-100 µL blood.
- Parasites concentrate below the granulocyte layer in the tube.
- More sensitive than light microscopy, 18% more positive are reported than conventional film.
- It can detect as low as one parasite per microliter of blood.
- Useful for screening large numbers of samples.
- Quick, saves time.
- The test is 5–7% more sensitive than Giemsa's thick film.

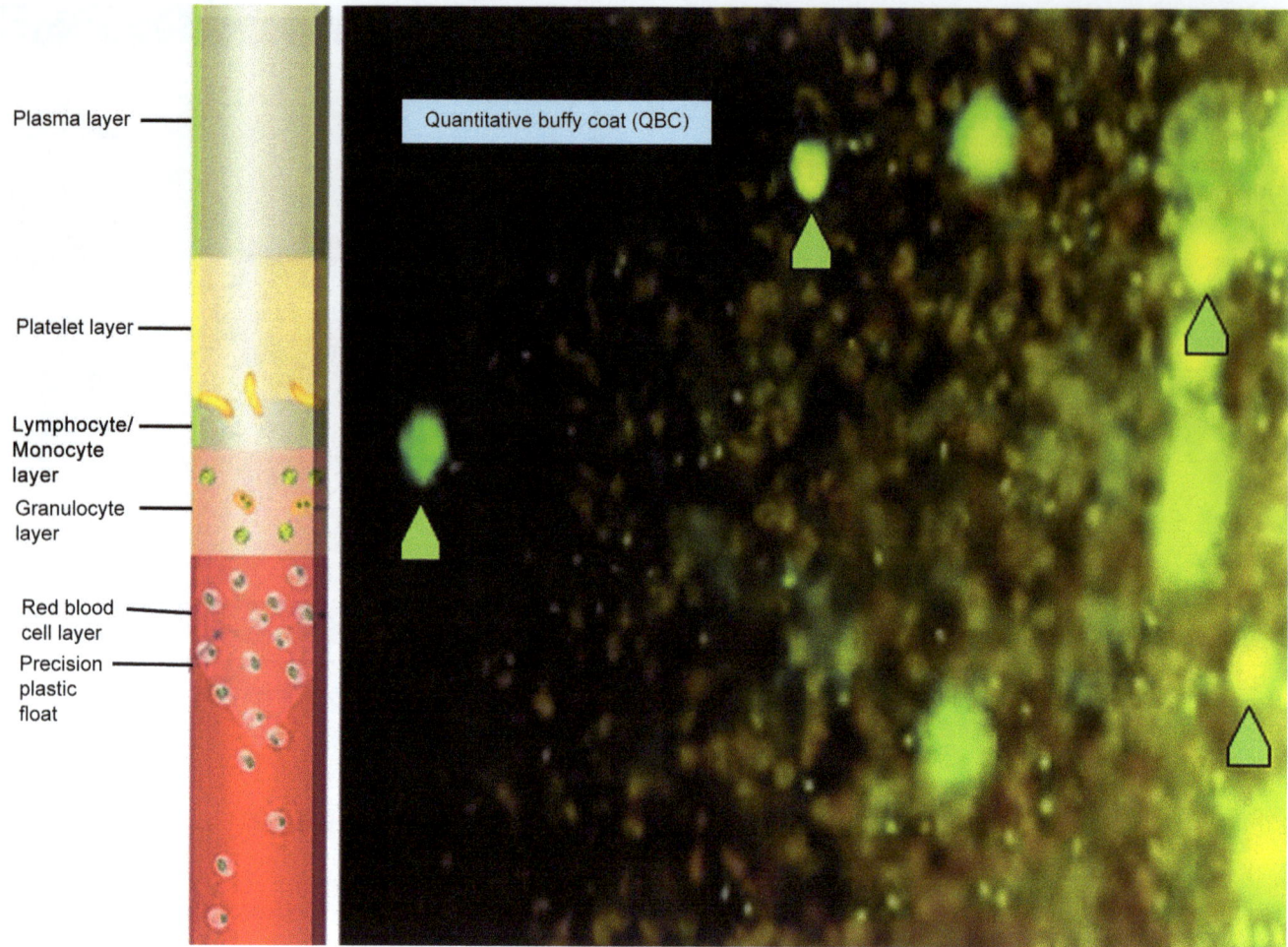

Main Disadvantages of QBC
- Requires centrifuge, capillaries coated with special stain
- High cost of capillaries and equipment
- Cannot store capillaries for later reference.

D. Malaria Serology–Antibody Detection
- Immunologic assays to detect host response.
- Antibodies to asexual parasites appear some days after the invasion of RBCs and may persist for months.
- Positive test indicates past infection.
- Not useful for treatment decisions.
- Valuable epidemiologic tool in some settings particularly.
  - Investigating congenital malaria, especially if mother's smear is negative
  - Diagnosing, or ruling out tropical splenomegaly syndrome.

E. Malaria Serology–Antigen Detection
- Immunologic assays to detect specific antigens.
- Commercial kits now available as immunochromatographic rapid diagnostic tests.
- Monoclonal and polyclonal antibodies used in antigen (Ag) capture test.
- Species-specific and pan-specific antibody.
- Cross-reactivity with other immunological conditions.

Principles of Detection of Plasmodium Antigens
- HRP-2 (histidine-rich protein 2) (ICT)
- pLDH (parasite lactate dehydrogenase) (Flow)
- HRP-2 (histidine-rich protein 2) (PATH).

Malaria antigen detection – RDTs		
Features	PfHRP-2 tests	pLDH tests
Test principle	Use of monoclonal (Ab) Detects a histidine rich protein of *P. falciparum*	Use of monoclonal and polyclonal Ab Detects a parasite enzyme, lactate dehydrogenase
Advantages	Threshold for parasite detection as low as 10 parasites/μl Does not cross-react with other species– *Plasmodium ovale, Plasmodium vivax, Plasmodium malariae*	Threshold for parasite detection ≥ 100 parasites/μl Can detect all species which infect humans Can differentiate between *Plasmodium falciparum* and nonfalciparum malaria
Disadvantages	Sensitivity and specificity decreases < 100 parasites/μL May remain positive up to 14 days posttreatment, in spite of asexual and sexual parasite clearance, due to circulating antigens	Cannot detect mixed infections Sensitivity and specificity decreases < 100 parasites/μL
Sensitivity Specificity	Sensitivity 94–100% Specificity 88–100%	Sensitivity *Plasmodium falciparum* 88–98%, *Plasmodium vivax* 89–94% Specificity *Plasmodium falciparum* 93–99%, *Plasmodium vivax* 99–100%

F. Polymerase Chain Reaction (PCR)

- Molecular technique to identify parasite genetic material.
- Whole blood collected in an anticoagulated tube (200 μL) or directly onto filter paper.
  - 100% DNA is extracted.
- Threshold of detection 0.1 parasite/μL, if whole blood in a tube and 2 parasites/μL, if filter paper is used.
- Definitive species—Specific diagnosis possible.
- Can identify mutations–Correlate to drug resistance.
- Requires specialized equipment, reagents, and training.
- Parasitemia not quantifiable.

Real-Time PCR

- New technique based on fluorescence
- Can quantify parasitemia
- Detect multiple wavelengths in the same tube identifying multiple species in one run.

G. Automation Based Malaria Detection

As complete blood count (CBC) is a baseline investigation ordered for patients with fever, there has been a growing focus on the utility of automated hematology analyzers in the presumptive diagnosis of malarial infection, even in unsuspected cases.

- Hematological parameter such as hemoglobin, total count, platelet count, and their different combination can predict the presence of acute malaria.
- Low platelet count has emerged as the strongest predictor of malaria.
- Leukopenia and anemia also occur.
- Autoanalyzer can detect various hematological parameters which can help in the early and easy diagnosis of malaria.
- Common findings in malaria are normocytic or microcytic anemia with low Hb, decreased RBC count, raised ESR, normal or low MCV, normal MCH, normal or reduced MCHC, normal to increased RDW in most of the cases.
- Total WBC count may be increased or decreased. Leukopenia is more common.
- Differential shows increased monocytes.
- Platelet parameter: Thrombocytopenia, variable mean platelet volume (MPV), normal or low plateletcrit, and PDW.
- Automated analyzer can detect malarial pigment in neutrophil and monocyte.
- The intracellular malarial pigment in white blood cells (WBCs) can be detected by DLL (Depolarize Laser Light).
- Some of the advanced hematology analyzers are designed to detect specific abnormalities in the WBCs of the patient infested with the malaria parasite. They detect malaria hemozoin in monocytes according to their abnormal depolarizing pattern.
- Sometimes hemozoin-containing neutrophils are misidentified as eosinophils with abnormal scattergram by the automated cell counters, resulting in the pseudoeosinophilia. Variation of the manual smear review of eosinophil count from pseudoeosinophilia of cell counter can be used as a suspicion indicator of a malarial infestation.
- The Cell-Dyn analyzers use laser light scatter at various angles, the so-called multiple-angle polarized scatter separation for WBC analysis.

- Multiple-angle polarized scatter separation is used to distinguish eosinophils from neutrophils based on the light depolarizing properties of their granules but has also been found to detect hemozoin-containing monocytes and granulocytes
- These malaria-related events are shown in a scatter-plot with 90° side-scatter on the x-axis and 90° depolarized side-scatter on the y-axis, usually labelled as lobularity/granularity scatter-plot.

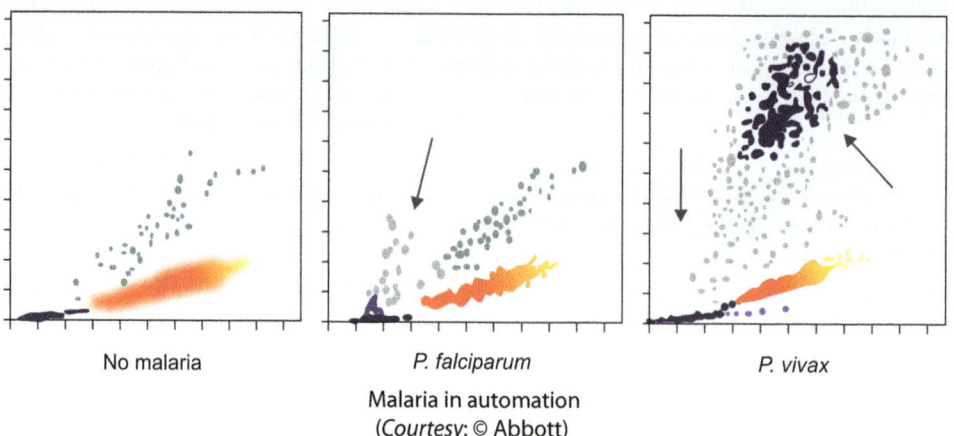

Malaria in automation
(*Courtesy*: © Abbott)

- Mindray (CUBE Technology) provides dedicated flags called "infected RBC?" and "InR"(#, %) parameters to represent the number and ratio of the infected RBC respectively.
- With the rising number of infected RBC with MP (malaria parasite), the number of dots in the "InR" increase proportionately, indicating the possible presence of Plasmodium parasite.
- WBC/BASO scattergram abnormalities are useful in the presumptive diagnosis of *P. vivax* when combined with presence of thrombocytopenia.
- This helps the pathologists and technicians who handle these autoanalyzers to pick up all suspicious cases and subsequently confirm the same on a peripheral smear and with other rapid diagnostic tests
- Other observations include thrombocytopenia with pseudoeosinophilia which is defined as a difference in automated and manual eosinophil count of >5%.
- It was also noted that all the scattergram abnormalities reversed after two days of initiation of antimalarial treatment.

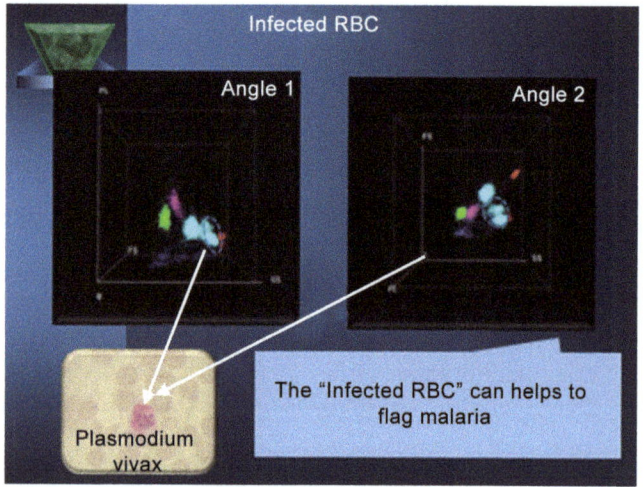

Mindray (CUBE technology)
Courtesy: © Mindray

Sysmex Scatter-plots Normal and with P. vivax-related Findings

Malaria-related findings that appear in the high SSC range of both the DIFF and WBC/BASO scatter-plot could be caused by hemozoin crystals in mature parasites.

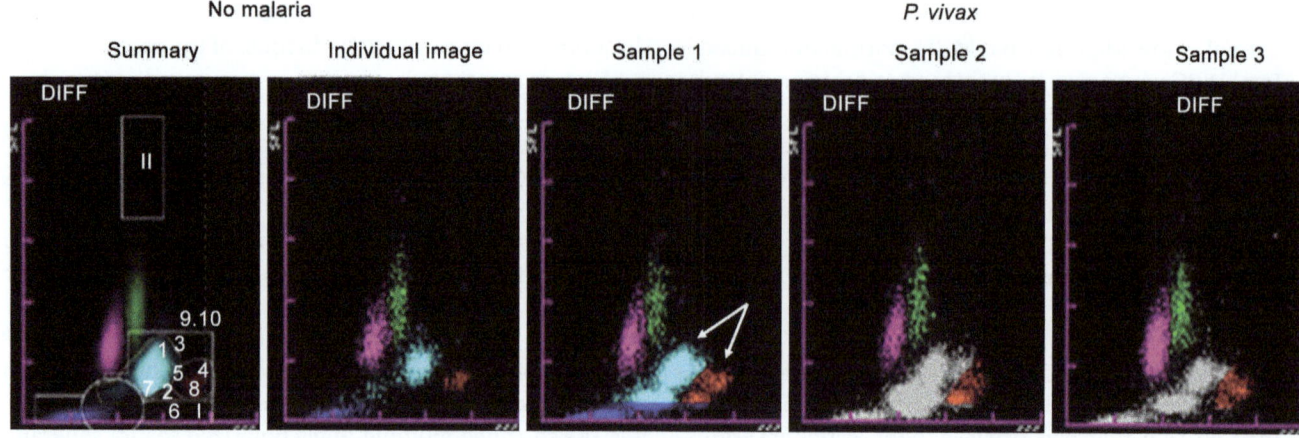

Courtesy: © Sysmax

FILARIASIS

Filariasis is a parasitic disease that is caused by thread-like filarial nematodes in the superfamily Filarioidea, also known as "filariae". There are 8 known filarial nematodes that use humans as the host. These are divided into 3 groups according to the niche within the body that they occupy:

- **Lymphatic filariasis** is caused by the worms: *Wuchereria bancrofti, Brugia malayi,* and *Brugia timori*. These worms occupy the lymphatic system, including the lymph nodes, and in chronic cases, these worms lead to the disease elephantiasis.
- **Subcutaneous filariasis** is caused by loa loa (the African eye worm), *Mansonella streptocerca, Onchocerca volvulus,* and *Dracunculus medinensis (the guinea worm)*. These worms occupy the subcutaneous layer of the skin, in the fat layer.
- **Serous cavity filariasis** is caused by the worms; *Mansonella perstans and Mansonella ozzardi*. These occupy the serous cavity of the abdomen.

Blood film examination: Microfilaria shows nocturnal periodicity, the blood should be collected between 10 pm to 4 am because the greatest number of microfilariae can be found in the blood during this peak biting time of the mosquito vectors.

The pattern of periodicity can be reversed by changing the patient's sleep-wake cycle. Thick blood smear and concentration techniques are used.

Eosinophilia is marked in all forms of filarial infection.

Concentration techniques: Usually microfilariae are scanty in peripheral blood, so concentration techniques may be necessary to demonstrate.
- Membrane filtration.
- Microhematocrit tube or capillary tube method.
- Lysed capillary blood method.
- **Lysed venous blood method**: 1 mL blood mixed with 9 mL of 2% formalin—Centrifuged for 5 min, smear prepared from sediments and stained.

Appearance of microfilaria in thick films
- Microfilariae measures 290 µm × 7 µm.
- Covered with a hyaline sheath projecting beyond the extremities (359 µm)
- Nuclei or somatic cells seen as granules in central axis of the body, extending from head to tail end but not up to the tip of tail
- The granules are broken at definite places, serving as landmarks for species identification
- Few G cells present posteriorly.

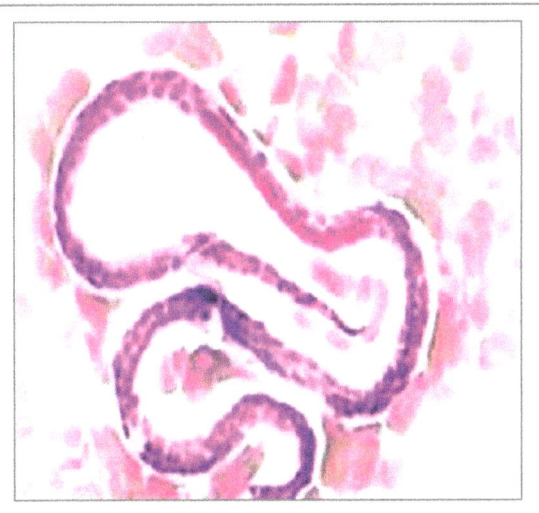

Leishmaniasis
- Leishmaniasis is a disease caused by parasites that belong to the genus *Leishmania*, transmitted by the bite of certain species of sand fly (subfamily Phlebotominae).
- Their primary hosts are vertebrates (man).
- Parasite is always intracellular, occurring in amastigote forms. It is essentially the parasite of RE System.
- Leishmaniasis is diagnosed by direct visualization of the amastigotes (Leishman-Donovan bodies).

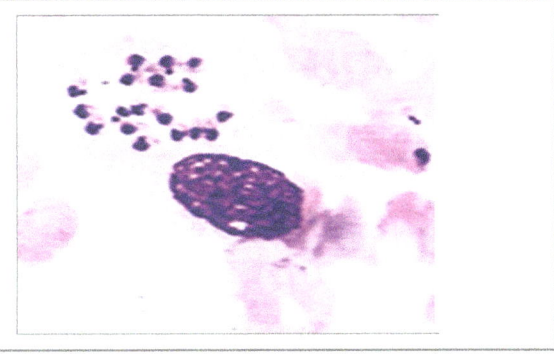

- Buffy-coat preparations of peripheral blood or aspirates from marrow, spleen, lymph nodes or skin lesions should be spread on a slide to make a thin smear, and stained with Leishman or Giemsa stain (pH 7.2) for 20 minutes
- Amastigotes are seen with monocytes or, less commonly in neutrophil in peripheral blood and in macrophages in aspirates
- They are small, round bodies 2–4 μm in diameter with indistinct cytoplasm, a nucleus, and a small rod-shaped kinetoplast
- Occasionally amastigotes may be seen lying free between cells.

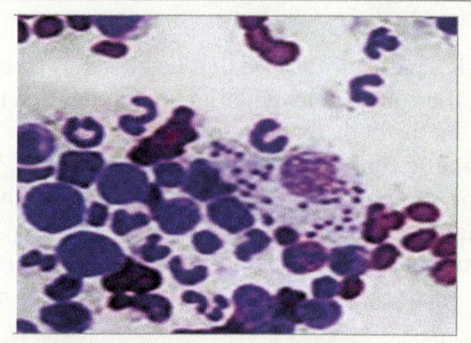

Babesiosis

- *Babesia microti* is a protozoan that infects mice
- It is transmitted between hosts by ticks
- Infected humans may be asymptomatic, but, especially in asplenic hosts, fever, myalgias, and hemolytic anemia can occur
- The organisms are intraerythrocytic, winged parasites that are 2–3 μm in diameter, have 1–2 chromatin dots, and may assume basket shapes.
- More than one organism can be present in a red cell; when four have their ends in contact, they form pathognomonic maltase cross appearance.
- *Babesia* organisms differ from those of malaria in that the ring forms are smaller pigment is absent, and schizonts and gametocytes do not exist.

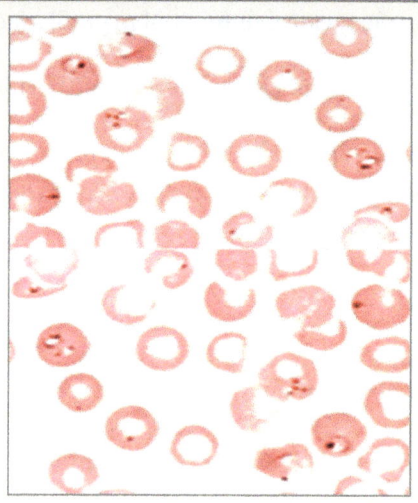

Trypanosoma Brucei

- Also known as "African sleeping sickness"
- Trypomastigotes found in peripheral blood
- When stained with Leishman stain, cytoplasm and the undulating membrane appear pale blue the nucleus reddish-purple or red. Kinetoplast and flagellum dark red.

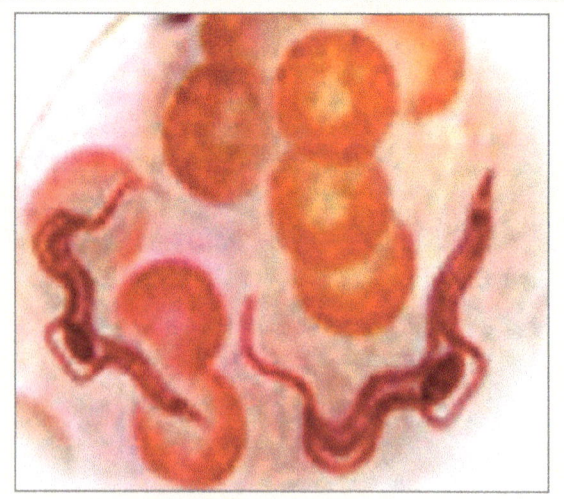

Trypanosoma Cruzi – (Chagas Disease)

Two forms are found:
- Trypomastigote form (peripheral blood)
- Amastigote form (in striated muscles)
  - Trypomastigote form appears as C or U shaped
  - Staining characters are same as that of other trypanomsomes.

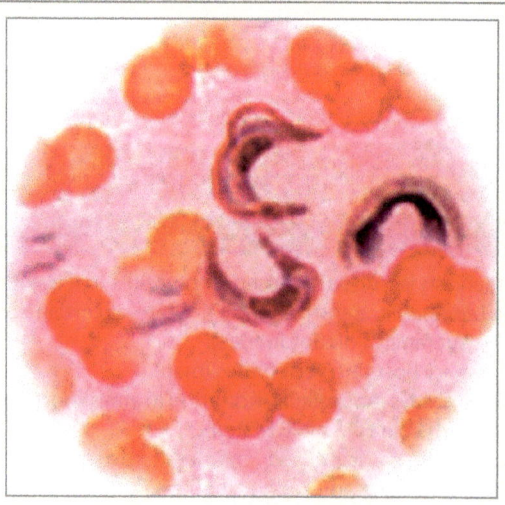

CHAPTER 4

White Blood Cells

WHITE BLOOD CELL COUNT

The name "white blood cell (WBC)" is derived from the fact that after centrifugation of a blood sample, these cells accumulate in the buffy coat, a thin, typically white layer of cells between the sedimented red blood cells and the blood plasma. The scientific term leukocyte directly reflects this description, derived from Greek λευκό (white), and κύτταρο (cell).
- White blood cells or leukocytes, are cells of the immune system involved in defending the body against both infectious disease and foreign materials.
- Blood plasma may sometimes be green if there are large amounts of neutrophils in the sample, this happens due to the heme-containing enzyme myeloperoxidase that they produce.

	Age	Leukocyte count
Normal WBC count	Birth	4–40 × 10⁹/L
	4 years	5–15 × 10⁹/L
	Adult	4–11 × 10⁹/L

Increase in count – *LEUKOCYTOSIS*, Decrease in count – *LEUKOPENIA*

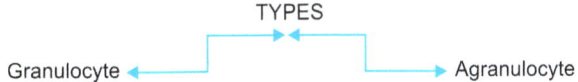

- **Granulocytes (polymorphonuclear leukocytes):** Leukocytes are characterized by the presence of differently staining granules in their cytoplasm when viewed under a light microscope. These granules are membrane-bound enzymes that primarily act in the digestion of endocytosed particles. There are three types of granulocytes: neutrophils, basophils, and eosinophils, which are named according to their staining properties.
- **Agranulocytes (mononuclear leukocytes):** Leukocytes are characterized by the apparent absence of granules in their cytoplasm. Although the name implies a lack of granules these cells do contain non-specific azurophilic granules, which are lysosomes. The cells include lymphocytes, monocytes, and macrophages.

LEUKOCYTOSIS—HIGH WBC COUNT

Leukocytosis, is an increase in disease-fighting cells (leukocytes) circulating in the blood. The significant numerical threshold of leukocytosis is relative to baseline leukocyte counts of an individual in healthy status.
A high white blood cell count usually indicates:
- Increased production of white blood cells to fight an infection
- Reaction to a drug that enhances white blood cell production
- Disease of bone marrow, causing high production of white blood cells
- An immune system disorder that increases white blood cell production.

Causes of High White Blood Cell Counts

- Acute and chronic bacterial infections
- Viral infections
- Stress, such as severe emotional or physical stress
- Tissue damage, such as from burns

- Polycythemia vera
- Rheumatoid arthritis
- Drugs
- Allergy, especially severe allergic reactions
- Acute lymphocytic leukemia
- Acute myeloid leukemia (AML)
- Smoking
- Chronic lymphocytic leukemia
- Chronic myelogenous leukemia
- Hairy cell leukemia
- Lymphoma spillage
- Measles
- Myelofibrosis

Causes of Low White Cell Counts

- Chemotherapy and radiation therapy
- Sepsis
- Typhoid
- Malaria
- Tuberculosis
- Dengue
- Enlargement of the spleen
- Leukemia (as malignant cells overwhelm the bone marrow)
- Folate deficiencies
- Psittacosis
- Drugs like various antipsychotic
- Myelofibrosis
- Aplastic anemia (failure of bone marrow production)
- Human immunodeficiency virus infection (HIV) and acquired immunodeficiency syndrome (AIDS)
- Influenza
- Systemic lupus erythematosus (SLE)
- Hodgkin's lymphoma
- Some types of malignancies
- Rickettsial infections

Pseudoleukopenia

May develop at the onset of infection. The leukocytes (predominately neutrophils, responding to injury first) are marginalized in the blood vessels so that they can scan for the site of infection. Although there is increased WBC production, it will appear low in a blood sample, since the blood sample is of core blood and does not include the marginalized leukocytes.

STAGES OF LEUKOCYTE MATURATION

The white cell series encompasses those cells that are distinguished by their granules and those that are agranular. In all, there are five maturation stages for neutrophils, four for eosinophils and basophils, and three each for monocytes and lymphocytes.

Distinguishing features of immature and mature stages of leukocytes are: • Cell size • Nucleus-to-cytoplasm ratio (N:C) • Chromatin pattern • Cytoplasmic quality • Presence of granules	The stages of maturation for the neutrophilic series immature to mature are: • Myeloblast • Promyelocyte or progranulocyte • Myelocyte • Metamyelocyte • Band • Segmented neutrophil

Myeloblast

Size: 12–20 μm

N:C: 4:1 with round, oval, or slightly indented nucleus

Chromatin: Light red-purple with a fine mesh like texture with 2 to 5 nucleoli

Cytoplasm: Blue, nongranular

Differentiating characteristic: Nucleus has thin velvety chromatin
Cluster designation (CD) 45, CD38, CD34, CD33, CD13, (HLA)-DR

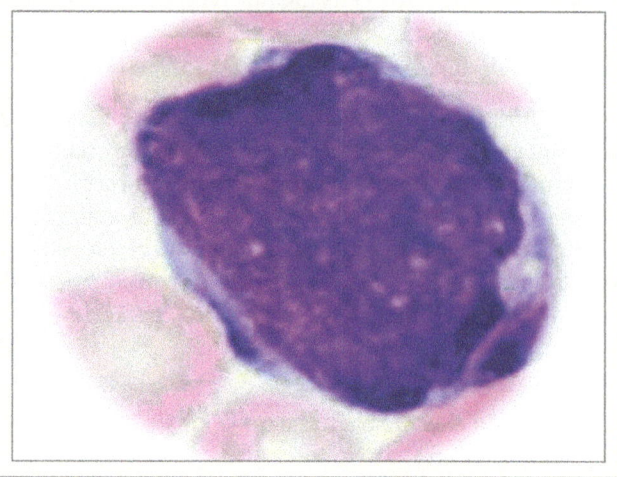

Promyelocyte (Progranulocyte)

Size: 15–21 µm

N:C: 3:1, oval, round, or eccentric flattened nucleus

Chromatin: Light red-purple of medium density, may see single nucleoli.

Cytoplasm: Moderate blue color but difficult to observe because fine to large blue-red azurophilic granules are scattered throughout the chromatin pattern; granules are nonspecific.

Differentiating characteristic: Cell is larger in size than the blast with large prominent nucleoli, nuclear chromatin is slightly coarse. CD45, CD33, CD13, CD15 positive.

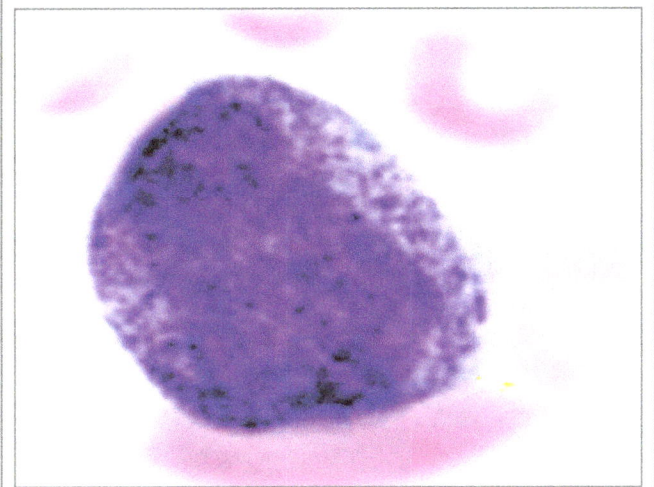

Myelocyte

Size: 10–18 µm

N:C: 2:1

Chromatin: Oval indented nucleus, denser, red-purple with slight granular appearance, coarser, clumped appearance.

Cytoplasm: Specific granules present, neutrophilic granules are dusty, fine, and red-blue; eosinophilic granules are large red-orange, and last stage capable of dividing.

Differentiating characteristic: Small pink-purple granules for the neutrophilic myelocyte, nucleus stains deeper color, granular pattern of the chromatin. Positive for CD45, CD33, CD13, CD15, CD11b/11c.

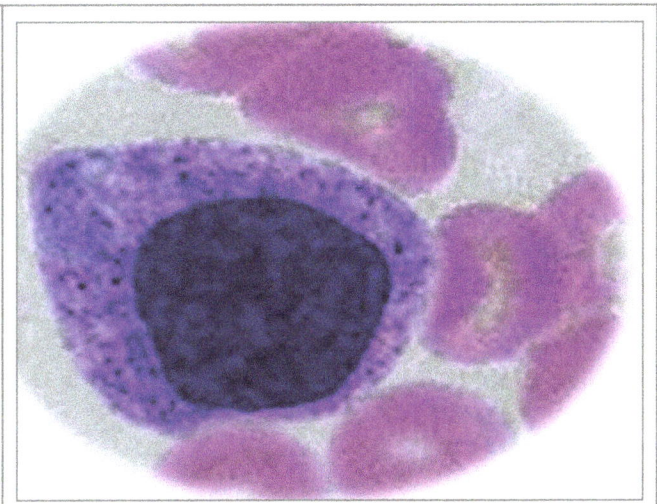

Metamyelocyte

Size: 10–15 µm

N:C: 1:1

Chromatin: Indented-shaped nucleus resembling a kidney structure, patches of coarse chromatin in spots.

Cytoplasm: Pale blue to pinkish-tan with moderate specific granules.

Differentiating characteristic: Nuclear indentation and condensed chromatin with no nuclei.

CD markers are the same as for the myelocyte.

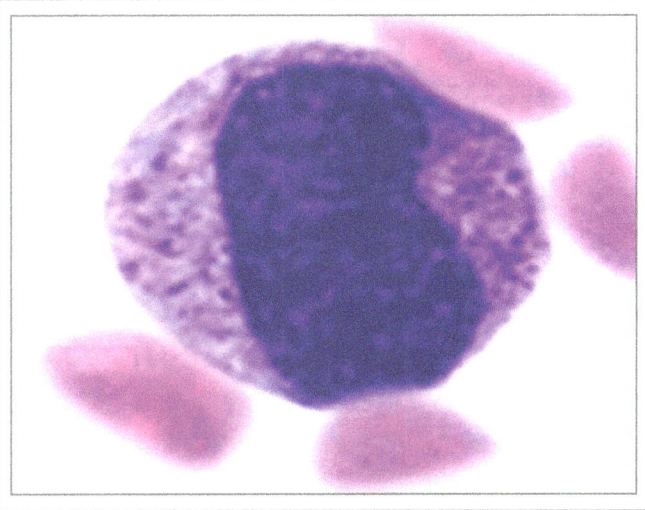

Chapter 4: White Blood Cells

Band (Juvenile or Stab Forms)

Size: 9–15 µm
Chromatin: Band-shaped like a cigar band, C or S-shaped, coarsely clumped
Cytoplasm: Brown-pink, with many fine secondary granules
Differentiating characteristics: Filament may resemble a metamyelocyte but indentation is more severe and chromatin is more clumped
Positive for CD45, CD13, CD15, CD11b/11c
Normally, bands constitute <5–10% of the white cells
An increase in the number of bands and other immature neutrophils is called a "shift to the left" and can occur in many situations, including
- Severe infections, sepsis
- Non-infectious inflammatory diseases
- Pregnancy

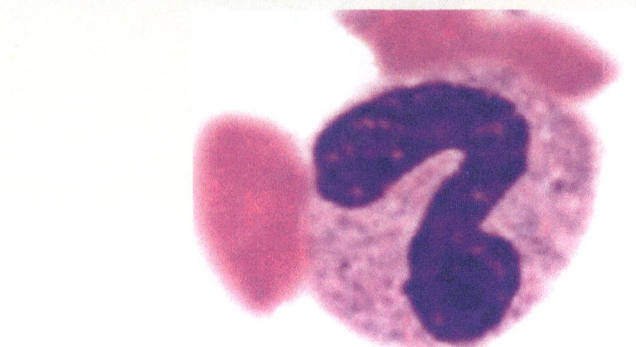
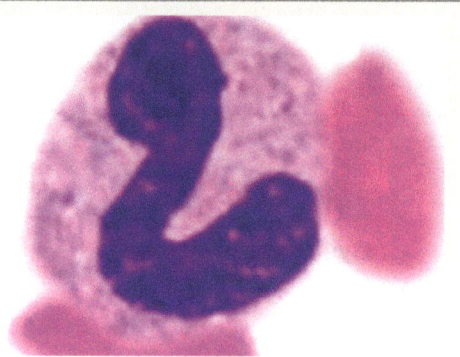

POLYMORPHS

- Polymorphonuclear (PMN) "Poly—Many" "morpho—Shape"
- "Neutro—Neutral"; have no preference for acidic or basic stains
- **Diameter:** 12-16 µm
- **Cytoplasm:** Pink
- **Granules:** Primary, secondary
- **Nucleus:** Dark purple to blue with dense chromatin, 2-5 lobes

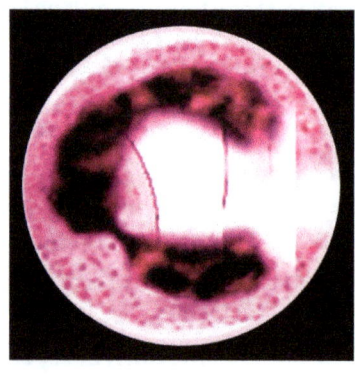

Causes of Increased Neutrophil (Neutrophilia): ANC >7,500/mm³

A. Physiologic increase (demargination)
- Release of cells in marginal pool
- Mediated by stress (stress leukocytosis)
- Exercise seizures
- Anxiety
- Epinephrine

B. Acute bacterial infection (and other infections)

C. Tissue injury and inflammation
- Myocardial infarction
- Burn injury
- Collagen vascular disease
- Hypersensitivity reaction

D. Metabolic condition
- Acute renal failure
- Eclampsia
- Ketoacidosis

E. Myeloproliferative disorder
- Myelocytic leukemia
- Myeloid metaplasia
- Polycythemia vera

F. Miscellaneous causes
- Hemolytic anemia
- Acute hemorrhage
- Splenectomy (leukocytosis may persist months)

G. Neoplasms
Metastatic cancer

H. Medications
- Corticosteroids
- Lithium
- Beta agonist

Causes of Neutropenia	
Decreased or ineffective production	*Increased removal from circulation*
• Aplastic anemia • Drugs • Disorders–vitamin deficiencies (B_{12}, folate) • Myelodysplastic syndromes • Post chemotherapy • Inherited disorder—Kostmann syndrome (defective genes of granulocyte differentiation)	• Immunological – SLE, drugs • Hypersplenism • Cyclical neutropenia • ↑ utilization—infections (mainly bacterial) <5,000/µL <1,50,000/µL

Hematological Scoring System and Early Diagnosis of Neonatal Sepsis

Neonatal Sepsis
- Neonatal sepsis or sepsis neonatorum or neonatal septicemia is the systemic response to infection in newborn infants.
- Hematological scoring system (HSS) can be a useful test to distinguish the infected from the non-infected infants.
- Higher score is indicative of sepsis. It has high sensitivity and specificity.
- An immature to total neutrophil ratio (I : T) along with degenerative changes followed by an immature to mature neutrophil ratio (I : M) is the most sensitive indicator in identifying infants with sepsis.
- Immature neutrophils include promyelocyte, myelocyte, metamyelocytes, and band cells.
- Degenerative changes in neutrophils include vacuolization, toxic granules, and Döhle bodies.
- The diagnosis of sepsis is confirmed by positive results of blood culture.

Hematological Scoring System

Criteria	Abnormality	Score
• Total WBC count	<5,000/µL³	1
	>25,000 at birth	1
	>30,000-(12–24 hours)	1
	>21,000 day 2 onwards	1
• Total PMN count	No mature PMN seen	2
	Increased/destruction	1
• Immature PMN count	Increased	1
• Immature: Total PMN ratio	Increased	1
• Immature: Mature PMN ratio	>0.3	1
• Degenerative changes in PMN	Toxic granules/cytoplasmic vacuoles	1
• Platelet count	<1,50,000/µL	1

Minimum Score is 0 and Maximum Score is 8

Interpretation of hematological scoring system

Score	Interpretation
<2	Sepsis is unlikely
3 or 4	Sepsis is possible
>5	Sepsis or infection is very likely

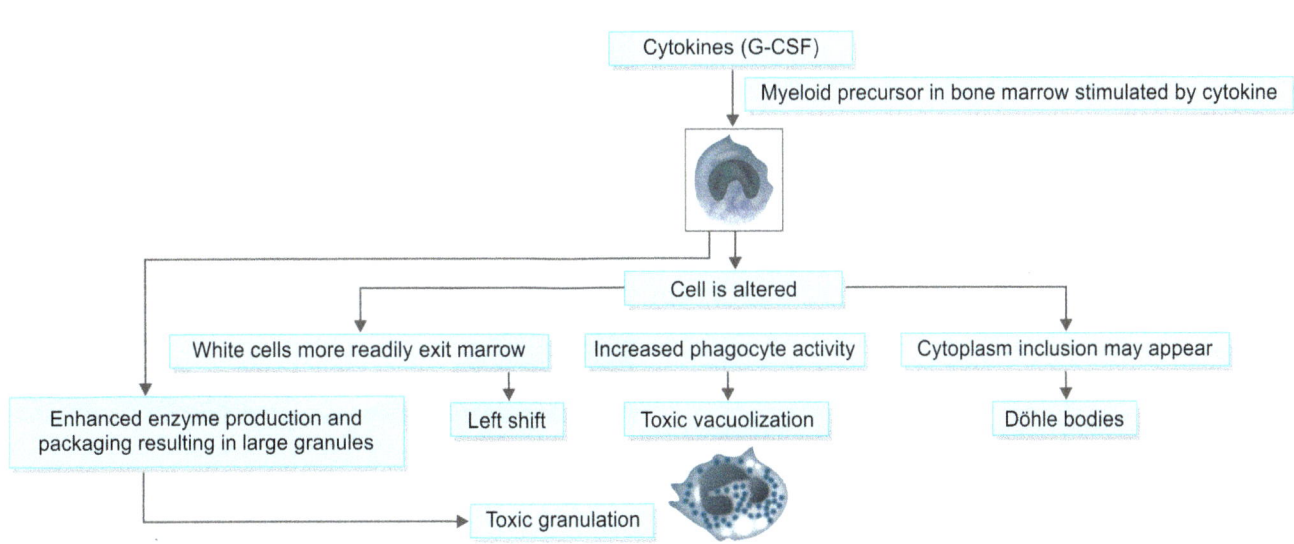

Toxic Granulation and Vacuolization

Toxic granulation indicates the presence of an increased number of granules that are larger and more basophilic than normal. It may occur in
- Severe infections (especially bacterial)
- Treatment with colony-stimulating factors
- During pregnancy
- Burns
- Malignancies
- Drug reactions
- Aplastic anemia
- Hypereosinophilic syndrome

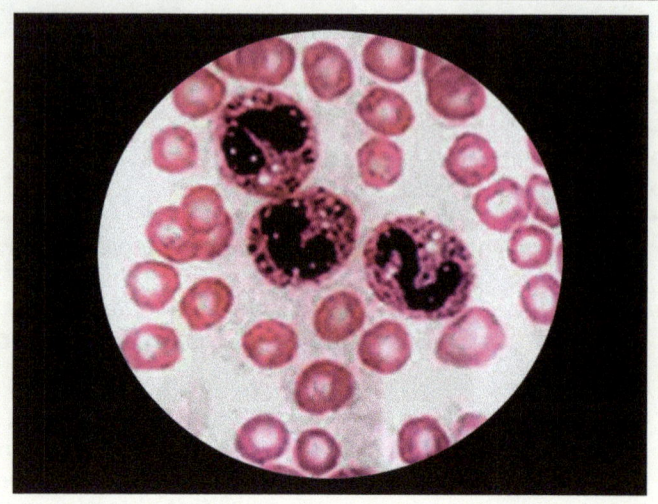

Döhle Body

- Composed of rough endoplasmic reticulum and glycogen granules.
- Döhle bodies are single or multiple, small blue-gray inclusions in the cytoplasm of neutrophils, often at the periphery.
- They may occur in several settings, including uncomplicated pregnancy, infections, inflammatory disorders, burns, myeloproliferative disorders, myelodysplastic syndromes, pernicious anemia, and cancer chemotherapy.

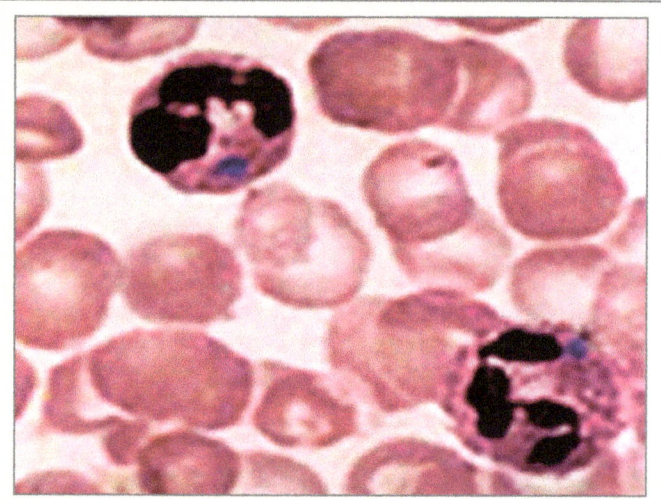

Hypersegmentation

- Exists when >5% of neutrophils have five lobes or more lobes.
- Such hypersegmentation is common in folate and vitamin B_{12} deficiency.
- Can be present in myelodysplastic and myeloproliferative disorders.

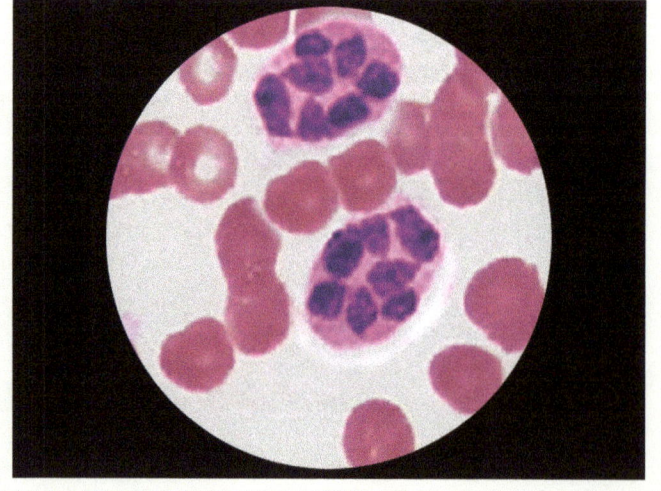

Pelger–Huët Anomaly

- About 70–90% of the neutrophils have hypolobulated, rounded nuclei with condensed chromatin.
- A thin strand of chromatin may connect the lobes, creating a pincenez (spectacle) shape, or a larger bridge can give the nucleus a peanut appearance.
- A few neutrophils have only one nucleus, but they differ from immature forms (myelocytes) by the presence of small nuclei, condensed chromatin, and mature cytoplasm.
- This hereditary hypolobulation has no clinical significance, and no other hematologic abnormalities coexist.
- An acquired (pseudo-Pelger–Huët) anomaly, common in myelodysplastic and myeloproliferative syndromes is distinguishable from the inherited disorder in that the percentage of affected neutrophils is smaller, the cytoplasm is often hypogranular, neutropenia is frequent, and Döhle bodies may be present.

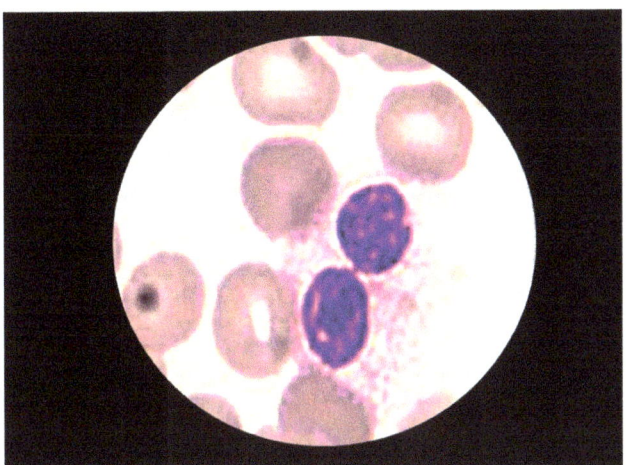 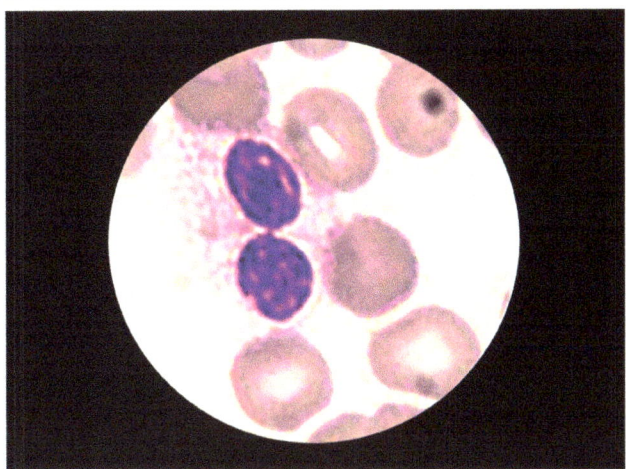

Chédiak–Higashi Syndrome

- Abnormal large irregular neutrophil granules
- Impaired lysosomal digestion of bacteria
- Associated with pigment and bleeding disorders
- Can be serious, especially in kids.

Auer Bodies (Auer Rod)

- Auer rods are classically seen in myeloid blasts of acute leukemias, but they are never seen in lymphoblasts or lymphocytes.
- Auer bodies are clumps of azurophilic granular material that form elongated red needle-like inclusions seen in the cytoplasm of leukemic blasts.
- They are composed of fused lysosomes and contain peroxidase lysosomal enzymes, and large crystalline inclusions.
  Their presence is virtually pathognomonic of myeloid leukemia.

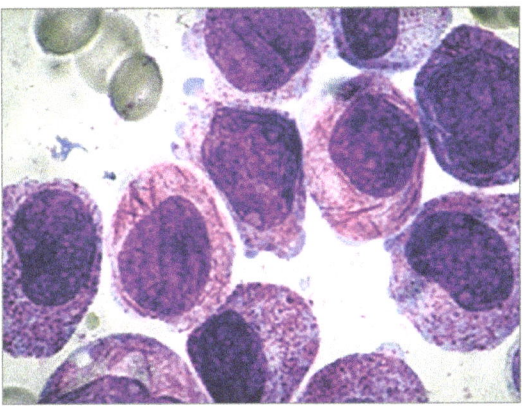

Left Shift

Left shift: Increased bands and other precursors in peripheral blood indicates rapid production of new neutrophils. Usually caused by excessive demand of defence system during acute processes like an acute infection.

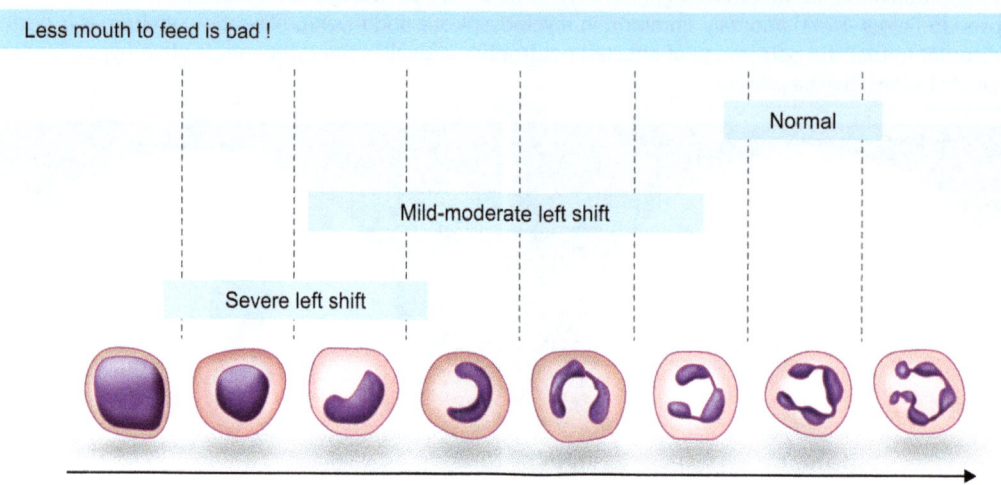

Right Shift

Right shift: Increased PMNs indicates increased mature neutrophils caused by chronic processes, such as pernicious anemia, hepatic disease, etc.

			Number of lobes		
	1	2	3	↑ 4	↑ 5
%	1%	10%	33%	34%	22%

LEUKEMOID REACTION

Leukemoid reaction is a hematological disorder that simulates leukemia due to high WBC counts and the presence of some premature leukocytes. In a leukemoid reaction, the circulating white blood cells are not clonally derived.

Persistent neutrophilia with cell counts of ≥30,000–50,000/μL is called myeloid leukemoid reaction.

Leukocyte alkaline phosphatase score (LAP-score) can differentiate leukemoid reaction from CML, the simulating condition. The LAP-score is raised in leukemoid reaction whereas decreased in CML.

Some Common Causes of Leukemoid Reaction			
Cause	*Myelocytic*	*Lymphocytic*	*Monocytic*
Infections	• Endocarditis • Pneumonia • Septicemia • Leptospirosis • Other	• Infectious mononucleosis • Infectious lymphocytosis • Pertussis • Varicella • Tuberculosis	Tuberculosis
Toxic conditions	• Burns • Eclampsia • Poisoning (e.g., mercury)		
Neoplasms	• Carcinoma of colon • Embryonal carcinoma of kidney	• Carcinoma of stomach • Carcinoma of breast	
Miscellaneous	• Acute hemorrhage • Acute hemolysis	Dermatitis herpetiformis	

Neutrophil Granularity Index

This parameter measures the intensity of neutrophilic granules and has its utility in **grading toxic granulations** in case of infections.
- It allows the detection of both the toxic granulation of infectious conditions and the hypogranularity of myelodysplastic syndromes.
- Reasonable correlation with microscopy to justify abandoning manual slide-based assessment of toxic granulation.

Immature Granulocytes (IG)

- With newer sophisticated cell counters, it is now possible to give the immature granulocyte count which can be an early indicator of infection
- Except for the neonatal blood samples, the appearance of immature granulocytes in the peripheral blood indicates an early-stage response to infection, inflammation, or other stimuli of the bone marrow.
- It enumerates metamyelocytes, myelocytes, and promyelocytes, but not bands.
- IG reflects the degree of a granulocytic left shift beyond bands.
- IG counts are relevant especially for patients who are **highly susceptible to infections** because of a suppressed immune system.
- Increased IG count indicates the severity of the early innate immune response.

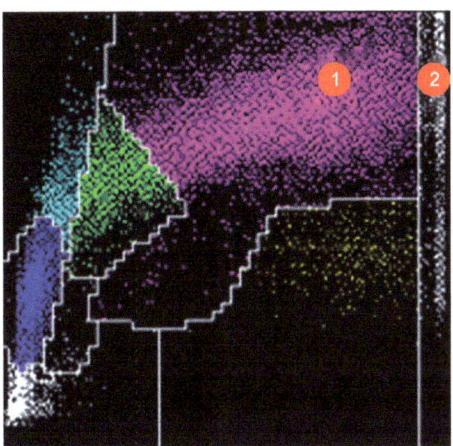
Location of immature granulocytes on PEROX cytogram

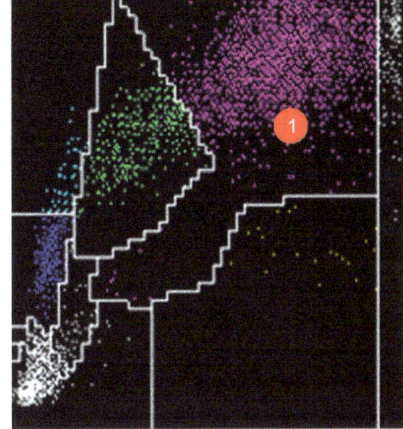
Location of bands on PEROX cytogram

Courtesy: © Siemens Healthcare GmbH 2020

Neutrophil Volume

Neutrophil volume (NV) gives the average size of circulating neutrophils in the peripheral blood. It is now being used for the diagnosis of neonatal sepsis. (Raimondi F, Ferrara T, Capasso L, et al.)
- It can be increased in immature or reactive neutrophils.
- Significant increases in NV correlate reasonably well with the likelihood of sepsis.
- The superior sensitivity over C-reactive protein levels makes it a useful screening tool.

Neutrophil Reactivity Intensity and Neutrophil Granularity Intensity

(Sysmex)
Neutrophil reactivity intensity (NEUT-RI) and neutrophil granularity intensity (NEUT-GI) parameters are an indicator of neutrophil activation and hence are the signs of immune response and inflammation. These are measured based on their fluorescence signal intensity.
NEUT-RI reflects the neutrophil reactivity intensity, representing their metabolic activity while NEUT-GI reflects the complexity of neutrophils
The understanding of neutrophil granulocytes' role in inflammation has changed essentially over recent years.
Now we know that:
- Important in monitoring patients with inflammatory diseases
- Helps to avoid the overuse of antibiotics.
- Activated neutrophils can perform most of the functions of macrophages.
- Activated neutrophils secrete a variety of proinflammatory cytokines and surface molecules (MHCII)
- They allow presentation of antigen to, and activation of, T cells.
- Neutrophil activation is an indicator of early innate immune response hence both, NEUT-GI and NEUT-RI, will be increased in such a condition
- These hematological inflammation parameters support an early diagnosis.
- Targeted treatment can be started, changed or modified faster.
- If the complexity of neutrophils increases upon a change in functionality, e.g., by toxic granulation or vacuolization, the position of the neutrophil cloud in the scattergram is also affected.
- The parameter NEUT-GI, expressed in the unit SI (scatter intensity), changes accordingly.

EOSINOPHILS

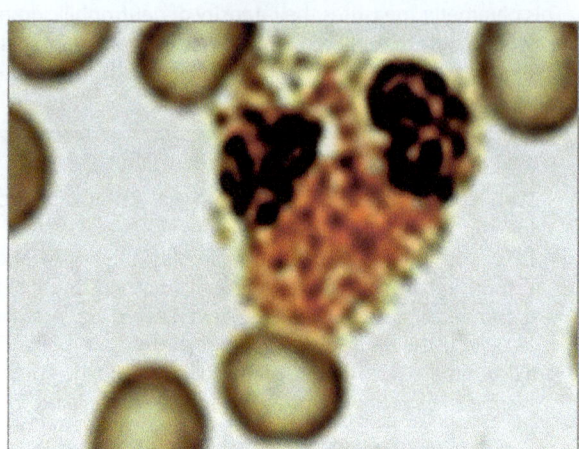

- "Eosin—Rose color", "-Phil—love"—Exhibit a rose color when stained
- Eosinophils can appear at the myelocytic stage and move through the maturation sequence
- **Size:** 10-16 µm
- **Cytoplasm:** Large, distinctive red-orange specific granules with orange-pink cytoplasm, granules are highly metabolic and contain histamine and other substances
- Granules are uniformly round, large, and individualized
- **Nucleus:** Blue dense chromatin, 2 lobes like a pair of glasses
- Lives 6 to 12 hours in circulation migrate into tissues.

Normal range
- Percentage of total WBC 1–4% of total white blood cells
- Absolute count 12–500 cells per microliter.

Diurnal variation (related to cortisol levels)
- Eosinophils lowest in the morning
- Eosinophils highest in the evening.

Eosinophilia

Mild (700–1,500 per µL)
Allergic rhinitis, extrinsic asthma, mild drug reaction, long-term dialysis, immunodeficiency

Moderate (1,500–5,000 per µL)
Parasitic disease, intrinsic asthma, pulmonary eosinophilia syndrome

Marked (> 5,000 per µL)
Trichinella, hookworm, *Toxocara canis*, eosinophilic leukemia, severe drug reaction.

Other causes
- Drug-induced eosinophilia
- Severe, long-standing rheumatoid arthritis
- Psoriasis
- Crohn's disease, ulcerative colitis
- Systemic lupus erythematosus
- Malignant disease
- Implies metastatic disease—poor prognosis
- Hypopituitarism (decreased steroids)
- No identifiable causes— hypereosinophilic syndromes

Eosinopenia

- Usually related to increased circulating steroids
- Cushing's syndrome
- Drugs
- ACTH, epinephrine, thyroxine, exogenous steroids
- Acute bacterial infection
- Normal diurnal pattern

BASOPHILS

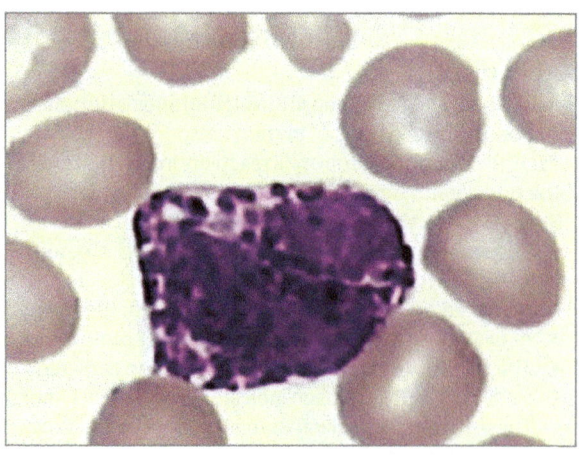

- Basophils can appear at the myelocytic stage and move through the maturation sequence
- Mediate allergic reactions
- Release proinflammatory chemicals bradykinin, heparin, serotonin, and histamine
- Circulate only a few hours then migrates into tissue
- **Size:** 10-14 µm
- **Chromatin:** Coarse, clumped bilobed
- **Cytoplasm:** Many large specific purple-black granules seem to obscure the large cloverleaf form nucleus, may decolorize during staining leaving pale areas within a cell; granules much larger than neutrophilic granules
- Lives 6–12 hours in circulation
- **Typical range:** 0.5–2%, Absolute count 6–200/µL

Distinguishing characteristics: Size and color of granules will obscure the nucleus.

Causes of Basophilia		
• Hypothyroidism, myxedema • Chronic myeloid leukemia • Ulcerative colitis	• Urticaria • Hodgkin's lymphoma/disease	• Chickenpox • Splenectomy

MONOCYTES

Monocyte

- **Size:** 12–20 μm
- **N:C:** 1:1
- **Nuclear chromatin:** Take different shapes from convolutions to lobulations and S-like shapes, chromatin is usually loose, lacy, open, and thin.
- **Cytoplasm:** Abundant gray-blue with granules
  - Lifespan in circulation 8 hours to 3 days
  - Migrate into tissue and become macrophages
    * Liver—Kupffer cells
    * Lungs—alveolar macrophages
    * First cells to pick up foreign organisms and present information to other WBCs.

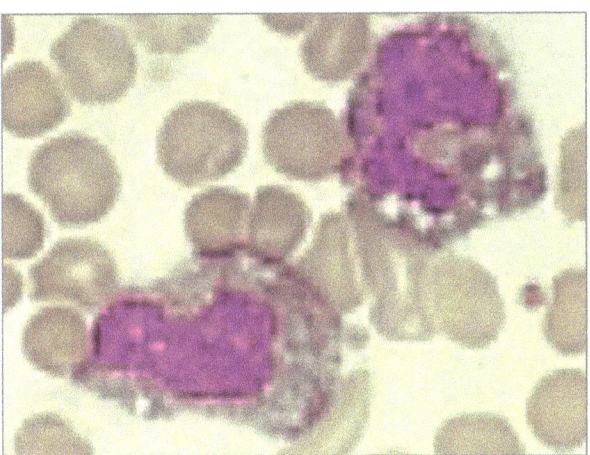

Monocytosis

- Monocyte levels >700 /μL or >12% of WBCs
- **Usual causes:**
  - Viral infections
  - Tuberculosis
  - Subacute bacterial endocarditis
  - Collagen diseases
  - Chronic inflammation
  - Stress response
  - Hyperadrenocorticism
  - Infectious mononucleosis
  - Sarcoidosis
  - Concomitant with neutrophilia
  - Autoimmune conditions
  - Crohn's disease
  - Rheumatoid disease
  - Systemic lupus erythematosus
  - Ulcerative colitis

Monocytopenia

- Very uncommon by itself
- **Usual causes:**
  - Hairy cell leukemia
  - Aplastic anemia

LYMPHOCYTES

Lymphoblast

Size: 10–20 µm
N:C: 4:1
Chromatin: One or two nucleoli with smudge chromatin
Cytoplasm: Little, deep blue staining at edge
Distinguishing characteristics: Nucleoli is surrounded by a dark rim of chromatin.

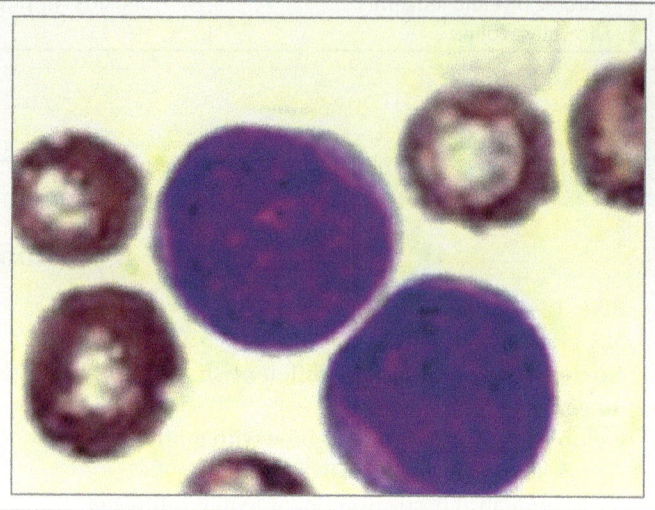

Prolymphocyte

Size: 9–18 µm
N:C: 3:1
Chromatin: Nucleoli present, slightly coarse chromatin
Cytoplasm: Gray-blue, mostly blue at edges
Diameter: Small 7–9, large 12–16
Granules: Small-agranular
Large-few primary granules

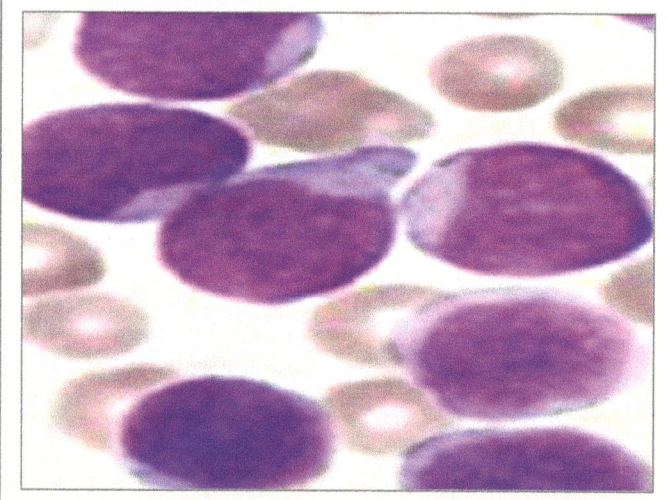

Small Lymphocyte

- About 90% of the circulating lymphocytes are small cells (9–12 µm in diameter) with a purplish nucleus approximately 8.5 µm in diameter that contains dense chromatin clumps. A thin rim of cytoplasm devoid of granules surrounds it
- About two-thirds of these cells are T-lymphocytes and most of the remainder are B-lymphocytes, but these two types are indistinguishable on routine smears

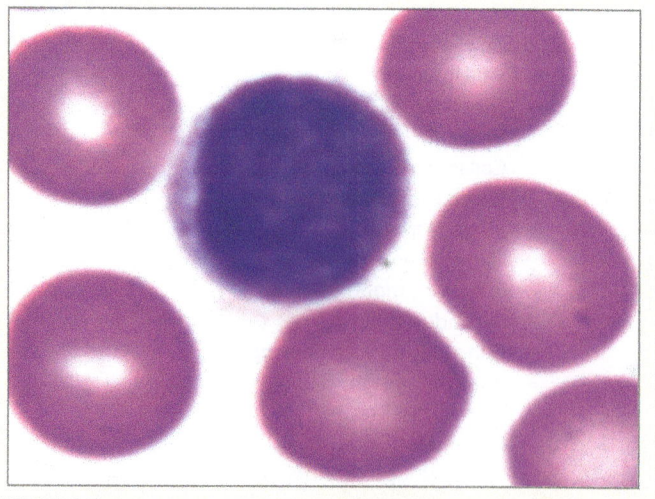

Large Lymphocyte

About 10% of the circulating lymphocytes are larger (12–16 μm in diameter) than the small lymphocytes, have more abundant cytoplasm, possess a less condensed nuclear chromatin, and often have a more irregular, less rounded shape

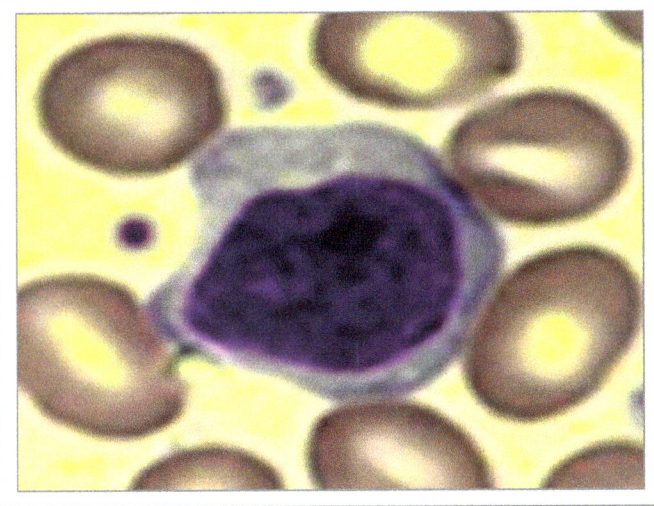

Large Granular Lymphocyte

- Large granular lymphocytes normally constitute about 5% of circulating white cells
- Abnormal elevations in large granular lymphocytes may occur in patients with viral infections, neutropenia, pure red cell aplasia, and rheumatoid arthritis

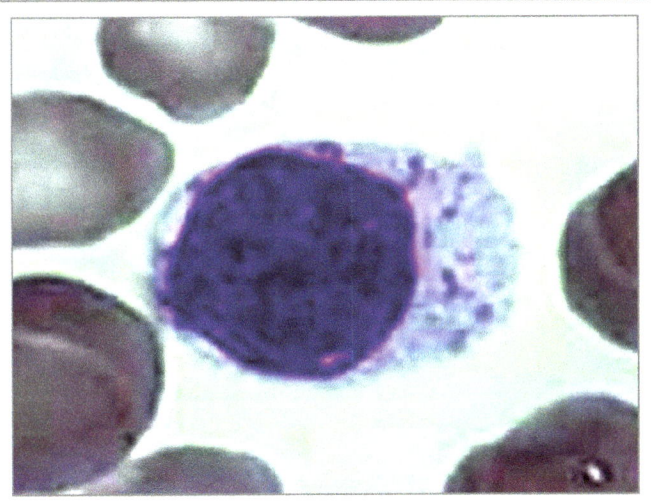

Plasma Cell

- Plasma cells, normally not seen on peripheral smears, may appear with bacterial or viral infections, drugs, and other allergies, immunizations, multiple myeloma, and systemic lupus erythematosus
- They have a diameter of about 14–18 μm, are oval, and possess eccentric nuclei with purple chromatin clumps.
- The deep blue cytoplasm commonly has vacuoles and is pale near the nucleus (perinuclear clear zone) where the Golgi apparatus is present and immunoglobulins are processed

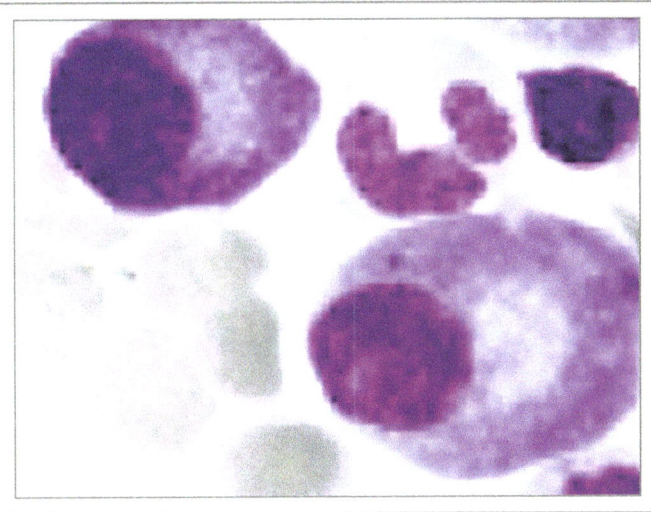

Atypical Lymphocyte

- "Atypical" lymphocytes, diverse in appearance, are usually larger than small lymphocytes and have an oval, kidney-shaped, or lobulated nucleus, which may appear folded.
- Nucleoli are sometimes prominent, and the chromatin is coarse, reticular, or clumped.
- The abundant cytoplasm, which often has a deep blue or gray color, lacks granules and is commonly vacuolated or foamy.
- Atypical lymphocytes are most common in viral diseases, especially with Epstein–Barr virus (infectious mononucleosis), but also with cytomegalovirus infection in normal hosts, and occasionally in acute human immunodeficiency virus (HIV) infection. They sometimes occur in drug reactions.

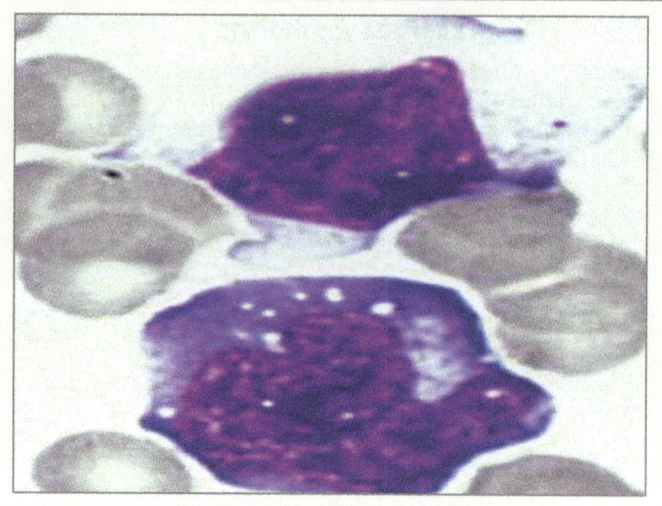

Plasmacytoid Lymphocyte

- The plasmacytoid lymphocyte resembles a plasma cell in its dark blue cytoplasm, but the nucleus is less eccentric, the cell is round, and the perinuclear clear space is absent or small.
- These cells may form in:
  - Viral infections
  - Lymphomas
  - Multiple myeloma
  - Waldenström's macroglobulinemia.

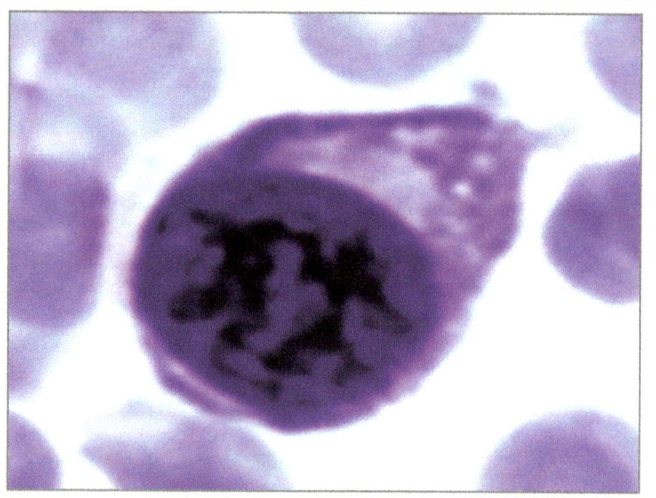

Smudge Cell

Fragile lymphocytes may rupture during the preparation of blood smears, creating smudge cells, in which the nucleus appears to spread out, its border hazy, and the cytoplasm is meagre or absent.

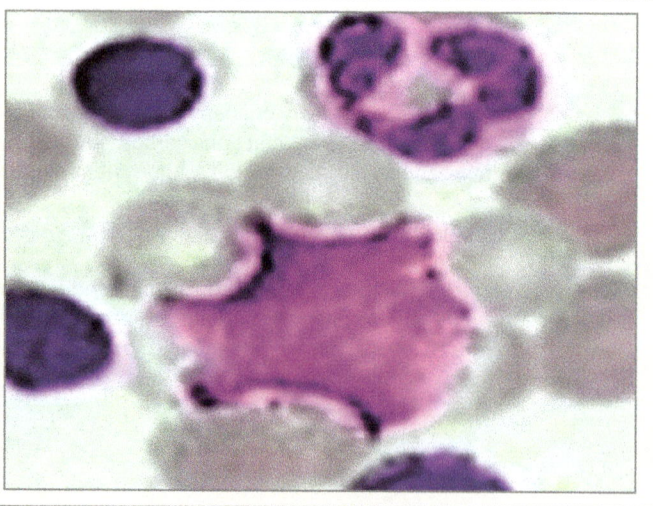

Lymphocytosis—causes

- Infectious mononucleosis
- *Mycobacterium tuberculosis*
- Acute lymphoblastic leukemia
- Brucellosis
- Burkitt's lymphoma
- Chronic lymphocytic leukemia
- Cytomegalovirus
- Epstein–Barr virus
- Hairy cell leukemia
- Hepatitis A
- Hepatitis B
- Myeloma
- Non-Hodgkin's lymphoma
- Phenytoin
- Rubella
- Secondary syphilis
- Serum sickness
- Syphilis, congenital
- Toxoplasma
- Waldenström macroglobulinemia
- Whooping cough
- X-linked lymphoproliferative disease

Lymphopenia—causes

- Viral infection
- HIV
- COVID-19 infection*
- Severe acute respiratory syndrome (SARS)
- Drugs, such as vinblastine, chloramphenicol, doxorubicin
- Marrow suppression
- Pancytopenia.

*COVID-19 and Lymphopenia

At the time of publication of this edition, various studies suggested that LYM% can be used as a reliable indicator to classify the moderate, severe, and critical ill types independent of any other auxiliary indicators.

Analysis of possible reasons for lymphopenia in COVID-19 patients

Lymphocytes play a guiding and decisive role in maintaining immune homeostasis and inflammatory response in the body. Understanding the mechanism of reduced blood lymphocyte levels is expected to provide an effective strategy for the treatment of COVID-19. Multiple studies hypothesized, four potential mechanisms which lead to lymphocyte deficiency in a COVID-19 patient (these hypotheses need to be confirmed in the future).

- The virus might directly infect lymphocytes, resulting in lymphocyte death. Lymphocytes express the coronavirus receptor ACE2 and may be a direct target of viruses.
- The virus might directly destroy lymphatic organs such as the thymus and spleen cannot be ruled out.
- Disordered inflammatory cytokines leading to lymphocyte apoptosis. The role of tumor necrosis factor-alpha (TNFα), interleukin (IL)-6, and other pro-inflammatory cytokines inducing lymphopenia cannot be ruled out.
- Inhibition of lymphocytes by metabolic molecules produced by metabolic disorders, such as hyperlactic academia, suppressing the proliferation of lymphocytes.

Lymphopenia occurs more frequently, especially in severe cases. **An increased neutrophil-to-lymphocyte ratio (NLR) with a cut-off of 3.5 is found to be correlated with disease severity and poor prognosis.**

Lymphocyte activation: Reactive lymphocytes (RE-LYMP) and antibody-synthesizing lymphocytes (AS-LYMP)

- The new diagnostic RE-LYMP and AS-LYMP parameters are used for the quantitative assessment of activated lymphocytes.
- They help clinicians to diagnose, treat and monitor patients with inflammatory conditions by providing additional information about activation of the immune response.

Reactive Lymphocytes (RE-LYMP)

- Reflects all lymphocytes that have a higher fluorescence signal than the normal lymphocyte population.
- The parameter is reported as an absolute count and percentage.
- The population of AS-LYMP always includes the RE-LYMP count.

Antibody-synthesizing Lymphocytes (AS-LYMP)

- This parameter quantifies the activated B lymphocytes (plasma cells) that synthesize antibodies.
- It reflects the lymphocyte subpopulation with the highest fluorescence signals.
- It is reported as absolute count and percentage.
- The combination of the RE-LYMP and AS-LYMP parameters provide information about the cellular activation of the innate and adaptive immune response.
- The change of value in these parameters depends on the nature of the inflammatory stimulus, severity, and stage of the infection.
- The concentrations of these two cell populations indicate whether there is a cell-mediated or humoral immune response to pathogens.
- Differentiate between various indications like viral or bacterial infections, acute or subsiding infections, or whether there is an inflammatory condition without an infection.

RE-LYMP and AS-LYMP parameters help to differentiate between:

- Bacterial and viral pathogenic causes of infection
- Early innate immune response, cellular or humoral immune response
- Inflammation and infection

Courtesy: @sysmax

CHAPTER 5

Platelets

- These are smallest cells of the cellular component of blood carry the great responsibility of hemostasis.
- Their role in thrombosis, hemorrhage and inflammatory processes resulting in myocardial infarction (MI), stroke, disseminated intravascular coagulation (DIC), like a life-threatening crisis, attracts the attention of practitioners belonging to all clinical disciplines.
- Polypoid megakaryocytes and their non-nucleated progeny "platelets" are found only in mammals, others have nucleated cells for hemostatic function.

PLATELET COUNT

Thrombocytes: "Thrombo— means clot". (They help in clot formation).
- Platelets are manufactured in the bone marrow by megakaryocyte
- Platelets are fragments of cytoplasm of megakaryocyte
- 1 megakaryocyte produces about 4,000 platelets.

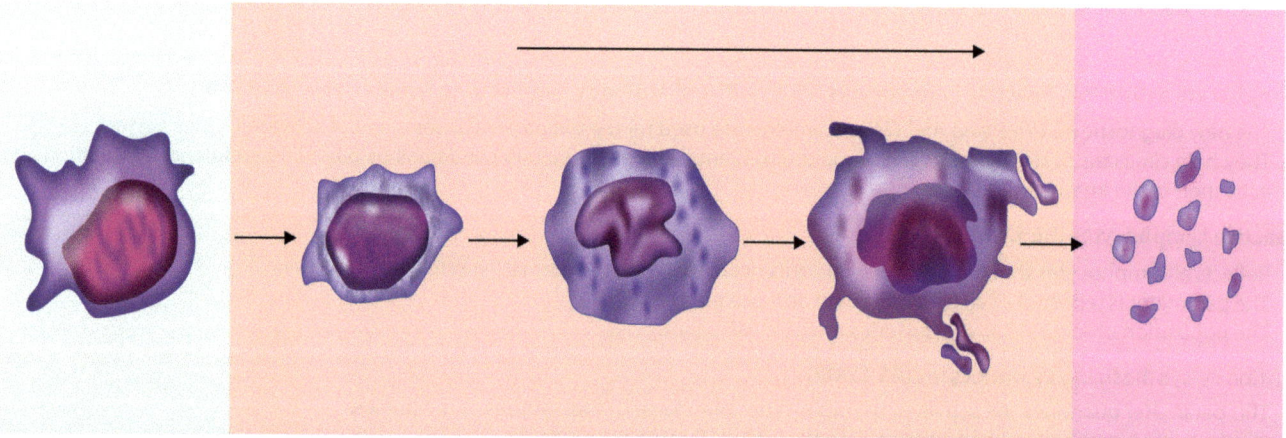

- Normal platelets are about 1–3 µm in diameter, blue-gray, and contain fine, purple to pink granules that may be diffuse or concentrated in the center of the cells, they resemble
- Normally, the ratio of red cells to platelets is about 10–40:1, and approximately 7–20 platelets are present in each oil immersion field
- Lifespan of platelets is about 9–12 days
- Production of platelet is regulated by a hormone called thrombopoietin (produced in the liver)
- They are removed by the spleen when they are old or damaged.

Platelets normal range	Men and women
	1,500,00–4,500,00/µL

Thrombocytopenia (TCP): Decreased Platelet Count

- Grade 1 TCP: Platelet counts of 75,000 to 150,000/microL
- Grade 2 TCP: 50,000 to <75,000/microL
- Grade 3 TCP: 25,000 to <50,000/microL
- Grade 4 TCP: Below 25,000/microL

CAUSES OF THROMBOCYTOPENIA

1. Decreased Platelet Production

- Thrombocytopenia with absent radii (TAR) syndrome
- Amegakaryocytic thrombocytopenia
- Aplastic anemia
- Myelodysplastic syndrome (MDS)
- Bone marrow hypoplasia due to:
  - Chemotherapy
  - Radiation
  - Toxins
  - Immune
- Bone marrow infiltration by:
  - Fibrosis
  - Malignancy – leukemias, metastasis
  - Granulomas
- Selective marrow suppression of platelet production due to:
  - Drugs
  - Infections
    - Viral: Human immunodeficiency virus (HIV), hepatitis B and C, Epstein-Barr virus (EBV), cytomegalovirus (CMV)
    - Parasitic: Malaria, Babesia
  - Ethanol
- Ineffective thrombopoiesis due to:
  - Folate or B_{12} deficiency
- Hereditary disorders
  - May–Hegglin anomaly
  - Wiskott–Aldrich syndrome

2. Increased Destruction

Immune mediated

- Systemic lupus erythematosus
- Lymphoproliferative disorders
- Drugs-induced thrombocytopenia:
  - Quinine, penicillins, abciximab, heparin, gold
  - Severe thrombocytopenia (<20 × 10^9/L)
  - Bleeding manifestation can vary from immediate use to 10 days post use
- Infections including HIV related
- Post-transfusion purpura:
  - Seen when PlA 1 negative patients receive PlA 1 positive blood
  - Severe thrombocytopenia upto 10 × 10^9/L
  - Starts 5–10 days post-transfusion
  - Commonly seen in multiparous females
- Idiopathic/immune thrombocytopenia (ITP):
  - Platelet count <100 × 10^9/L
  - No secondary causes
  - No gold standard test for diagnosis

Nonimmune mechanisms

- Severe bleeding
- Disseminated intravascular coagulation (DIC)
  - Presents as microangiopathic hemolytic anemia (MHA) with thrombocytopenia with deranged coagulation parameters
  - Thrombosis, arterial, may lead to organ failure
  - Seen secondary to sepsis, malignancy, trauma, obstetric complications and transfusion reactions.
- Abnormalities in small vessels
- Vasculitis
- von Willebrand disease (vWD)
- Thrombotic thrombocytopenic purpura (TTP)
  - Seen in deficiency of ADAMTS13, von Willebrand factor (VWF) cleaving enzyme.
  - Causes microvascular occlusion and impaired perfusion of tissues
  - Presents in classic pentad features (in <35% cases)
    - Microangiopathic hemolytic anemia (MAHA)
    - Thrombocytopenia
    - Fever
    - Renal insufficiency
    - Neurological involvement from headache or seizures to stroke
- Hemolytic uremic syndrome (HUS)
  - Caused by enterotoxin producing, shiga toxin producing *E. coli* or *Shigella dysenteriae*
  - Presents with:
    - MAHA
    - Thrombocytopenia
    - Bloody diarrhea
    - Renal failure due to microthrombi

3. Abnormal Distribution

- Dilutional, from massive transfusion
- Hypersplenism

4. Artifactual (Pseudothrombocytopenia)

Thrombocytopenia in asymptomatic patients alarms the possibility of artifactual or "pseudothrombocytopenia" as the etiology. This is caused by in vitro clumping of platelets due to various causes which include:

A. EDTA-induced Platelet Agglutination (EIPA)
- This *in vitro* phenomenon is due to the presence of naturally occurring autoantibody against a crypt antigen on the GPIIb/IIIa platelet receptor. When calcium is chelated by EDTA, the GPIIb protein undergoes a change that exposes the crypt antigen. The autoantibody then binds to the exposed site and crosslink to other platelets causing agglutination.
- The condition occurs in approximately 1% of hospitalized patients.
- This condition may persist for decades without any evidence of abnormal hemostasis.
- EDTA-platelet clumping needs to be recognized and documented in the patient's history to prevent unnecessary treatment for thrombocytopenia.
- Confirmed by evaluating a repeat blood specimen drawn into Sodium Citrate (NaCitrate), revealing normal platelet count.

B. Platelet Satellitism
- In this phenomenon platelets rosettes are formed around neutrophils or rarely around other cells. The satellite platelets are not counted by automated cell counters, resulting in spurious thrombocytopenia.
- Platelet satellitism is caused by EDTA-dependent antiplatelet and antineutrophil IgG antibodies in the patient's plasma. The diagnosis is made by making a blood smear and looking at platelet rosettes. The phenomenon has not been associated with any disease state or drug and is thought to be benign.

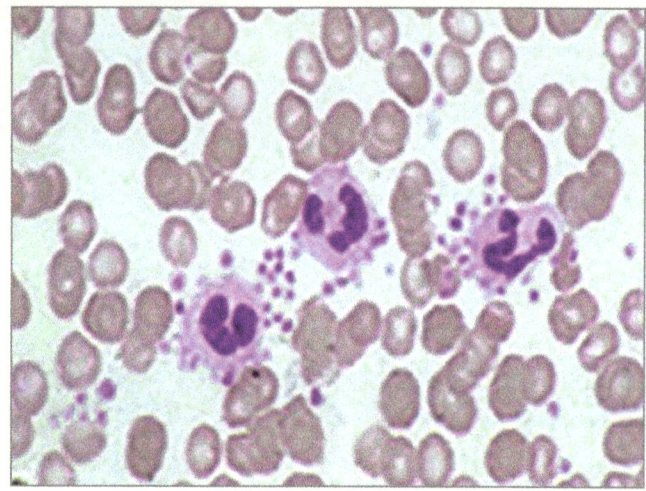

C. Cold Agglutinins
- This phenomenon is temperature-dependent. Agglutination occurs in citrate and heparin as well as EDTA anticoagulants
- The specimen should be maintained at 37°C or warmed to 37°C to obtain an accurate platelet count.

D. Giant Platelets or Megathrombocyte
- Platelets that are 36 fL or larger will be counted as red cells in most automated counters, resulting in spuriously low platelet counts.
- Low platelet counts along with instrument flagging of giant platelets should prompt the technocrat to confirm the abnormal platelet count by finger-prick blood smear review or perform a manual platelet count.
- Mean platelet volume (MPV) increases when many large platelets are present.
- Young platelets are usually big.

Causes of large platelets include:

Hereditary
Bernard–Soulier syndrome, benign Mediterranean macrothrombocytopenia

Acquired
- Immune thrombocytopenia purpura
- Myeloproliferative disorders
- Myelodysplasia (MDS)
- Disseminated intravascular coagulation (DIC)
- Thrombotic thrombocytopenic purpura (TTP)
- Infections, such as dengue and other peripheral challenges of platelet destructions

E. Partially Clotted Specimen
- When blood clots, platelets adhere to the clot and are removed from the fluid blood
- Examine a finger prick smear for the presence of platelet clumps if clumping is seen, repeat with a fresh specimen.

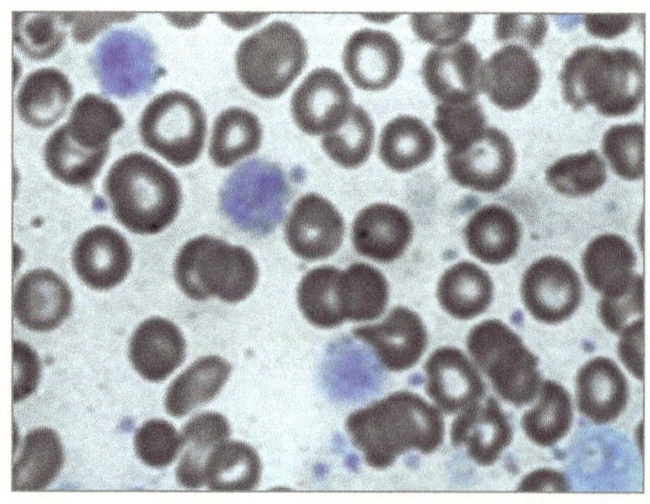

Mild Thrombocytopenia

Diagnostic entities to consider are:
- Viral infection (of which HIV is most common)
- Gram-negative bacterial infection
- Medication (antibiotics, anti-inflammatory agents, antineoplastic, cardiac medications and certain psychotropics)
- Environmental toxin
- Chronic alcoholism
- Occult cirrhosis
- Adult Gaucher disease
- Autoimmune disease (systemic lupus erythematosus or rheumatoid arthritis)
- Chronic lymphocytic leukemia
- Portal hypertension
- Hypersplenism

Thrombasthenia (Platelet Function Defects)

A platelet function disorder, where platelets are numerically in normal range but they are incapable of performing normal hemostatic function and may result into bleeding disorder despite normal to increase platelet count. Causes are:

A. Inherited: Aggregation defects
- Glanzmann thrombasthenia
- Congenital afibrinogenemia

Platelet adhesion defects
- Bernard–Soulier syndrome
- von Willebrand disease

Signalling pathway defects
- Defects in calcium mobilization
- Thromboxane synthetase deficiency
- Cyclooxygenase deficiency
- Lipoxygenase deficiency

Agonist receptor defects
- Thromboxane A_2 receptor deficiency

Secretion defects
- Chédiak–Higashi syndrome
- Storage pool disease
- Wiskott–Aldrich syndrome
- Gray platelet syndrome

B. Acquired
- Essential thrombocythemia
- Uremia
- Drugs and other agents
- Myeloproliferative disorders
- Chronic myeloid leukemia
- Polycythemia vera
- Antiplatelet antibodies
- Acute leukemias and myelodysplastic syndromes
- Dysproteinemias
- Acquired von Willebrand disease
- Acquired storage pool deficiency
- Liver disorders

Causes of Increased Platelet Count—Thrombocytosis

Myeloproliferative disorders
- Essential (primary) thrombocythemia—clonal overproduction
- Idiopathic myelofibrosis
- Polycythemia vera
- Chronic granulocytic leukemia

Transfer from extravascular pools into circulation
- Splenectomy (over 70% of platelets stored in spleen)
- Exercise
- Epinephrine
- Parturition

Thrombocytosis secondary to
- Iron deficiency anemia
- Malignancy
- Infections
- Non-infectious inflammation
- Acute blood loss
- Hemolysis
- Recovery from thrombocytopenia

Besides the absolute number of platelets the size and appearance of the platelets, on the smear help to differentiate the causes of thrombocytosis and might suggest a specific diagnosis.

Platelets are large in myeloproliferative disorders and after splenectomy, but they tend to be small in reactive thrombocytosis due to hemorrhage, trauma, iron deficiency, inflammation, infection, or malignancy.

In myeloproliferative disorders, hypogranular, agranular, or markedly misshapen platelets may appear.

DISORDERS OF PLATELETS

Essential (Primary) Thrombocythemia

- Essential thrombocythemia (ET) is clonal overproduction of megakaryocytes and in turn platelet count usually over 6.0 lacs/cumm
- Diagnosis of ET may be during routine blood count or on a blood count that is ordered on a patient who has a blood clot, unexpected bleeding, or an enlarged spleen and there is no other cause for the increased numbers of platelets
- ET occurs mostly in adults
- Most common complication of ET is blockage of blood vessels by excess platelets (thrombosis)
- Janus kinase 2 (JAK2) mutation in blood cells.
- Bone marrow will show a significant increase in megakaryocytes and masses of platelets.

Thrombotic Thrombocytopenia Purpura

- Thrombotic thrombocytopenic purpura (TTP) is characterized by platelet thrombi formation in the arterioles and capillaries throughout the body.
- Five major clinical features occur in this disease—fever, neurologic abnormalities, renal failure, thrombocytopenia, and microangiopathic hemolytic anemia (the last two are essential to the diagnosis)
- LDH level is markedly elevated
- Indirect bilirubin rises
- Haptoglobin level diminishes because of the intravascular hemolysis
- Hemosiderin and hemoglobin may be present in the urine.
- Peripheral blood smear reveals low platelets, polychromasia, nucleated red cells, and schistocytes.
- Bone marrow samples demonstrate hyperplasia of megakaryocytes and red cell precursors.

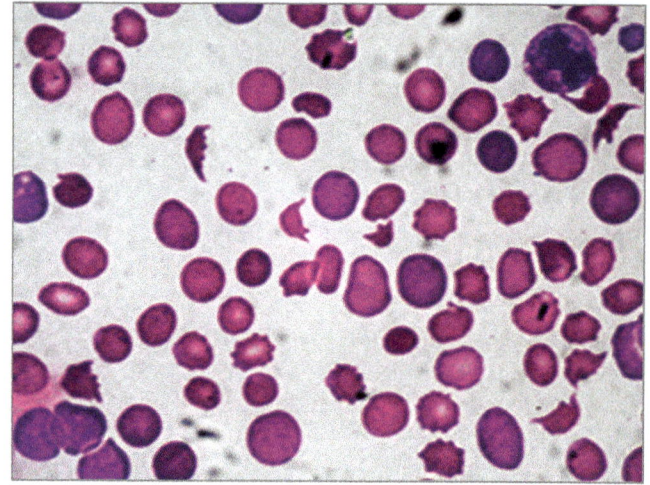

Gray Platelet Syndrome (α-granule Deficiency)	Bernard–Soulier Disease	May–Hegglin Disease
The platelets are characteristically larger than normal and are pale gray forms. Thrombocytopenia may also occur.	Large platelets, some with a range from slightly enlarged (one-third the diameter of a red cell) to enormous giant-sized platelet.	• Giant platelets of the size of a red cell • There may be a presence of gray-blue giant neutrophil inclusion. • The neutrophil inclusions are precipitates of nonmuscle myosin heavy-chain type IIA.
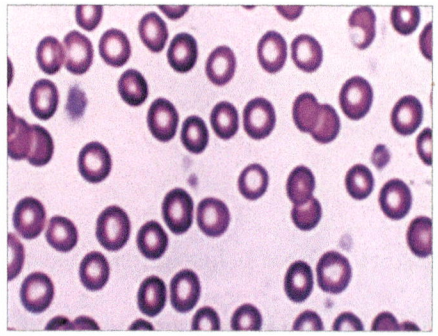	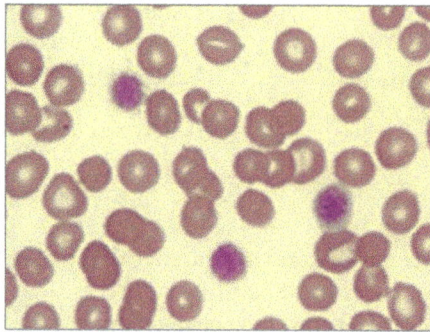	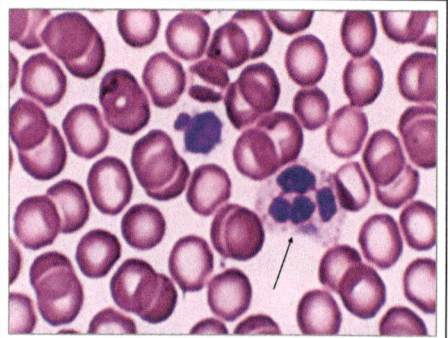

MEAN PLATELET VOLUME

Mean platelet volume (MPV) is a measurement that describes the average size of platelet in the blood. This parameter provides an indicator as to whether the bone marrow is manufacturing platelets normally or there is some kind of production pressure from the periphery like excessive destruction, etc. MPV is inversely proportional to the degree of PLT maturity. Normal to decreased MPV is seen in thrombocytopenia of hypoproliferative bone marrow.

An increased MPV is a sign of larger platelet size, and is indicative of compensated bone marrow, under the challenge of peripheral platelet destruction/sequestration.

MPV normal range	Men and women
	7.4–10.4 fL

- MPV as measured with an automatic blood cell counter increases when many large platelets are present.
- The MPV is calculated by dividing the plateletcrit (PCT) by the total number of platelets.
- In impedance analyzers, the MPV and PDW are derived from the platelet volume distribution curve.
- Young platelets are usually big.
- MPV has usually an inverse relationship with platelet number, with larger platelet volumes seen in thrombocytopenic patients in whom platelets are decreased due to peripheral destruction (as in idiopathic thrombocytopenia purpura).
- Although platelet count is the most basic measure of platelet health, but at places, the MPV measurement, may enable a physician to detect a problem even before the recordable thrombocytopenia sets in.
- Change in MPV without any change in platelet count may be an early indicator of a serious bone marrow problem.
- Platelets are considered large when about 4–8 μm in diameter and giant when wider and equal to or larger than a normal erythrocyte.
- Platelets tend to swell during the first 2 hours in EDTA anticoagulant, shrinking again with longer storage.
- The platelet volume is found to be associated with cytokines (thrombopoietin, interleukin-6, and interleukin-3) that regulate megakaryocyte ploidy and platelet number and result in the production of larger platelets.
- During activation, platelets' shapes change from biconcave discs to spherical, and a pronounced pseudopod formation occurs that leads to MPV increase during platelet activation.
- MPV variation is an important risk factor in cases of arterial thrombosis, venous thromoembolism, acute myocardial infarction, etc.

Increased MPV	Decreased MPV
It means the platelets are larger than normal. They are now known as megathrombocytes. Causes include: • Idiopathic thrombocytopenic purpura • Bernard–Soulier disease • May–Hegglin anomaly • Sepsis (recovery phase) • Heart valve prosthesis • Myeloproliferative disorders, CML • Myelodysplasia • DIC • TTP • Sickle cell anemia • Following splenectomy • Hyperthyroidism • Infection-related thrombocytopenia, such as dengue, malaria, etc.	It means the platelets are smaller than normal. They are now known as microthrombocytes. This may indicate the following disorders: • Aplastic anemia • Wiskott–Aldrich syndrome • Thrombocytopenia-absent radii (TAR syndrome) • Storage Pool disease • Megaloblastic anemia • Chemotherapy • Hypersplenism • Megakaryocytic hypoplasia

In general, platelets are large when thrombocytopenia results from increased destruction and small with disorders of diminished production. If the platelet count is low and MPV is high the risk of bleeding is comparatively less as larger platelets have multifold better hemostatic capacity than normal size platelet. Guidance during crisis roughly may be:

High MPV + Stable platelet count ------------------ Recovery from disease
High MPV + Falling platelet count ---------------- Active disease*
Low MPV + Low platelet count -------------------- Risk to hemostasis*
*Warrants consideration for platelet transfusion depending on clinical status.

PLATELET DISTRIBUTION WIDTH

PDW normal range	Men and women
	9–13 fL

Platelet distribution width (PDW) is analogous to the red cell distribution width. It compares the uniformity and heterogeneity of platelet size. PDW is numerically equal to the coefficient of platelet volume variation, which is used to describe the dispersion of platelet volume and is increased in the presence of platelet anisocytosis.

Increased values are observed in:
- Essential thrombocythemia
- Aplastic anemia
- Megaloblastic anemia
- Chronic myelogenous leukemia
- Chemotherapy
- Fragmented erythrocytes
- PDW directly measures variability in platelet size, changes with platelet activation, and reflects the heterogeneity in platelet morphology and size.
- A high value of PDW suggests a large range of platelet size due to swelling, destruction, and immaturity.
- In sepsis, PDW increases due to activation and destruction of platelets.
- It is measured in percentage (%).
- Under physiological conditions, there is a direct relationship between MPV and PDW; both usually change in the same direction.

Actual causes for increased PDW values are not known but may be due to dysfunctional megakaryocyte development. If erythrocyte fragments are being counted as platelets, the PDW will be falsely elevated because it broadens the platelet volume distribution curve.

The PDW is a reasonably good tool to distinguish essential thrombocythemia (PDW increased) from reactive thrombocytosis (PDW normal).

PLATELETCRIT

The plateletcrit (PCT) is the volume percentage that platelets match on a total volume of blood, and it is directly related to the total number of platelets and MPV.

PCT normal range	Men and women
	0.110–0.280

- PCT is the volume occupied by platelets in the blood as a percentage.
- PCT is influenced by the number and the size of platelets, and has a positive relationship with the platelet count.
- The plateletcrit nonlinearly correlates to the platelet count.
- The normal range for PCT is 0.22–0.24%.
- Under physiological conditions, the amount of platelets in the blood is maintained in an equilibrium state by regeneration and elimination.
- In healthy subjects, platelet mass is closely regulated to keep it constant, while MPV is inversely related to the platelet.
- PCT is the volume occupied by platelets in the blood as a percentage and calculated according to the formula PCT = platelet count × MPV/10,000.

IMMATURE PLATELET FRACTION (IPF)

- **Immature platelet fraction (IPF) is a parameter used to assess thrombopoiesis. This parameter is increased in the setting of platelet destruction or consumption and decreased with bone marrow failure.**
- Immature platelets or immature platelet fraction are identified as high-fluorescing, large platelet area of the scattergram. The immature platelet fraction (IPF), or reticulated platelets, contains RNA and can be detected using nucleic acid dyes.

- IPF is the percentage of the total optical platelet count. The reference range is 1.1–6.1%
- It indicates the percentage of immature platelets in the total platelet population.
- The IPF percentage increases as the production of platelets increases, and low values indicate suppressed thrombopoiesis.
- It is a sensitive marker for assessing regenerating bone marrow post-chemotherapy or transplant.
- Immature platelets are found to be increased approximately 1–2 days before platelet recovery in patients with chemotherapy induced or post stem cell transplant thrombocytopenia.
- In allogeneic bone marrow transplants, the rise in IPF is seen 4–5 days before the rise in platelet counts. This ability reduces prophylactic platelet transfusions in transplant patients.
- Patients with **essential thrombocythemia** and polycythemia vera show increased reticulated platelets compared with healthy individuals
- Patients with **reactive thrombocytosis** show higher reticulated platelets than patients with myeloproliferative disorders.
- It is a useful marker to predict recovery of platelet counts in **dengue**. Attainment of peak IPF and rise in IPF helps to predict platelet recovery within 1–2 days, this predictive capacity of IPF can be used to rationalize/streamline platelet transfusions in dengue.
- Immature platelet fraction (IPF)$_{(Sysmex)}$ or Reticulated platelet (rPLT) $_{(Abbot)}$, may have potential clinical utility in assessing disease activity, predicting treatment response in:
  - Sepsis with thrombocytopenia
  - Acute coronary syndrome
  - Immune thrombocytopenia (ITP)
  - Disseminated intravascular coagulation (DIC)
  - Thrombotic thrombocytopenic purpura (TTP)
  - Myelodysplastic syndrome (MDS).

Benefits of the Immature Platelet Fraction

- Differentiate between consumptive versus productive reasons for thrombocytopenia. (IPF increases in the former but not in the latter).
- Immature platelet fraction (IPF) can better discriminate between the causes of thrombocytopenia than the mean platelet volume (MPV) since younger platelets are not necessarily larger
- Reported reliably even with very low platelet counts.
- Avoid a bone marrow biopsy with obvious benefits for the patient.
- IPF is very useful in cardiovascular, hemato-oncological, pediatric/neonatology patients with low platelet counts for differential diagnosis and monitoring the course of thrombocytopenia.
- IPF$_{(sysmex)}$ verses rPLT$_{(Abbot)}$, despite the fact that both parameters deliver information about platelet turnover, but cannot be used interchangeably due to weak correlation.

Mean Platelet Component

- Mean platelet component (MPC) is a measure of the mean refractive index of the platelets by modified two-angle light scatter.
- It is useful in determining changes in the status of platelet activation.
- Measured in gram/deciliter (g/dL).

Platelet-Large Cell Ratio

- Platelet large cell ratio (P-LCR) is a surrogate marker for the platelet volume, which identifies the largest-sized fraction of platelets. It is an indicator of circulating larger platelet (>12 fL), which is presented as a percentage.
- The normal percentage range is 15–35%.
- It has also been used to monitor platelet activity. An increase in PLCR usually signifies that there is an increase in new platelets (which are larger in size).
- P-LCR increases in destructive thrombocytopenia in severe sepsis.
- P-LCR is significantly decreased in patients with thrombocytosis than in normal while it was increased in thrombocytopenia.
- Strong association with coronary artery disease.
- P-LCR is inversely related to platelet count and directly related to platelet volume distribution width (PDW) and MPV.

Mean Platelet Mass

Mean platelet mass (MPM) is calculated from the platelet dry mass histogram picogram (pg).

Platelet Component Distribution Width
Platelet component distribution width (PCDW) is the measure of the variation in platelet shape, measured in gram/deciliter (g/dL)

Composite Platelet Index
- Composite platelet index (CPLI) is a conceptual index derived by multiplying platelet count (as decimal value) with MPV.
- Any result beyond 1.5 is considered in the safe zone hemostatically.

Peripheral Smear Examination in Thrombocytopenia

RBC Lineage
- Schistocytes/fragmented RBCs .... Microangiopathic hemolytic anemia, DIC, HUS
- Malaria parasite .... Thrombocytopenia due to *Pl. falciparum*
- Spherocytes .... AIHA + TCP (Evans syndrome)
- Normoblast and polychromasia .... HELLP syndrome
- Autoagglutination .... Cold antibodies

WBC Lineage
- Increased polymorphs .... Infection/septicemia
- Toxic granulation/band cells .... Septicemia
- Precursor cells/blast .... Leukemia
- Dysplastic cells .... MDS

Platelet Lineage
- Giant platelets .... ITP, Bernard–Soulier syndrome, May–Hegglin anomaly, Gray platelet syndrome, Montreal platelet, Fechtner syndrome, Sebastian syndrome, Epstein syndrome
- Scattered platelet in direct smear .... Glanzmann's thrombasthenia

- While examining the smear of thrombocytopenic patient, make sure to examine the edges of the smear since the platelet clumps may migrate there.

Thrombocytopenia in Pregnancy
- Thrombocytopenia is the second most common hematological disorder in pregnancy after anemia. It affects about 10% of all pregnancies.
- In most cases the course and severity are usually benign.
- There are many causes of thrombocytopenia in pregnancy. Gestational thrombocytopenia is the most common cause. This is incidental thrombocytopenia of pregnancy.
- Change in platelet count during pregnancy may be due to:
  - Hemodilution
  - Increased platelet consumption
  - Increased platelet aggregation is driven by increased levels of thromboxane A2
  - Fetal thrombocytopenia may occur due to transplacental passage of maternal IgG.

Causes of thrombocytopenia in pregnancy
- Pregnancy-specific:
  - Gestational (70%)
  - Pre-eclampsia (20%)
  - HELLP
  - Disseminated intravascular coagulopathy (DIC)

- Other causes:
  - Peripheral destruction
    - Idiopathic thrombocytopenic purpura (ITP) (3–5%)
    - Microangiopathies: TTP, HUS, DIC
    - Hypersplenism
    - Antiphospholipid syndrome
    - Drug-induced
    - Viral infections: HIV, HCV, EBV, CMV
  - Production disorders
    - Nutritional deficiency
    - Liver disease
    - Bone marrow disease

Gestational thrombocytopenia (GT)

- This is incidental thrombocytopenia of pregnancy.
- Mechanism is not clearly defined; two main factors are associated with gestational thrombocytopenia:
  - Accelerated platelet activation at placental circulation.
  - Accelerated consumption due to reduced lifespan of platelets during pregnancy
  - Hemodilution

The HELLP syndrome

The hemolysis, elevated liver enzymes, and low platelets (HELLP) syndrome is a form of severe pre-eclampsia and can be fulminant. Criteria Include:

- Thrombocytopenia with coagulopathy
- Hypertension
- Hemolysis MAHA—schistocytes on peripheral smear (PS)
- Deranged Liver function
- Serum AST elevated
- Total bilirubin elevated
- Serum LDH elevated

CHAPTER 6

Manual versus Automation in Hematology

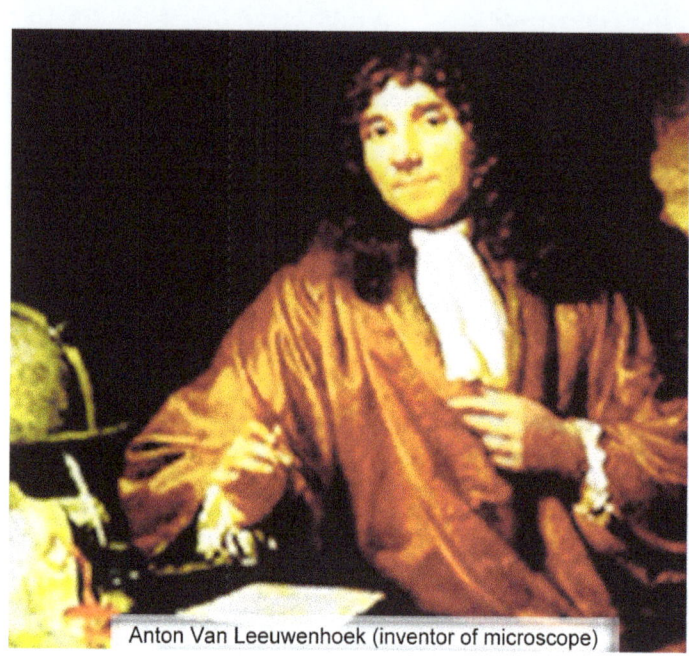
Anton Van Leeuwenhoek (inventor of microscope)

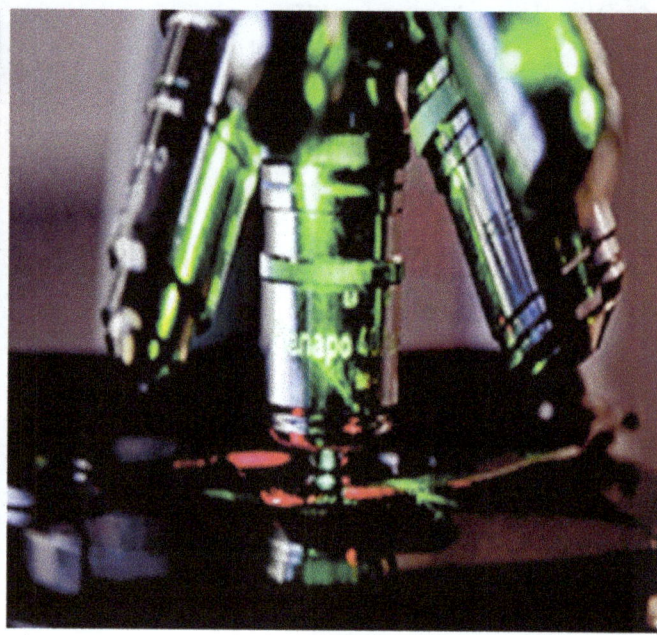

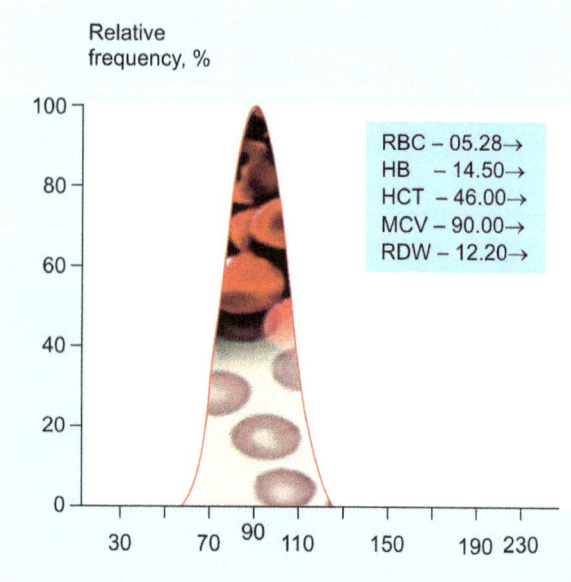

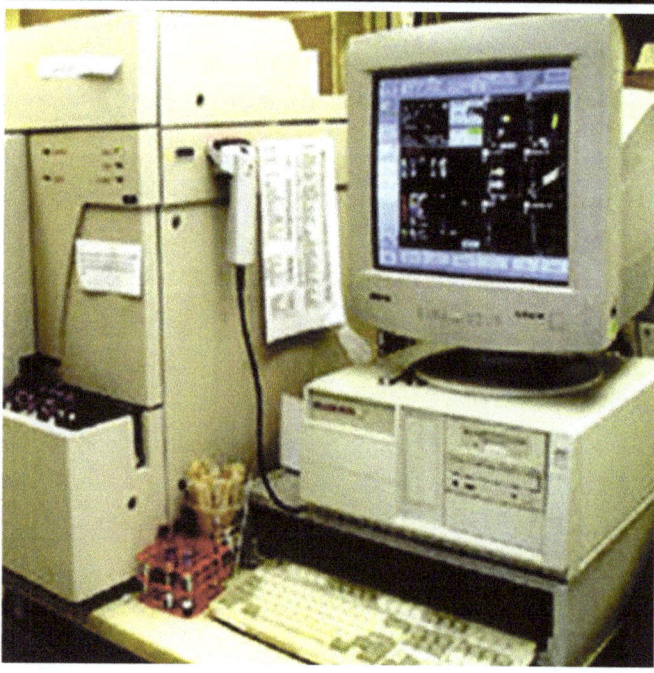

INTRODUCTION

Even though automation is indispensable given accuracy and efficacy, the manual age-old complete blood cell (CBC) methodology with the help of the Neubauer chamber is not yet obsolete due to economic considerations and nonavailability of automation (cell counters), particularly in the smaller laboratory setups in underdeveloped, and developing countries.

Calculating the RBC, WBC, and platelet counts using diluting fluid in various squares of the Neubauer chamber has a very high risk of subjective variation and artifacts, resulting in, not only the spuriously low and high counts but also significant variations in the RBC count dependent indices, and in turn, leading to a wrong diagnosis. Awareness and changing attitude of laboratory services is replacing the manual methodology with automation.

SAMPLE COLLECTION FOR COMPLETE BLOOD CELL

Proper specimen collection is required for reliable and accurate laboratory data to be obtained on any hematologic specimen.
- Data such as patient age, sex, and time of specimen collection should be noted. Correlative clinical information is extremely important in evaluating hematologic specimens. For example, a patient who has had severe diarrhea or vomiting before may be sufficiently dehydrated to have an erroneous increase in red blood cell concentration.
- Most often, blood is collected by venipuncture into tubes containing anticoagulants. The three most commonly used anticoagulants are tripotassium or disodium salts of ethylenediaminetetraacetic acid (EDTA), trisodium citrate, and heparin.
- EDTA and disodium citrate act to remove calcium, which is essential for the initiation of coagulation, from the blood. EDTA is the preferred anticoagulant for blood cell counts because it produces complete anticoagulation with minimal morphological and physical effects on all types of blood cells. Trisodium citrate is the preferred anticoagulant for platelet and coagulation studies.
- The concentration of the anticoagulant used may affect cell concentration measures if it is inappropriate for the volume of blood collected and may also distort cellular morphology. Most often, blood is collected directly into commercially prepared negative-pressure vacuum tubes (vacutainer tubes), which contain the correct concentration of anticoagulant (1–2 mg/mL) when filled appropriately, thereby minimizing error.
- Anticoagulated blood may be stored at 4°C for 24 hours without significantly altering cell counts or cellular morphology. However, it is preferable to perform hematologic analysis as soon as possible after the blood is obtained to minimize anticoagulant effects on cell morphology.
- Smears for the microscopic examination should preferably be prepared from the sample before mixing to anticoagulant (or finger prick smear for better morphological detail and platelet studies).

COLLECTION OF BLOOD SMEAR DIRECT FROM FINGER
- The second or third finger is usually selected and cleaned
- Puncture at the site of the ball of the finger
- Gently squeeze toward the puncture site
- Slide must always be grasped by its edges
- Touch the drop of blood to the slide from below.

Traditional Hematology: CBC—Manual Procedure

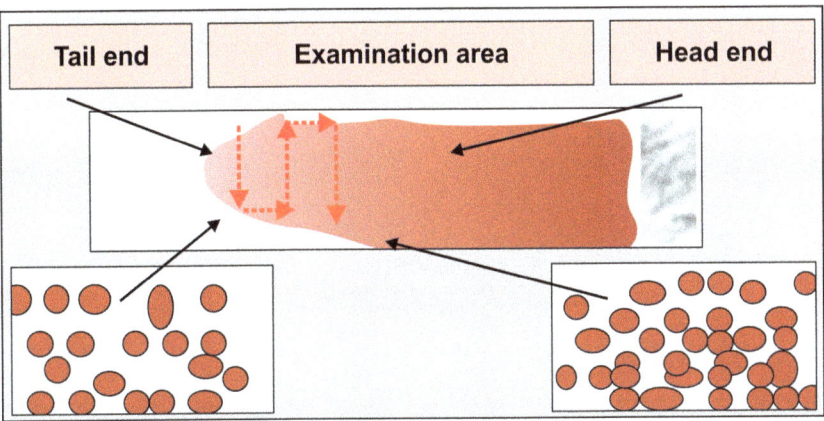
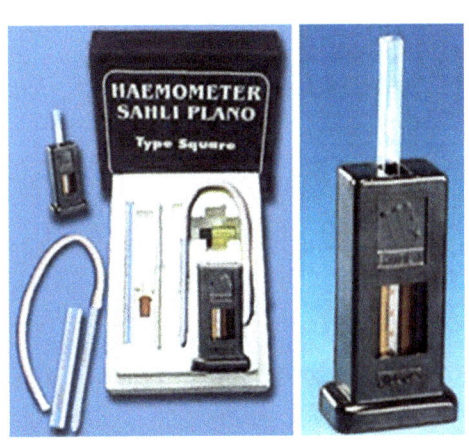

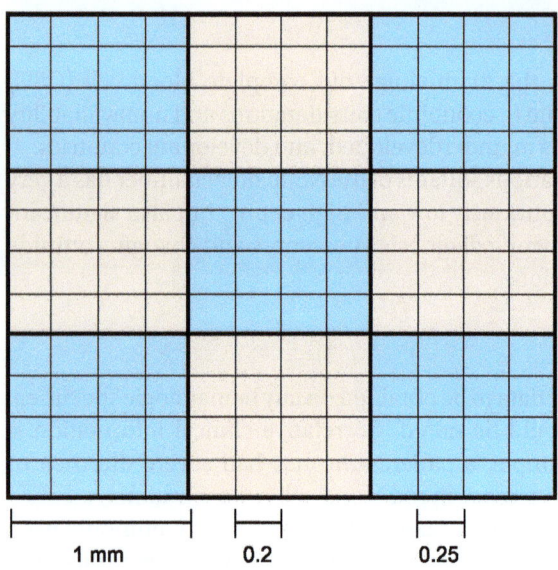
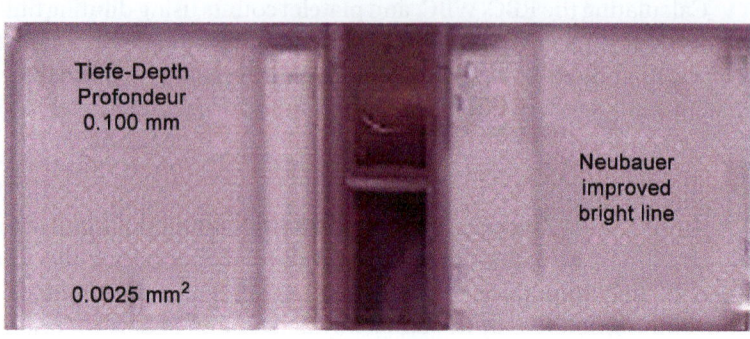

MANUAL CELL COUNTING (WBC, RBC AND PLATELET)

Charging of Hemocytometer
- The collected blood sample is diluted and loaded in a pipette.
- The hemocytometer is carefully charged with the diluted blood by gently squeezing the reservoir.
- The tip of the pipette is placed at the glass interface the contents should be released till the chamber is properly filled without air spaces.
- Be careful not to overcharge the chambers.

Precautions
- Specimen should be properly mixed and have sufficient volume of blood so that there is no dilution of the anticoagulant.
- The capillary tube must be filled and should be free of any air bubbles.
- After the hemocytometer is charged, it should be placed in a premoistened Petri dish to prevent evaporation while the cells are settling out.
- The light adjustment is critical. It is important for both WBCs and especially the platelets. If the condenser is not in the correct position, it will fade out platelets.
- Debris and bacteria can be mistaken for platelets.
- Clumped platelets cannot be counted properly; in that case, the specimen must be recollected. The anticoagulant of choice is EDTA for preventing platelet clumping.
- Avoiding overloading of hemocytometer chamber.

A WBC count is performed with a Neubauer hemocytometer.
- Using the 10 × microscope magnifications, WBC is counted using all nine squares of the counting chamber. Count both sides of the chamber and the average of the count is taken.
- When counting, the cells that touch the extreme lower and the extreme left lines are not included in the count.
- Use the following formulas to calculate the WBC.

$$\text{Cells/mm}^3 = \frac{(\text{average no. of cells}) \times (\text{depth factor 10}) \times (\text{dilution factor 100})}{\text{Area}}$$

Example: Side 1 = 85 cells and side 2 = 95 cells
  90 cells average/all 9 squares counted 90 × 10 × 100 ÷ 9 = 10,000 WBCs

Observing and Recording Nucleated Red Blood Cells (nRBCs)
If nRBCs are observed while performing the differential leucocyte count, they should always be reported. These elements in a peripheral smear are indicative of increased erythropoietic activity and usually a pathologic condition. Additionally, the presence of nRBCs per 100 white cells will falsely elevate the white cell count and is clinically significant.

Correct the WBC count if the nRBC count is >5 nRBCs/100 WBC. The following formula is applied for correcting nRBCs:
Corrected WBC count = WBC count [100 ÷ (nRBC + 100)]
Example: If WBC = 5,000 and 10 NRBCs have been counted
Then 5,000/10 + 100 = 4,545.50, the corrected white count is 4,545.50.

Estimated WBC Count from Peripheral Smear

WBC/High-Power Field	Estimated WBC Count
2–4	4.0–7.0×10^9/L
4–6	7.0–10.0×10^9/L
6–10	10.0–13.0×10^9/L
10–20	13.0–18.0×10^9/L

Platelet counts are performed with a Neubauer hemocytometer:
- Counting is done using × 40 dry phase contrast objectives. Platelets will have a faint halo. The middle square of the hemocytometer chamber is counted. It contains 25 small squares.
- Count 5 of the 25 squares if the platelet count is <100,000. Take the average of both sides.
- To calculate platelets, use the following formula:
  – If 5 squares of the middle square counted number of platelets × 5000 = No. of platelets/mm^3
  – If 25 squares of the middle square are counted (if the platelet count is <100,000, count all 25 squares of the middle square) number of platelets × 1000 = No. of platelets/mm^3.

Observations Under 100 × (Oil Immersion): Platelet Estimation

- Platelet estimation is done under 100 × objective (oil) in the field where the RBCs barely touch each other. On average there are 8 to 20 platelets per field.
- Ten fields are counted using the zigzag method. This method of counting is done by going back and forth, lengthwise or sidewise.
- After the 10 fields are counted, the total number of platelet is divided by 10 to get the average. The average number is now multiplied by a factor of 20,000 for wedge preparations. For monolayer preparations, use a factor of 15,000.

Example: 120 platelets/10 fields = 12 platelets per field = 12 × 20,000 = 240,000 platelets (approx.)

Platelet Estimate from Peripheral Smear

Average No. of platelets per 100 × objective (oil field)	Platelet count estimate (approx.)
0–1	< 20,000
1–4	20,000–80,000
5–8	100,000–160,000
10–15	200,000–300,000
16–20	320,000–400,000
>21	>400,000

Disadvantages of Manual Cell Counting

- Cell identification errors in manual counting:
  – Mostly associated with distinguishing lymphocytes from monocytes, bands
  – From segmented forms and abnormal cells (variants of lymphocytes from blasts)
  – Lymphocytes may be overestimated and monocytes may be underestimated.
- Slide cell distribution error:
  – Increased cell concentration along edges and also bigger cells are found there, i.e., monocytes, eosinophils, and neutrophils.
- Statistical sampling error.

HEMATOLOGY AUTOMATION

General Principles of Hematology Automation

Over the years, the components of the CBC have expanded, as the instrumentation has become more and more sophisticated. The CBC test menu on basic instruments usually includes red cell count (RBC), white cell count (WBC), platelet count (PLT), mean platelet volume (MPV), hemoglobin (Hb) concentration, and the mean red cell volume (MCV). From these measured quantities, the hematocrit (Hct), mean cell hemoglobin (MCH), mean cell hemoglobin concentration, and the red cell distribution width (RDW) are calculated. The newer analyzers include white cell differential counts, relative or percent and absolute number, and reticulocyte analysis. The most sophisticated instruments also provide:

- Flagging systems when data fall out of range
- Embedded quality control programs
- Delta checks
- Preparation, examination, and reporting of white cell differentials
- Automatic maintenance in some instruments

Automated methods for white cell count and differentials use several distinct technical approaches, including those that measure changes in electrical impedance and those that use differences in light scatter or optical properties, either alone or in combination. Another recent advancement in hematology analyzers is the incorporation of optical scatter, using both argon laser and no laser light technology, allowing integration of some flow cytometric data using specific fluorochrome stains, such as T-cell subsets (CD4:CD8) or CD34 positive cells, with routine hematologic analyses.

Each instrument presents a pictorial representation of the hematological data registered as either a histogram or a scatterogram. A histogram is a graphic representation of blood cells, produced from thousands/millions of signals generated by the cells passing through detector where they are differentiated by their size, and frequency of occurrence in the population thus provides an objective record of variation in cell sizes within the population under study.

Automated Counters Provide a Three-Part or Five-to Seven-Part Differential Count

3-part differential	5-part differential—Classify cells to	7-part differential

Usually count
• Granulocytes or large cells
• Lymphocytes or small cells
• Monocytes (mono-nuclear cells) or (mid cell population)
	• Neutrophils
	• Eosinophils
	• Basophils
	• Lymphocytes
	• Monocytes
	• A sixth category designated "large unstained cells" include cells larger than normal and lack the peroxidase activity. This includes:
	  – Atypical lymphocytes
	  – Various other abnormal cells
		Includes 5 part plus
		• Large immature cells (composed of blasts and immature granulocytes)
		• Atypical lymphocytes (including blast cells)

Automated Hematology Cell Counter

History

- **1852:** Karl Vierodt published first procedure of counting red cells by spreading blood on a slide and counting the cells.
- **1874:** Louis Charles started microscopic analysis of blood cells.
- **1891:** Paul Ehrlich and Dimitri Romanovasky develop technique of staining red cells.
- **1929:** Maxwell Wintrobe introduced Hematocrit method.
- **1953:** Wallace Coulter patented coulter principle which was a landmark in automation.

Basic Principles

Coulter's Concept of Electronic Impedance

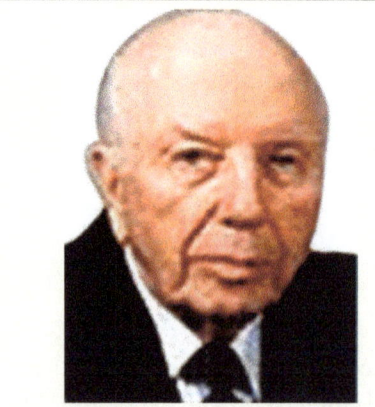

In 1953, Wallace Coulter patented the Coulter principle in which particles are counted in fluid which is passed through a hole.

The incredulous attorneys who had told him "You can't patent a hole" were proven wrong

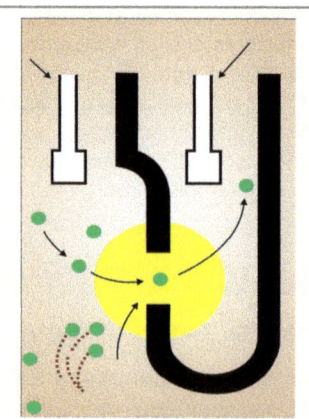

Most hematology instruments operate under several basic principles. Using this technology, cells are sized and counted by detecting and measuring changes in the electrical resistance when a particle passes through a small aperture. This is called the electrical impedance principle of counting cells. A blood sample is diluted in saline (a good conductor of electrical current) and the cells are pulled through an aperture by creating a vacuum. Two electrodes establish an electrical current. The external electrode is located in the blood cell suspension. The second electrode is the internal electrode and is located in the glass hollow tube, which contains the aperture. A low-frequency direct current is applied to both electrodes. Electrical resistance or impedance occurs as the cells pass through the aperture causing a change in voltage.

Mathematically V = R × C where V = Voltage, C = Current, R = Resistance

This change in voltage generates a pulse. This weak pulse is amplified and measured, the number of pulses is proportional to the number of cells counted as cell count, and is displayed on a screen. The size of the cell will determine the amount of interruption (also called resistance) and can be correlated to cell size. The size of the voltage pulse is also directly proportional to the volume or size of the cell. This information can be transmitted to a microprocessor of a computer and is used to provide an accurate cell count and identification of the types of cells. This concept is employed by Coulter cell counters (Coulter), some Cell-Dyn instruments (Abbott), Sysmex counting instruments (Baxter), and COBAS cell counters (Roche).

The Coulter-type cell counters are probably the most widely-used example of hematology analyzers that use electrical impedance methods, with the following principle and process of cell counting:

- The counting of the cellular elements of the blood (erythrocytes, leukocytes, and platelets) is based on the method of electrical impedance.
- There are two chambers one measures Hb and WBCs and the second chamber counts RBCs + PLTs. The aspirated whole blood specimen is divided into two aliquots and mixed with an isotonic diluent.
- The first dilution is delivered to the RBC aperture bath, and the second is delivered to the WBC aperture bath.
- In the RBC chamber, both the RBCs and the platelets are counted and discriminated by electrical impedance.
- Particles between 2 and 20 fL are counted as platelets, and those greater than 36 fL are counted as RBCs.
- A reagent to lyse RBCs and release hemoglobin is added to the WBC dilution before the WBCs are counted by impedance in the WBC bath.
- After the counting cycles are complete, the WBC dilution is passed to the hemoglobinometer for hemoglobin determination (light transmittance read at a wavelength of 535 nm).
- The electrical pulses obtained in the counting cycles are sent to the analyzer for editing, coincidence correction, and digital conversion.
- With the variation of "make and technology" there will be some variations in the above principle, and process.

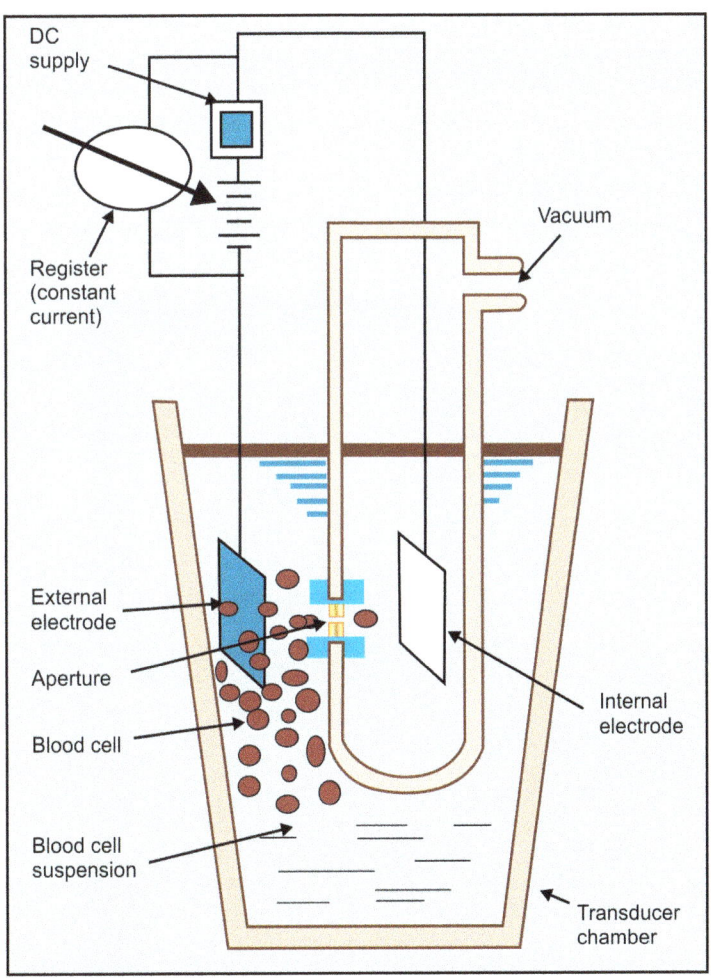

The Basic Components of the Hematology Automated Cell Analyzer
• The electrical system consists of circuitry, sequence controls, transformers. • Hydraulic system consists of an aspirating unit, dispensers, diluters, mixing chambers, flow cells, aperture baths, and a hemoglobinometer. • The pneumatic system consists of vacuum and pressure devices (to assure the movement of fluids through the analyzer system). • Computer systems (microprocessors and software applications) that perform complicate calculations (RDW, graphs, QC, critical value alerts), start-up and shut-down capability, internal self-checks, storage of QC and patient data, delta checks, selected self-maintenance capability.

ROLE OF FLOW CYTOMETRY IN LABORATORY MEDICINE

The Principle of Light Scattering to Characterize Blood Cells

The blood cell is subjected to fluid dynamics which leads them to flow in a single line. Each cell will pass through a detection device called a flow cell. This flow cell will have a laser device focused on it and as the cell passes through the laser light path, it will scatter light in several directions. The unit has one detector that captures the forward scatter light (FSL) and a second detector that captures the light that is scattered (side scattered or SS) at 90° or orthogonal angle. This principle allows for differentiating between granulocytes, lymphocytes, and monocytes.

APPLICATION OF LASER LIGHT TO IDENTIFY CELL TYPES

Laser light is a monochromatic light focused on a detection device through the use of mirrors and prisms. Laser light is preferred because of its properties of intensity, stability, and monochromatism. The leukocytes are forced to move past this laser light beam in a single file arrangement. The light that strikes each WBC can be measured as reflected or scattered light. This phenomenon is called "optical scatter". The detector used to collect the light scattered by each cell is called a photomultiplier tube. The cell with its internal and external features determines the quantity and character of the light scatter. The light that strikes the cell is scattered at angles proportional to its structural features. Each cell as it passes into the laser beam is measured according to its cell size, the number of nuclear lobules and distribution of dye in the cell if present.

Multiple Angle Polarized Scatter Separation

Each cell is analyzed through a flow cytometry cell as it is subjected to a variety of angled light scatter. Five subpopulations of cells are identified.

- 0° indicator of cell size
- 10° indicator of cell structure and complexity
- 90° polarized: indicates nuclear lobularity
- 90° depolarized: differentiate eosinophils

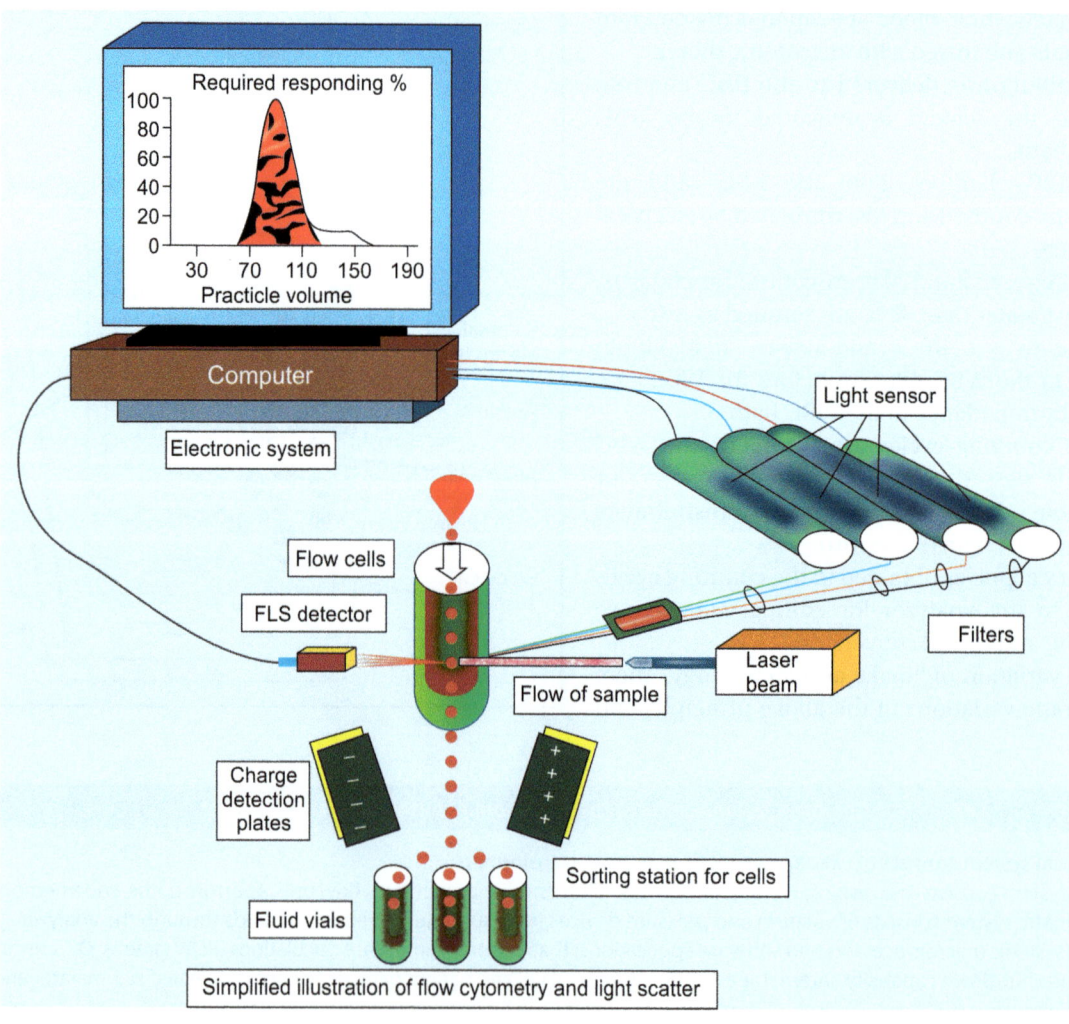

Simplified illustration of flow cytometry and light scatter

A light that is scattered 180° to the light source is called forward-angle light scatter (designated as FALS or FS). FALS is used to determine cell density or volume which relates to the cell size. A light that is scattered 90° to the light source is designated as side scatter or SS. This right-angle light scatter is a function of the cell contents revealing information about the nuclear complexity and cellular granularity. The information from these detectors is processed by a microprocessor and will appear in designated areas on a histogram screen.

The cell information posted to a screen is called a bitmap. The computer is the heart of this instrumentation coordinating all decisions regarding data collection, cell sorting, and analysis.

The characteristics of each type of blood cell determine the nature of the light scatter which can be designated as high, moderate, or low light scatter. If the FALS and SS from a leukocyte are low, then this would be interpreted as a lymphocyte. High FALS and high SS would indicate a neutrophil.

Flow cytometry employs low voltage DC electrical impedance, laser light technology, non-laser light technology, radiofrequency (high-voltage electromagnetic) current, fluorescence techniques. This technology can examine blood, bone marrow, body fluids, lymph nodes, needle aspirates, solid tumors, and splenic tissues. Flow cytometry has greatly affected the ability of the laboratory to provide data to diagnose hematological malignancies.

This technology may be applied in the following ways:
- Count and cell size (erythrocytes and leukocytes)
- Perform differential WBC counts
- Analyze up to 10,000 cells per second
- Count reticulocytes and platelets
- Immunophenotyping with monoclonal antibodies
- Perform basic lymphocyte screening panels
- Perform immunocytochemistry and immunofluorescence staining
- Cell sorting into subpopulations
- Detect fetal cells and hemoglobin
- Detection of malarial parasites
- DNA content analysis
- Enzyme studies
- RNA content

FLUORESCENT DYES AUGMENTATION OF FLOW CYTOMETRY

Fluorescent dyes can be used to stain certain components of the cell or may be bound to an immunological molecule that binds to a specific receptor on a cell membrane. Fluorochrome will become excited by different wavelengths of light. This permits the counting of specific tags independently. A flow cytometer with the capability to detect different types of dye tags can be used to perform a differential leukocyte count. This type of cytometry can analyze a single cell at the rate of 50,000 cells per minute.

Radiofrequency (RF) Principle of Cell Counter
This technology employs a high voltage electromagnetic current, which can estimate the cell size based upon its cellular density and nuclear volume. The RF pulse is a type of electromagnetic probe that is affected by the conductivity of the cell and other parameters. This pulse or conductivity can be attenuated, (i.e., weakened or made to fade in strength) by the nuclear to cytoplasmic ratio, nuclear density, degree of granulation of the cytoplasm. This information can be plotted into a two-dimensional graph or scatter diagram. This technology can be combined with other methodologies (such as optical scatter) to facilitate the separation of the leukocytes into their respective groups for a five-part differential. This technology is employed on the Sysmex cell analyzers.

The Concept of VCS Technology
This was developed by Coulter instruments and employs three principles of evaluating the leukocyte. VCS is "volume", "conductivity", and "scatter". These principles are: • **Direct current:** A low-frequency direct current measures the size of the leukocyte based upon its volume. • **High-frequency radio wave:** Emitted as an HF electromagnetic probe, it measures the conductivity of the cell, based upon its internal content. • **Laser light scatter**: This light beam evaluates the surface feature, structure, shape, granularity, and reflectivity. These features affect the scatter characteristics of the light beam.

Combined Impedance and Optical Counters

Some of the newer hematology analyzers have combined impedance and optical methods together within one instrument, thereby allowing for optimal use and integration of the data generated by each method.

Examples of combined impedance and optical method analyzers include the Beckman Coulter Gen-S (Hialeah, FL) and Cell-Dyn 4000. Many of these newer instruments also provide an automated reticulocyte count and have improved precision of automated differential counts to lower the need for manual reviews by a technician.

Laser Technology in Cell Counters

The blood is drawn into a buffered reagent that iso-volumetrically dilutes the cells and causes the platelets and RBCs to assume a spherical shape, and fixes the cells. As the erythrocytes and platelets are injected into the counter, the scattering phenomenon from the laser light will be measured at its high and low angles to measure the volume (fL) and hemoglobin concentration (g/dL) of each cell. The signal generated is transformed by the computer into cytograms and/or histograms.

Sophisticated high technology hematology analyzers use a **combination of:**
- **Light scatter**
- **Electrical impedance**
- **Fluorescence**
- **Light absorption**
- **Electrical conductivity**

Methods to produce RBC, WBC, and platelet analysis. Majority of the modern automated instruments are highly specialized flow cytometers.

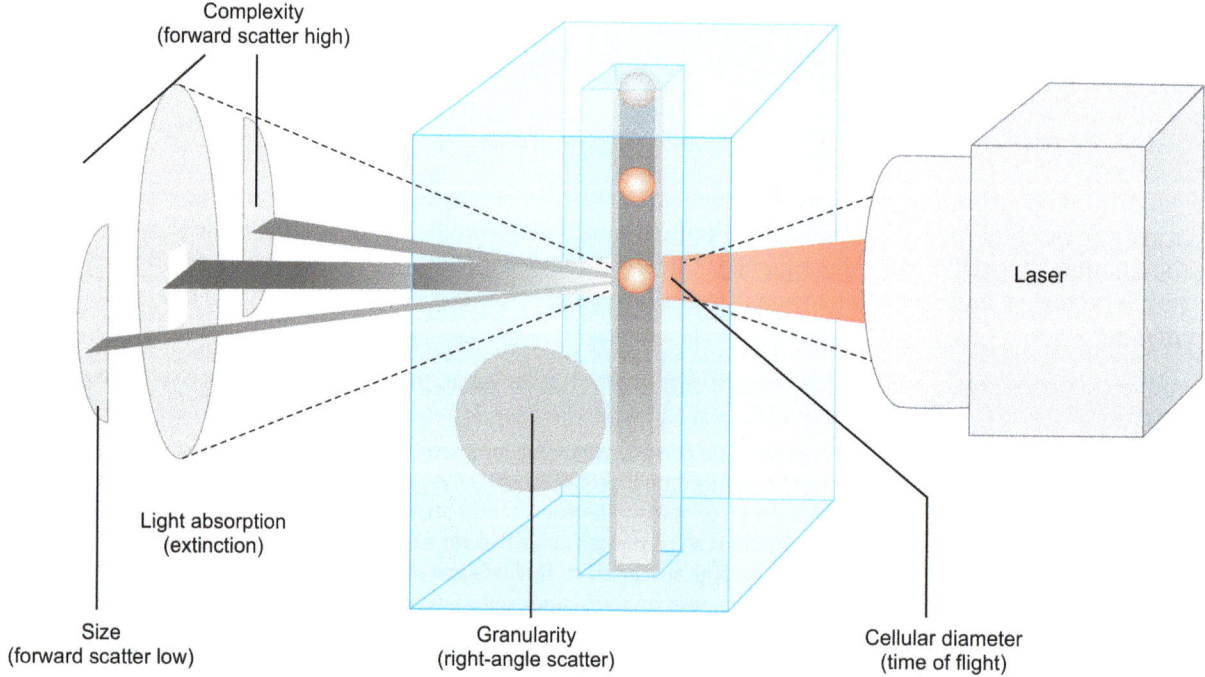

- **Light scatter**—detected at various angles determines **cell size and cellular characteristics**
- **Electronic impedance**—LW DC resistance determines **cell volume**
- **Conductivity/radio frequency (RF)**—determines internal **cell structure density**
- **Fluorescence with light scatter**—determine **RNA/DNA content**

Reticulocyte Count on Automation

- Automated reticulocyte counting is quickly becoming the standard for reticulocyte counting in clinical laboratories.
- For reticulocyte analysis, new methylene blue is incubated with whole blood samples.
- The dye precipitates the basophilic RNA network of the reticulocytes.
- Hemoglobin and unbound stain are removed by adding a clearing reagent, leaving clear spherical mature RBCs and darkly stained reticulocytes.
- Stained reticulocytes are differentiated from mature cells and other cell populations by light scatter, direct current measurements, and opacity characteristics.
- The normal reference range is 0.5–1.5%.
- Reticulocyte parameters (derived from advanced automation)
  - Reticulocyte count
  - MCVr
  - CHCMr
  - CHr (mean hemoglobin content of reticulocytes)
  - RDWr
  - HDWr

Recirculation and Coincidence Error

If more than one cell goes through the counting aperture at the same instant and is counted as one cell, this is called a coincidence error.

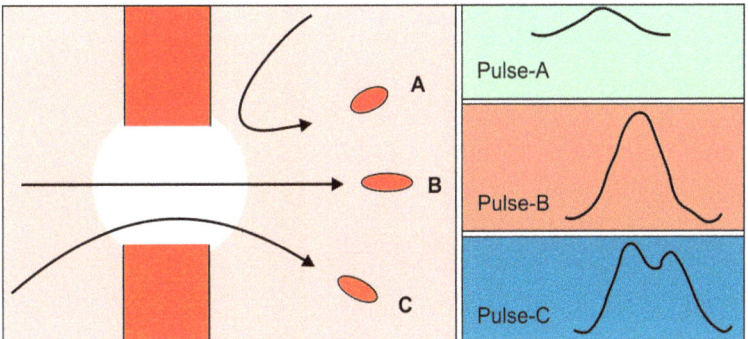

HYDRODYNAMIC FOCUSING

This is a technique that narrows the stream of cells to a single file, eliminating data above and below the focus points. Hydrodynamic focusing allows greater accuracy and resolution of blood cells. Diluted cells are surrounded by a sheath fluid, which lines up the cells in a single file while passing through the detection aperture. After passing through the aperture, the cells are then directed away from the back of the aperture. This process eliminates the recirculation of cells and the counting of cells twice.

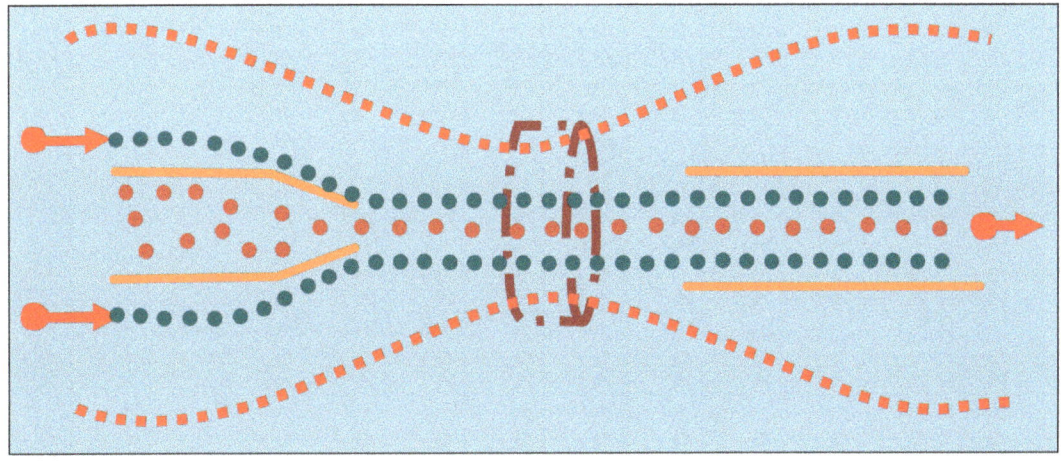

Role of Flow Cytometry in Laboratory Medicine

- Most hematology laboratories have now changed over from the labor-intensive manual methods of testing to 3- or 5- or 6- or 7-part differential automated hematology analyzers.
- Most of the sophisticated cell counters are equipped with modern technology using advanced flow cytometry.
- Although laboratory personnel and hematopathologists handling the automated data are familiar with the basic interpretation and benefits of numerical data, the seemingly complex graphical representation of the red cell data in the form of histograms and cytograms is often ignored.
- All automated cell counters are screening devices. Abnormalities must be verified by a blood film, staining, and scanning by an expert observer.

Advantage of Automated Cell Counters

- No interobserver variability
- No slide distribution errors
- Eliminates statistical variations
- Many parameters are not available on a manual count, e.g., red blood cell distribution width (RDW), histogram
- More efficient and time effective (high throughput)
- High level of precision and accuracy
- Aberrant results are "flagged" for subsequent review

CHAPTER 7

General Principle of Histogram Generation and Interpretation

GENERAL PRINCIPLE OF HISTOGRAM GENERATION

What is a histogram?

A histogram is a vertical bar chart that depicts the distribution of a set of data.

A histogram will make it easy to see where the majority of values fall in a measurement scale, and how much variation is present?

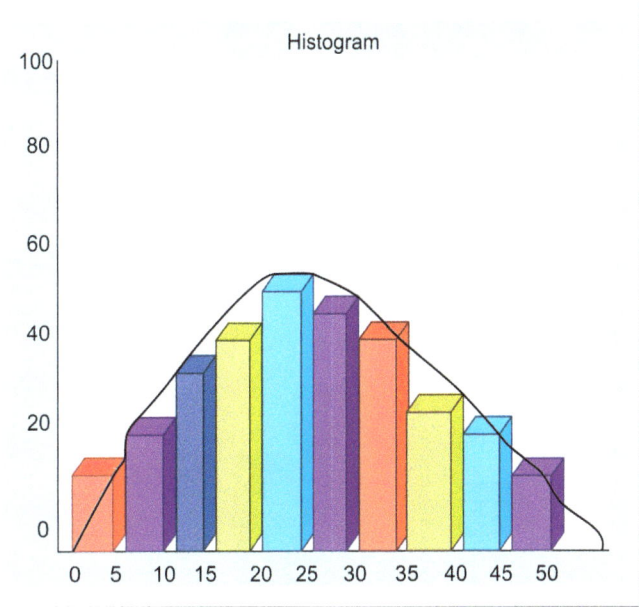

Histogram is made up of these parts:

1. **Title:** The title describes the information that is contained in the Histogram.
2. **Horizontal or X-axis:** The horizontal or X-axis shows the scale of values into which the measurements fit.
3. **Bars:** The bars have two important characteristics—height and width. The height represents the number of times the values within an interval occur. The width represents the length of the interval covered by the bar. It is the same for all bars.
4. **Vertical or Y-axis:** The vertical or Y-axis is the scale that shows you the number of times the values within an interval occurred.

The number of times is also referred to as "frequency."

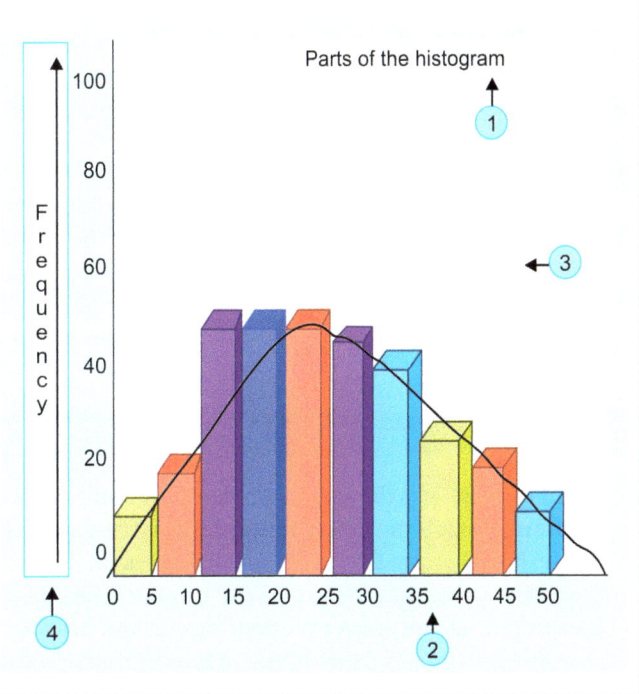

Interpretation of Histogram

A histogram provides a visual representation so you can see where most of the measurements are located and how spread out they are. Your histogram might show any of the following conditions.

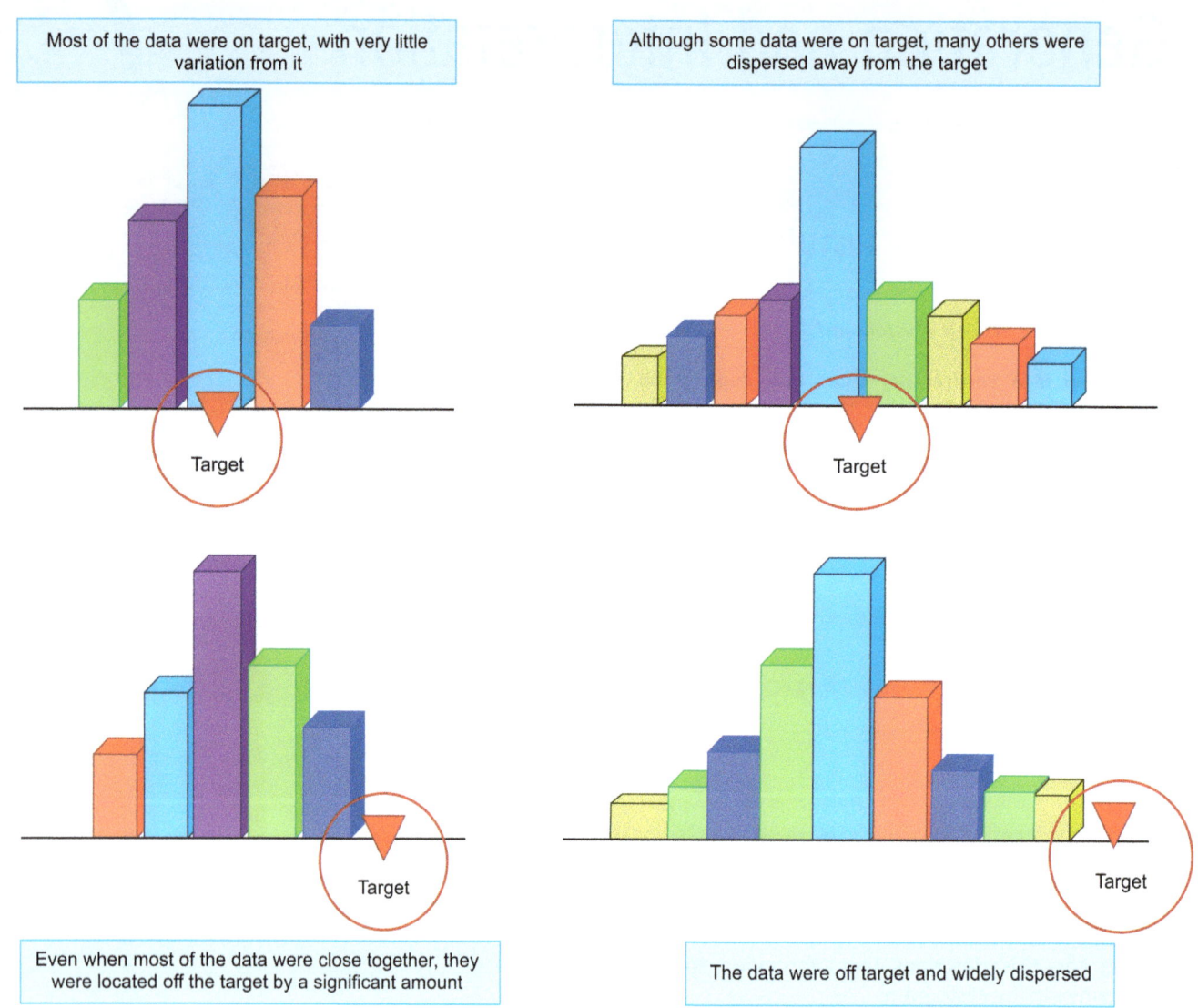

The basic principles behind the graphic displays of scatter plots, scattergrams, and histograms are fairly universal.

Scatter plots and scattergrams place a specific cell on a grid identification system while histograms measure size thresholds of white cells, red cells, and platelets compared to the normal data for each of these cell groups.

Scatter plots and scatter grams provide colorful imaging of normal and abnormal cells. A technocrat/an observer can immediately notice a particular deviation in numbers and distribution of a particular cell line by analyzing scatter plots.

STATISTICAL DEFINITIONS

- **Mean (X-bar):** It is the sum of all measurements divided by the number of measurements.
- **Median (m):** It is the point on the scale that has an equal number of observations above and below.
- **Mode:** It is the most frequently occurring result.
- **Standard Deviation (SD):** It is the measurement of the random variation or dispersion of data about the mean; the greater the SD, the greater the distribution and broader the curve; the smaller the SD, the narrower the curve.
  - One SD on either side of the mean encompasses about 60% of the population; two SD on either side of the mean encompasses about 95% of the population. Similarly, 99% of the population would be within 3 SDs.

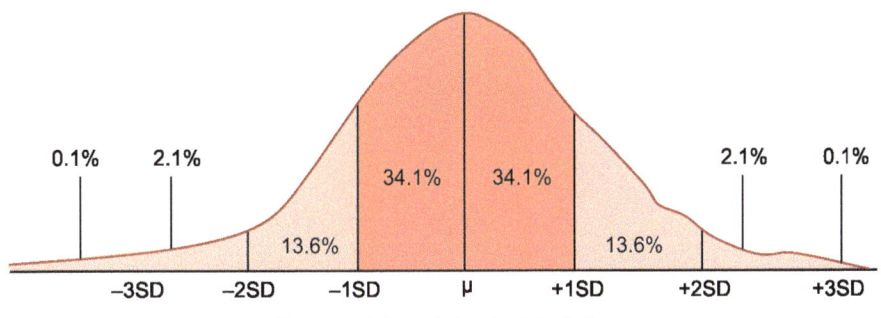
Representation of standard deviation

- **Coefficient of Variation (CV):** CV is the dispersion of data about the mean. It is a different way of expressing the SD. It is expressed as a percentage and takes into account the mean value. It is calculated as SD multiplied by 100 and divided by mean.
- **Gaussian Distribution:** Describes events or data which occur symmetrically about the mean. With this type of distribution, mean, median, and mode will be approximately equal.
- If data do not follow a Gaussian distribution a larger number of data are towards one side of the mean. Thus, data are asymmetric. The mean would be nearer to that side and the mean, median and mode would all differ. To calculate geometric mean and SD such data are converted to their logarithm and after calculating the mean and SD, the results are reconverted to the antilog. Thus log-normal distribution curves are used to describe shifted data.
- **Standard Error of Mean:** It is a measure of the dispersion of the mean of a set of measurements. It is used to compare the means of two sets of data.

HISTOGRAM IN HEMATOLOGY

HISTOGRAM CHARACTERISTICS

Histograms are graphic representations of cell frequencies versus size.

In a homogeneous cell population, the curve assumes a symmetrical bell-shaped or Gaussian distribution. A wide or more flattened curve is seen when the standard deviation from the mean is increased.

Histograms provide information about erythrocyte, leukocyte, and platelet frequency and distribution as well as depict the presence of subpopulations.

Shifts in one direction or another can be of diagnostic importance.

Cell counting and sizing are based on the detection and measurement of changes in electrical impedance (resistance) produced by a particle as it passes through a small aperture.

Particles such as blood cells are nonconductive but are suspended in an electrically conductive diluent. As a dilute suspension of cells is drawn through the aperture, the passage of each cell momentarily increases the impedance (resistance) of the electrical path between two submerged electrodes that are located on each side of the aperture.

The number of pulses generated during a specific period of time is proportional to the number of particles or cells.

The amplitude (magnitude) of the electrical pulse produced indicates the cell's volume.

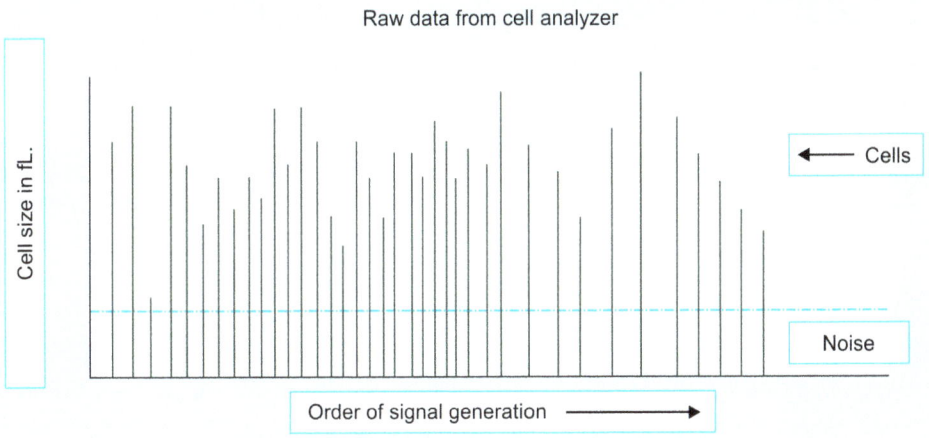

The output histogram is a display of the distribution of cell volume and frequency.
Each pulse on the X-axis represents the size in femtoliters (fL).
The Y-axis represents the relative number of cells.

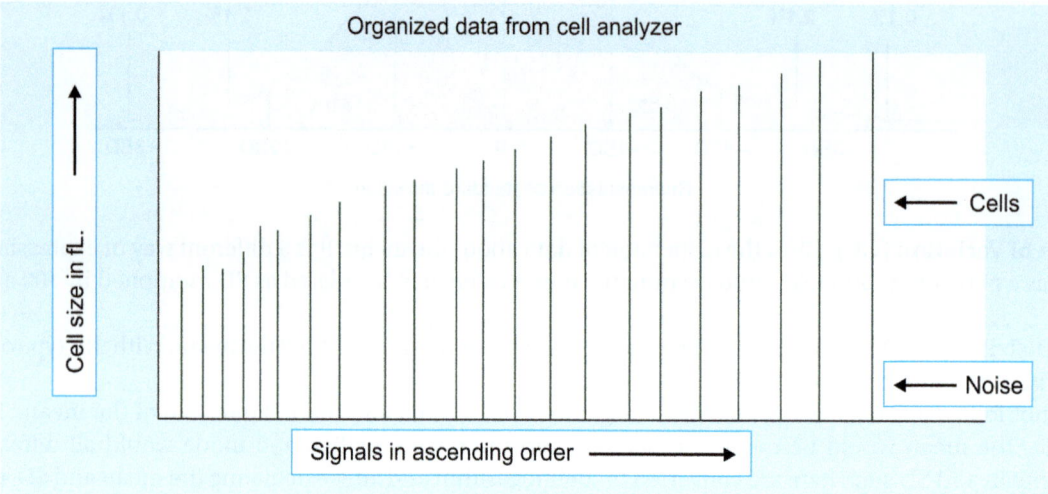

In the electrical impedance system, raw data is generated and the analyzer's computer classifies the raw data which is sorted and histograms are then smoothed (smooth curve). It is tested against mathematical criteria and finally fitted to a lognormal distribution curve.

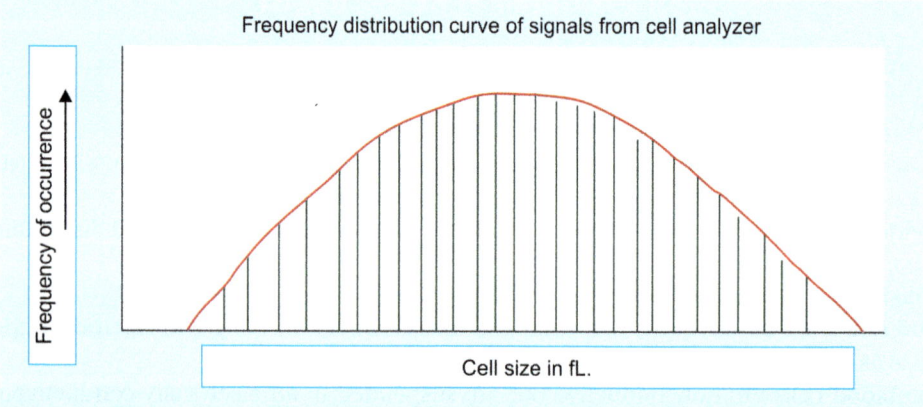

This general knowledge of histogram formation will facilitate better understanding of RBC, WBC and platelet histograms and their variations in disease in the following chapter.

CHAPTER 8

RBC Histogram and Cytogram

Over the past few decades, hematology analyzers have evolved from semi-automated to fully automated ones. Many additional parameters have become available now. From the earlier instruments that used electrical impedance as the sole counting principle for blood cells, modern-day analyzers, also use conductivity differences, cytochemical staining, light scatter and flow cytometric principles.

As the automated analyzers become more advanced, their precision has shown enormous improvement and manual blood smear review rates have been on a steady decline.

Graphical representation of results in the form of histograms or scatterplots has been largely ignored in favor of newer numerical parameters that have become available over the years. Some of these like the red cell distribution width, hemoglobin distribution width, and reticulocyte hemoglobin content provide very useful information in addition to the red cell indices that have been traditionally used.

Erythrocyte size and hemoglobin distribution cytograms provide very useful qualitative information, which is an adjunct to the numerical data but can sometimes be a very important pointer to a hematological condition no otherwise suspected.

Interpretation of histograms and scatterplots, in conjunction with the numerical data, can also be clinically useful in the diagnosis and follow-up of many hematological conditions.

For example, in patients with iron deficiency on treatment, sequential histograms can show the progressive appearance of a new well-hemoglobinized erythrocyte population far before the conventional numerical parameters.

Certain conditions like the presence of a significant population of **fragmented red cells or red cell agglutinate in cold agglutinin** disease that could not have been identified earlier without a blood smear examination can now be detected on the red cell cytogram.

In **iron deficiency anemia**, even before the red cell indices are affected, the **RBC cytogram** shows a shift to the microcytic zone.

Changes in the RBC indices, being a mean of many measurements, usually lag behind a direct representation of the microcytic population seen on the cytogram.

The uniform microcytosis seen in **heterozygous beta-thalassemia** is identified on the RBC cytogram as closely clustered sizing points, forming a typical **comma shape**.

Homozygous thalassemic, in contrast, owing to its inherent marked red cell anisocytosis, shows a much wider scatter pattern resembling an exaggerated version of the cytogram seen in iron deficiency anemia.

Double populations of red cells exist in patients on **hematinic treatment**, following **blood transfusion** or in **dual (vitamin B_{12}/folate and iron) deficiency anemia** due to their different size and hemoglobin concentration can be identified on the RBC cytogram and may not be reflected in the numerical data due to the averaging effect of macrocytes and microcytes on the MCV.

Non-megaloblastic macrocytosis can be seen in liver disease, aplastic anemia, hypothyroidism, etc.

Spherocytic pattern may be seen in hereditary spherocytosis, warm type auto-immune hemolytic anemia.

Red cell cytograms from automated hematology analyzers provide valuable information regarding common hematological conditions, hematopathologist and clinicians having a basic understanding of the graphical output while interpreting the numerical data can enhance the diagnostic utility of automated data.

"Interpretation of histograms and scatter plots, in conjunction with the numerical data, can be clinically useful in the diagnosis and follow-up of many hematological and nonhematological conditions".

THE VOLUME HISTOGRAM FOR ERYTHROCYTES

- The volume histogram reflects the size of erythrocytes or any other particle in the erythrocyte size range.
- The instrument counts the cells as erythrocyte with volume sizes between 25 fL and 250 fL.
- RBC histogram is a symmetrical bell-shaped curve. Under some situations, it is altered and then shows RBC flags on the calculated parameters.
- The area of the peak is used to calculate the MCV and RDW. This area represents 60 fL to 125 fL.
- If the RBCs are larger than normal (macrocytic), the curve will shift toward the right.
- If the RBCs are smaller than normal (microcytic), the curve will **shift to the left**.
- The extension of the lower end of the scale allows for the detection of erythrocyte fragments, leukocyte fragments, and large platelets.
- If the histogram curve is bimodal (Camel humps), then there are two populations of red blood cells as might be seen when a patient received a blood transfusion. Other conditions that will cause a bimodal distribution curve are cold agglutinin disease, hemolytic anemia with the presence of schistocytes, or anemias with different size cell populations.
- WBCs are present in the diluted fluid containing RBCs, but their numbers are statistically insignificant to cause any change in the histogram.
- If the leukocyte count is significantly elevated, the erythrocyte histogram will be affected as in the case of CLL.
- Variations in the shape and placement of the RBC histogram are an indicator of change in the size and/or shape of the erythrocytes.
- The mean corpuscular volume (MCV) is calculated from the area under the peak.
- The red blood cell distribution width (RDW) is also calculated from the data used to calculate the MCV.
- Interpretation of the RBC histogram, along with the numerical values of RBC count, Hgb, Hct, MCH, MCHC, and RDW can significantly assist in the diagnosis of various RBC disorders avoiding many expensive and invasive investigations.

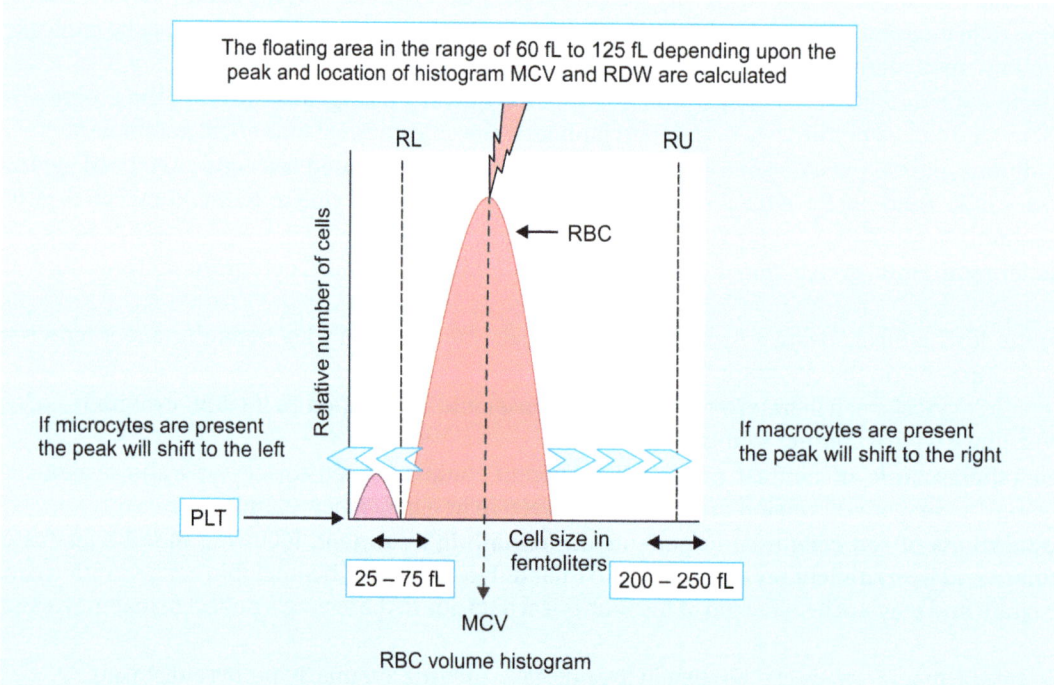

RBC volume histogram

- RBC detection: between 25 fL and 250 fL.
- Distribution curves are separated by flexible discriminators: RL and RU.
- The histogram curve should start and end at the baseline within the discriminators.
- The flag messages: RL; RU or MP are generated in case of abnormal histogram curves. The results must be manually checked.

The RBC histogram has fluctuating lower and upper discriminator. The lower discriminator fluctuates between 25 fL and 75 fL and the upper discriminator between 200 fL and 250 fL. RDW is an important parameter for the measurement of the degree of variation in red cell size.

The two important options available on the instrument are RDW-CV and RDW-SD. RDW-CV is calculated by SD/MCV × 100 and normally ranges between 11.5% and 14.5%.

RDW-SD is not a statistical SD, but measured by drawing an arbitrary line at a height of 20% on the y-axis in femtoliters, and is termed as RDW-SD. Its normal value is in the range of 35–45 fL.

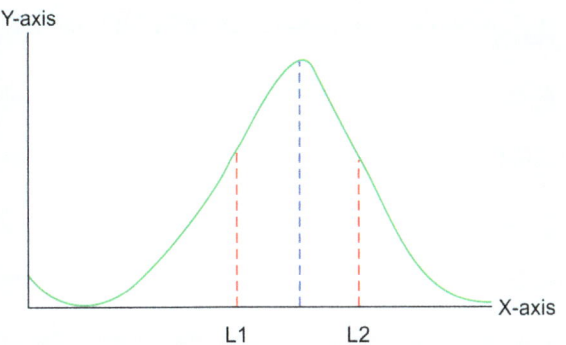
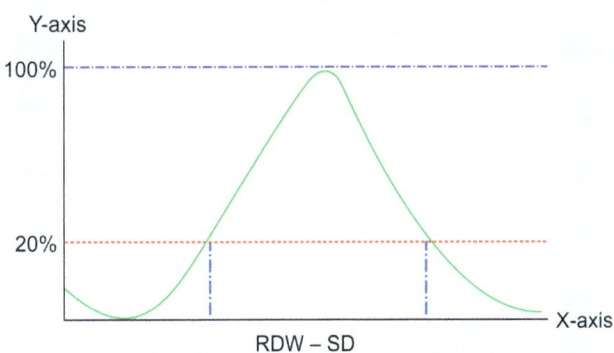

ABNORMAL RBC HISTOGRAMS AND RED CELL FLAGS

1. Abnormal Height at Lower Discriminator RL Flag

This flag is seen when the LD exceeds the preset height by greater than 10%.

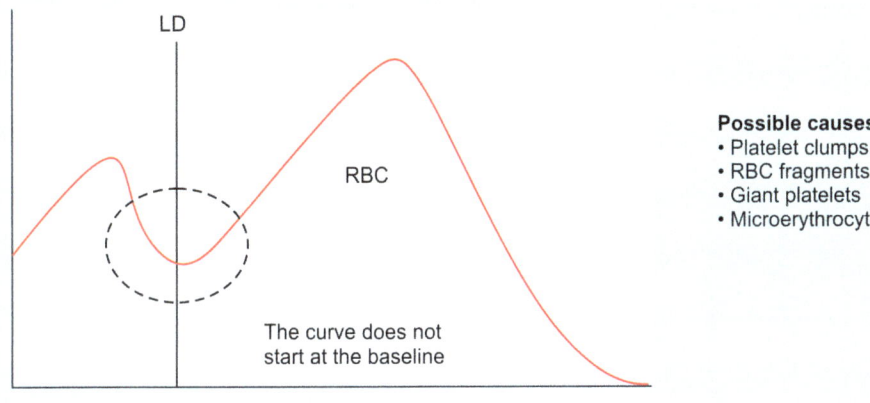

Possible causes:
- Platelet clumps
- RBC fragments
- Giant platelets
- Microerythrocytes

2. Abnormal Height at Upper Discriminator RU Flag

This flag is seen when the UD exceeds the preset height by greater than 5%.

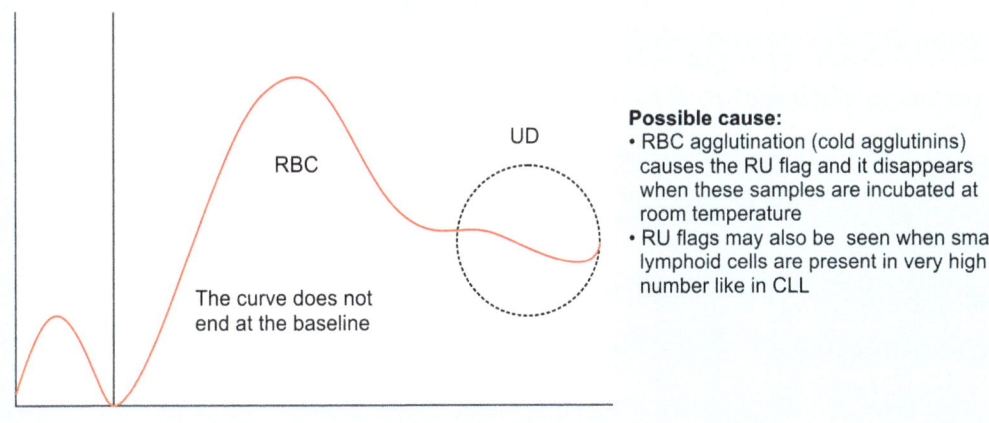

Possible cause:
- RBC agglutination (cold agglutinins) causes the RU flag and it disappears when these samples are incubated at room temperature
- RU flags may also be seen when small lymphoid cells are present in very high number like in CLL

3. Abnormal Distribution Width (DW)

Abnormal histogram distribution RDW - SD or RDW - CV is flagged.

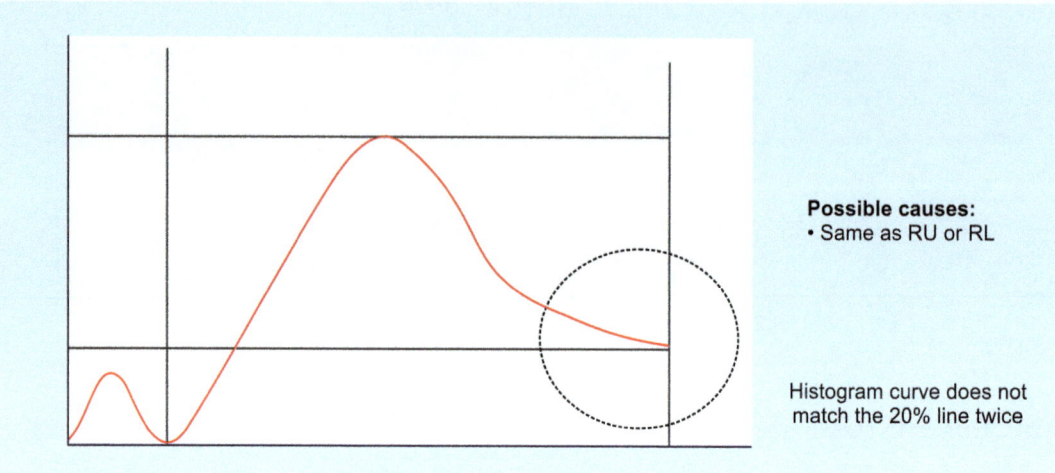

Possible causes:
• Same as RU or RL

Histogram curve does not match the 20% line twice

RBC Microcytosis

The % MICRO parameter indicates the percent of red blood cells that have a volume lower than 60 fL and is derived from the RBC volume histogram.

Severity levels are:

+   %MICRO = 2% to 6%

++   %MICRO = 6% to 10%

+++ %MICRO > 10%

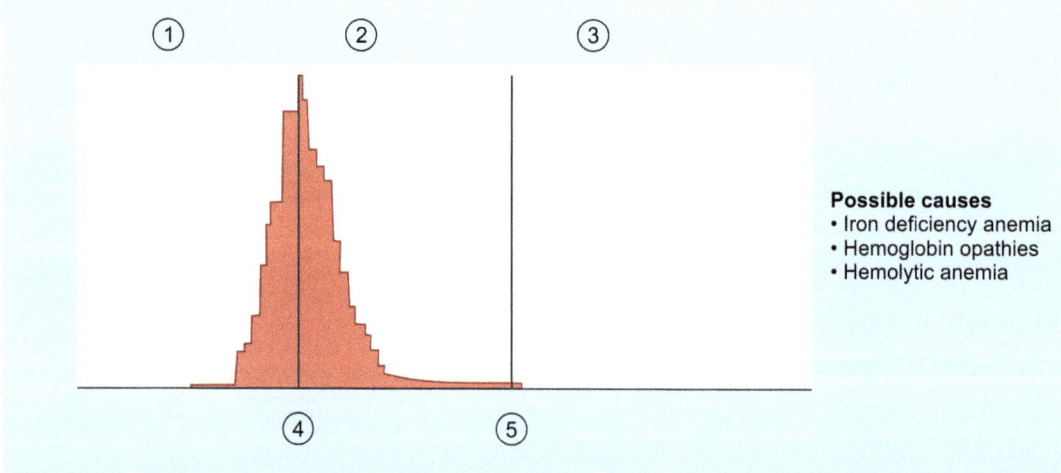

Possible causes
• Iron deficiency anemia
• Hemoglobin opathies
• Hemolytic anemia

In samples with increased numbers of microcytic red blood cells, the histogram curve shifts to the left, indicating an increase in the percentage of the cells with volumes less than 60 fL.

RBC Macrocytosis

The % MACRO parameter indicates the percent of red blood cells that have a volume greater than 120 fL and is derived from the RBC volume histogram.

Severity Levels

+   %MACRO = 2% to 6%

++   %MACRO = 6% to 10%

+++ %MACRO > 10%

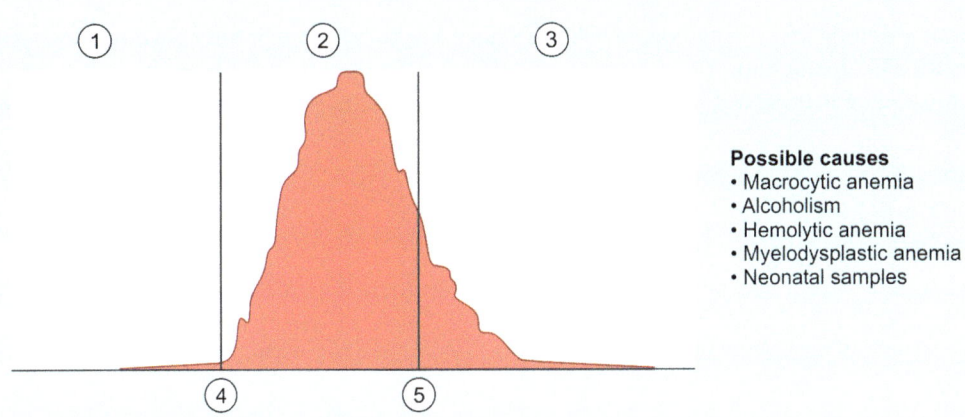

RBC Anisocytosis

RDW is monitored as an indication of anisocytosis, and the results are flagged if the RDW exceeds 16%.

Anisocytosis - Multiple Peaks (MP)

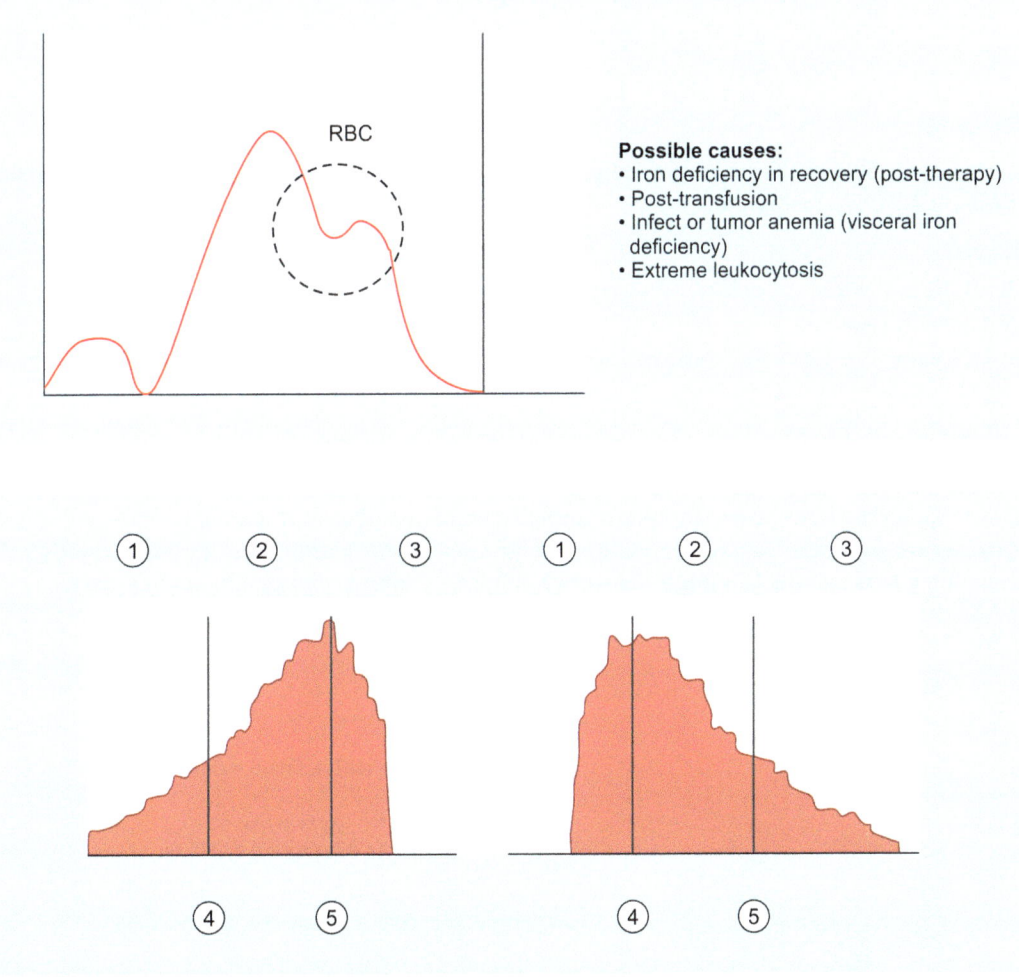

Note that two specimens with the same RDW value can have different degrees of microcytosis and macrocytosis.

RBC Hypochromia

The % HYPO parameter indicates the percent of cells that have a cellular hemoglobin concentration less than 28 g/dL and is derived from the RBC HC histogram.

The hypochromia flag is triggered if the percentage of cells with low cellular hemoglobin concentration (% HYPO) is greater than 5.0%.

Severity levels are:

+   %HYPO = 4.0% to 7.9%
++   %HYPO = 8.0% to 12.0%
+++   %HYPO = > 12.0%

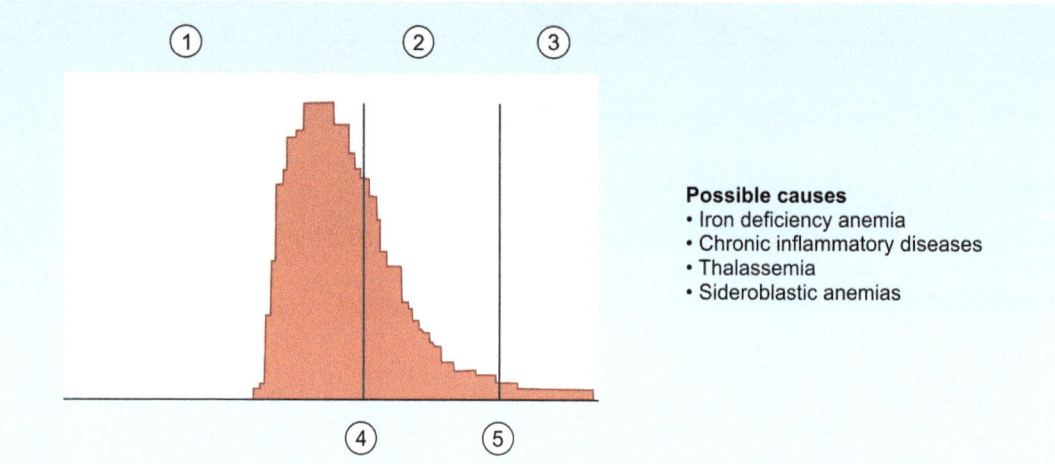

Possible causes
- Iron deficiency anemia
- Chronic inflammatory diseases
- Thalassemia
- Sideroblastic anemias

RBC Hyperchromia

The %HYPER parameter indicates the percent of cells that have a cellular hemoglobin concentration greater than 41 g/dL and is derived from the RBC HC histogram.

Severity levels are:

+   %HYPER = 4.0% to 7.9%
++   %HYPER = 8.0% to 12.0%
+++   %HYPER = > 12.0%

Possible causes
- Hereditary spherocytosis
- Sickle cell anemia
- Hemolytic uremic syndrome

RBC CYTOGRAM

- The sophisticated newer analyzers perform red cell analysis by **flow cytometry and laser technology.**
- The cells move through the laser beam, analysis is done based on the degree of scatter.
- The red cell **cytogram** is a graphical representation of 2 light scatter measurements; the **high angle (5–15°)** light scatter is plotted along the **x-axis** and the **low angle scatter (2–3°)** light scatter is plotted along the **y-axis**.

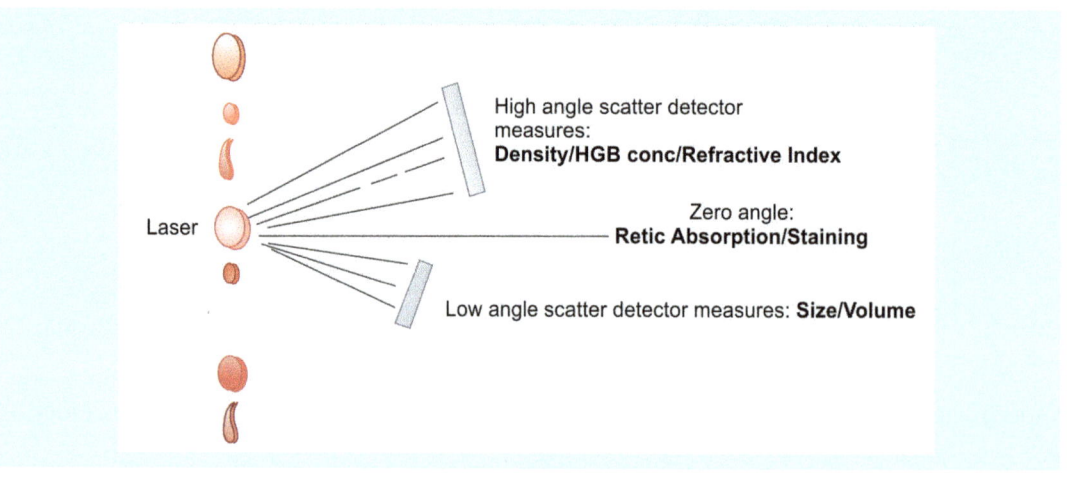

- The RBC volume/hemoglobin concentration (V/HC): Represents volume/Hb concentration. Data is a linear version of the RBC map for easy interpretation
- RBC V/HC cytogram pattern from a normal individual plotted with a 9-part grid showing the volume markers and hemoglobin concentration markers (x and y). Most RBC plots fall in the central zone (normocytic normochromic)
- On the V/HC cytogram, hemoglobin concentration is plotted along the x-axis and the cell volume along the y-axis.
- On the x-axis, hemoglobin concentration markers are set at 28 g/dL (x) and 41 g/dL (y).
- Red cells with a hemoglobin concentration of **less than 28 g/dL are hypochromic** while those with a concentration of **more than 41 g/dL are hyperchromic.**
- On the y-axis, RBC volume markers are set at 60 fL and 120 fL.
- Red cells with a **volume of less than 60 fL are microcytic**, while those with a **volume of more than 120 fL are macrocytic.**
- Normal red cells show most RBCs to fall in the central square of the V/HC cytogram because of their normal size and hemoglobin content.
- Abnormal red cells present in various disease conditions will deviate from the central square of the V/HC cytogram and will be plotted in specific shapes at specific locations.
- This specification is not absolute always but an understanding of these diversified cytograms along with histogram and numerical parameters become a great help in diagnosis and monitoring of disease process.
- Pictorial grid of cytogram with labelling of 9 squares is a base to understand cytograms which are exhibited along with histograms, smear pictures, and numerical values on subsequent disease-specific pages.
- RBC-related graphical pattern recognition is the key to clinical decision making and needs greater awareness.

Pictorial RBC Cytogram

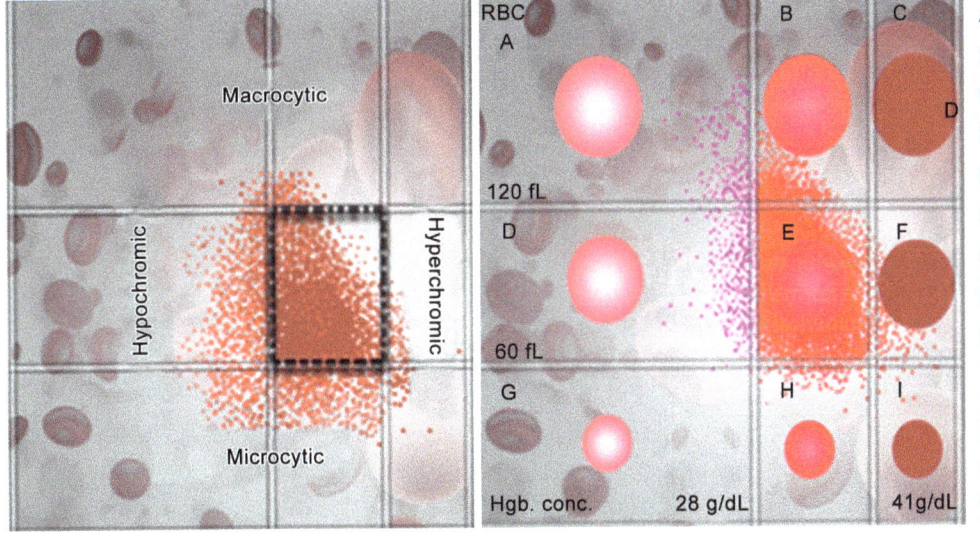

Pictorial grid of cytogram with labelling of 9 squares is a base to understand cytograms
Courtesy: © Siemens Healthcare GmbH 2020.

Utility of RBC Cytograms

- Contains valuable information
- Some plots are virtually diagnostic
- Pattern recognition is the key
- Can guide physicians on hematological status
- Clinical decision making is faster
- Aids thalassemia diagnosis
- Monitoring of EPO therapy
- Detects spherocytosis
- Unsuspected conditions may be diagnosed

The RBC Histogram

This is a diagrammatic representation of histograms designed for a better understanding of the interpretation of hematological disorders, with the help of variations of histograms seen in CBC reports, for learners.

This normal histogram will be repeated in subsequent figures, as a representative normal pattern against which variations of histograms in various disease conditions will be interpreted. Although such combinations are not generated by commercially available cell counters.

Variations of the programming of different instruments will result in variation of histogram design therefore each laboratory should know its machine's values in normal.

Normal RBC Histogram and Cytogram

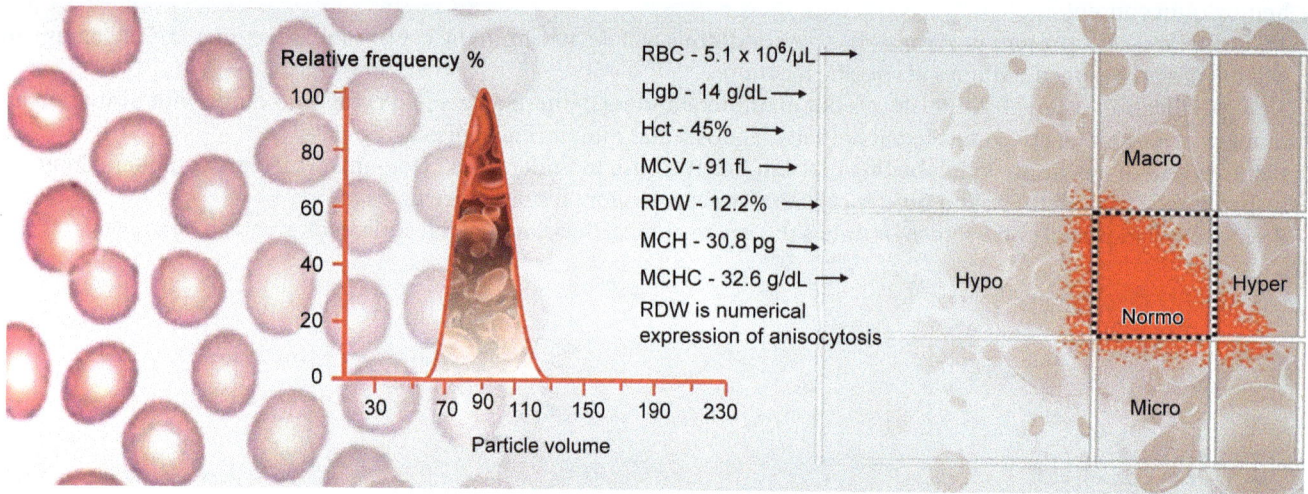

- This is a peripheral blood smear of a normal subject.
- Variation in cell size and shape is there but is within the acceptable range.
- The RBC-filled symmetrical histogram shows a normal degree of variation.
- The automated blood counter displays the numerical values of RBC, MCV, Hb, Hct, and RDW, which are within normal range.
- Normal red cells show most RBCs to fall in the **central square of the V/HC cytogram**.

Early Iron Deficiency

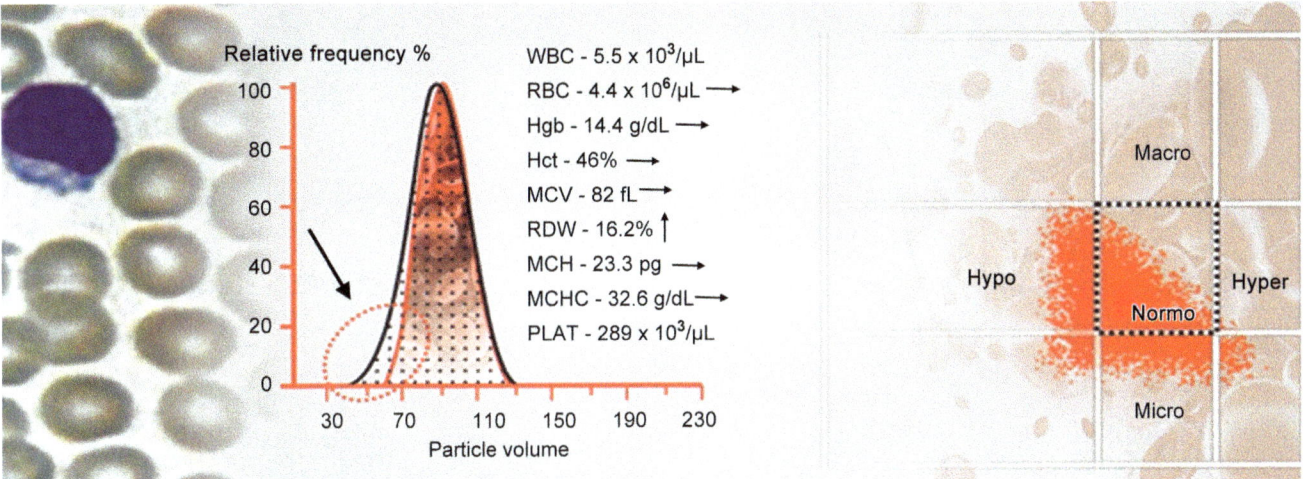

Increased RDW combined with normal RBC values (MCV, Hb, Hct) distinguishes iron deficiency from normal subjects	• RBC and Hb levels are within normal range. • Anemia is not yet apparent. • MCV and MCH still are in the normal range. • Peripheral smear hardly shows any anisocytosis. • RDW is increased (earliest indicator). • Histogram is unimodal, but is wider, extended toward the left side (microcytic population). • No expression of numerical hematological data that indicates anemia, yet the histogram and increased RDW are indicating the beginning of the process of iron deficiency anemia at a very early stage. • The diagnostic benefit of the knowledge of interpretation of histogram and RDW is that, even at 14.4 gm% Hb, the forthcoming event of iron deficiency is predicted. • **The RBC cytogram** shows a small red cell population in the microcytic hypochromic zone, appearing with a mild shift to the left and lower region.
Increased RDW combined with low MCV distinguishes iron deficiency from nonanemic heterozygous thalassemia	

Advanced Iron Deficiency

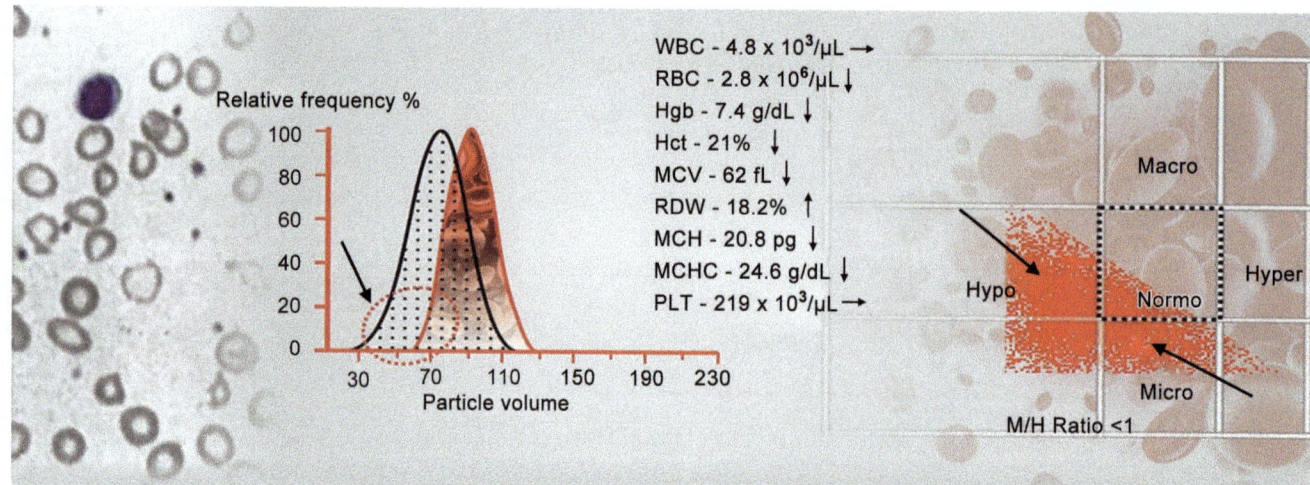

- Increased RDW is the first indication of iron deficiency
- Helps to distinguish iron deficiency from heterozygous thalassemia
- Hypochromia and microcytosis are proportional to the severity of anemia
- Target cells may be present but are more common in thalassemia
- MCV decreased (<79 fL), MCH decreased (<27 pg)
- Serum iron is decreased (usually <40 µg/dL)
- TIBC is increased (usually > 350 to 460 µg/dL)
- Transferrin saturation decreased (<15%)
- Serum ferritin is decreased
- Serum ferritin is the first test to reflect iron deficiency; it is decreased before anemia
- Decreased serum ferritin is the most sensitive and specific test and it returns to normal within few days after onset of oral iron therapy; failure of return suggests noncompliance, malabsorption, or continued iron loss
- Bone marrow: Normoblastic hyperplasia with absent iron

- RBC, Hb, Hct, MCV, MCH all are reduced showing microcytosis with hypochromia.
- Anemia is present.
- RDW is abnormally high due to the heterogeneity of cells.
- Histogram is abnormal with the shift to right indicating microcytosis and widening of the base of the graph indicating heterogeneity of cells
- The diagnosis is easily made at this point, but earlier identification would improve management.

- Red cell distribution width (RDW) and hemoglobin distribution width (HDW) both are raised in IDA contrast to thalassemia trait, where both the parameters tend to be normal.
- **RBC cytogram** appears characteristically a distinct 'wedge' or 'right-angled triangle' shape, that differs from other causes of microcytosis and hypochromia.
- The RBC cytogram shows the majority of the red cell population to be in the microcytic hypochromic zone, appearing with a shift to the left and lower region of the cytogram.
- Hypochromia is more than microcytosis, and the ratio of **microcytic% to hypochromic cell % (M/H Ratio) is usually less than 1**

Recovery from Iron Deficiency

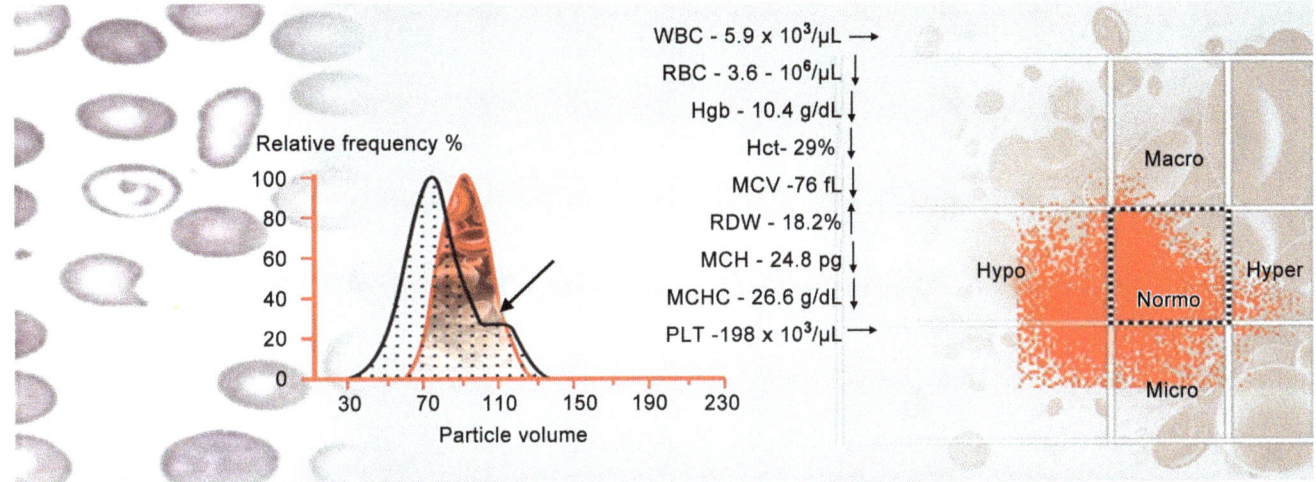

Anemia is not a disease, but a term indicating insufficient hemoglobin to deliver oxygen to the cells. It is always a secondary phenomenon

- The red cell count is increasing.
- MCV is not yet normal.
- Two populations of red cells are seen as pre-existing microcytes and newly-formed normocytes.
- The two populations are distinguished easily on the red cell histogram but not so easily on the peripheral blood smear.

- Double populations of red cells may exist in patients on hematinic treatment.
- Due to their different size and hemoglobin concentration leading to varying scatter properties, two populations (Hypo and Normo) can be identified on the RBC cytogram.
- Presence of a dual red cell population may only be visible on the scatterplot and may not always be reflected in the numerical data.

Mentzer Index
- It is used to differentiate iron deficiency anemia from beta-thalassemia
- It is calculated as MCV/RBC
- If MCV/RBC < 13, it signifies thalassemia trait
- MCV/RBC > 13 signifies iron deficiency anemia

Recovery from Iron Deficiency Bimodal Peak

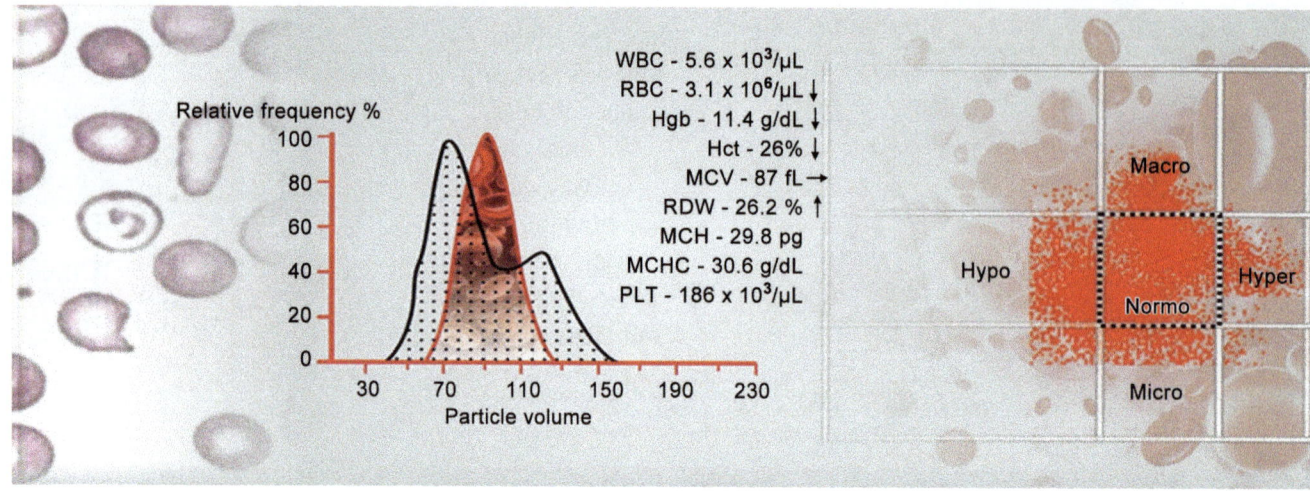

In patients with iron deficiency on treatment, sequential histograms can show the progressive appearance of a new well-hemoglobinized erythrocyte population well ahead of that indicated by the conventional numerical parameters.

- Double populations of red cells may exist in patients on hematinic treatment.
- Due to their different size and hemoglobin concentration leading to varying scatter properties, many populations (Hypo, Normo and Hyper) can be identified on the RBC cytogram.
- Presence of a such red cell population may only be visible on the scatterplot and may not always be reflected in the numerical data due to the antagonistic effect of macrocytes and microcytes on the MCV.

- In contrast to earlier figures, in this case as the second peak is on the right of the normal peak indicating that the new cells are macrocytic.
- Note the right peak has a mean value of 117 fL.
- This macrocytic response indicates an unmasking of the underlying macrocytic disorder leading to the diagnosis of dimorphic anemia of combined nutritional (iron and Vit B_{12}/Folic acid) deficiency.
- Only the correct interpretation of the histogram leads to this analysis, although the MCV is only 86.8 fL (due to the averaging of micro and macrocytosis).
- The two populations cannot be well-distinguished from the blood smear.

Anemia of Chronic Disease

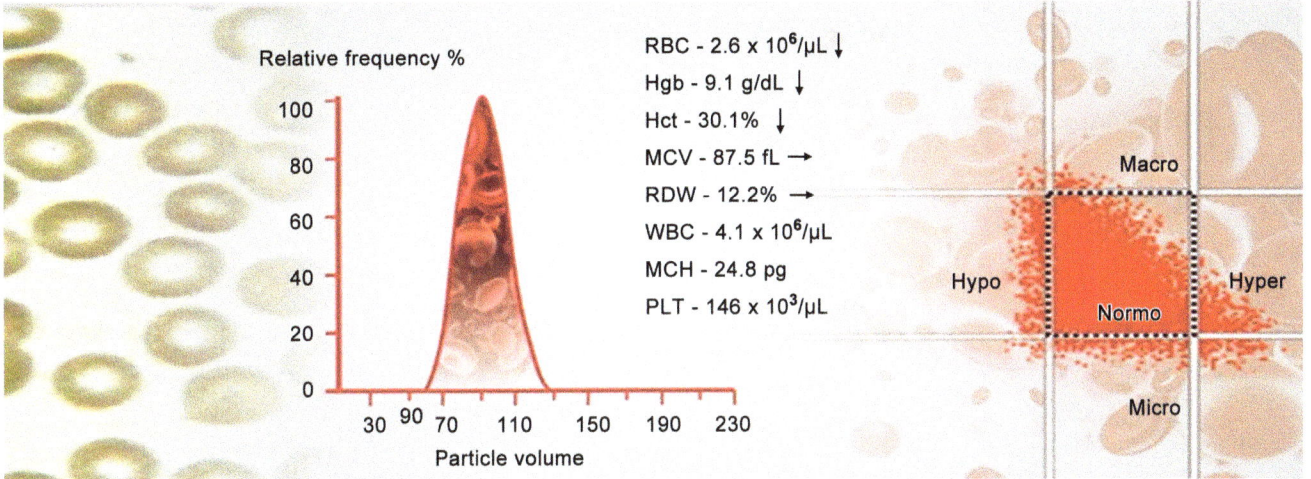

RBC - 2.6 x 10^6/μL ↓
Hgb - 9.1 g/dL ↓
Hct - 30.1% ↓
MCV - 87.5 fL →
RDW - 12.2% →
WBC - 4.1 x 10^6/μL
MCH - 24.8 pg
PLT - 146 x 10^3/μL

Anemia of Chronic Disease
- Anemia is usually caused by multiple mechanisms, e.g., hypoproliferative (failure of erythropoiesis), decreased RBC survival, iron deficiency of chronic inflammation, impaired erythropoietin, etc.
- Anemia is normocytic, normochromic in most cases.
- RDW and indices are usually normal.
- Anemia may be hypochromic and/or microcytic in 25 to 30% of the cases.
- Moderate anisocytosis and slight poikilocytosis may be seen.
- Low reticulocyte count.
- Polychromatophilia, and nucleated RBCs are absent.
- Serum ferritin is increased or normal in contrast to iron deficiency.
- Free erythrocyte protoporphyrin is increased.

Bone marrow sideroblasts are decreased; cellular elements are generally morphologically normal. Myeloid: Erythroid ratio is usually normal.

High serum ferritin differentiates IDA from iron-deficient erythropoiesis in inflammation, which increases two or three-fold in anemia of inflammation.

- All values are normal except for anemia and the peripheral blood smear and histogram resemble those seen in normal subjects.
- Almost similar picture may be seen in:
- Anemia of acute blood loss
- Hypothyroidism
- CRF
- Radiation or drug suppressed marrow
- Chronic liver disease (with variable MCV)

Anemia of chronic disorder can mimic the hematological parameters and cytogram seen in early iron deficiency anemia or closure to normal cytogram

Early Megaloblastic Anemia

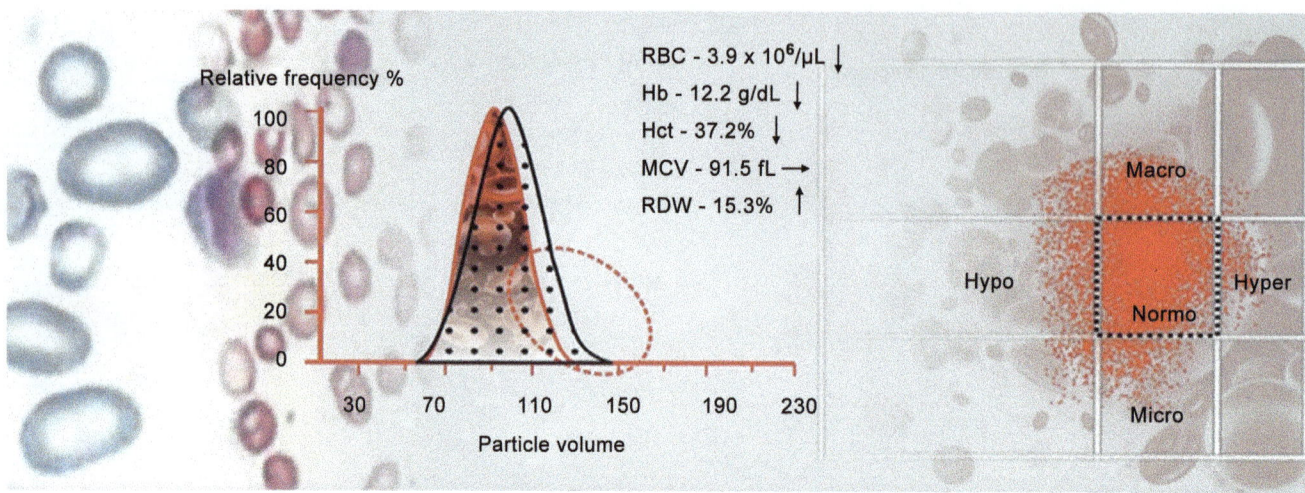

Advanced Megaloblastic Anemia

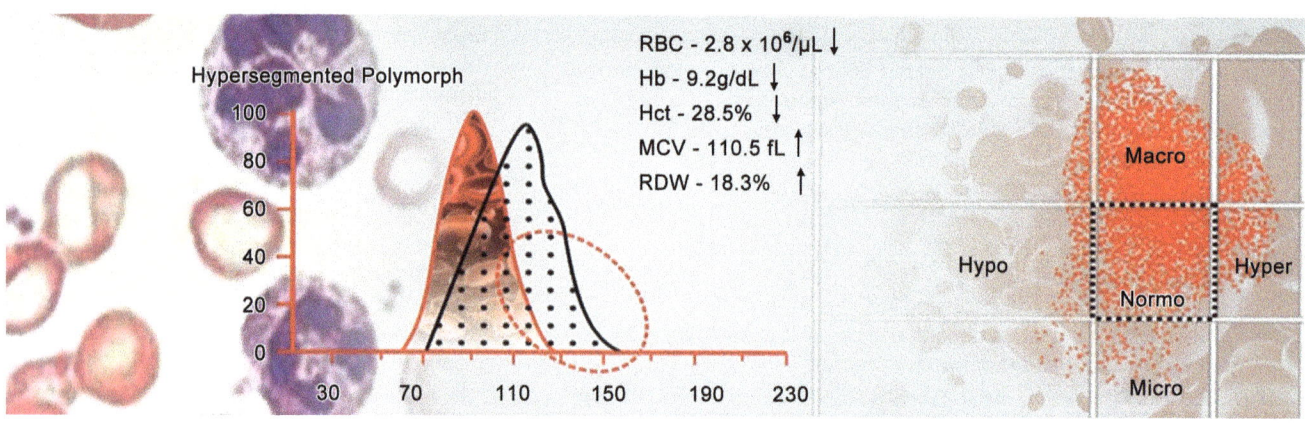

In Case of Early Megaloblastic Anemia
- The MCV is still normal RBC count and Hb slightly reduced.
- RDW is distinctly increased.
- Histogram is widened on the right side, indicating the appearance of macrocytic population, although not yet enough to increase MCV.
- Raised RDW with changes in the histogram may alert the clinician for the possibility of early megaloblastic anemia even before apparent anemia.

In case of advanced megaloblastic anemia with severe folate deficiency
- RBC count is low, MCV is high, and RDW is increased.
- Histogram is widened and shifted to the right distinctly, indicating macrocytosis.

Large hyper-segmented neutrophils with low Hb, increased MCV, raised RDW with presence of macro ovalocytes are considered diagnostic.

Most red cells have a larger volume (>100 fL) and show significant poikilocytosis (macrovalocytes).

The red cell cytogram, therefore, shows most cell plots in the macrocytic zone with a wider spread as compared to that seen in non-megaloblastic macrocytosis.

Source of folate is fruits and vegetables.
Source of vitamin B_{12} is meat and dairy products.

Recovery from Megaloblastic Anemia

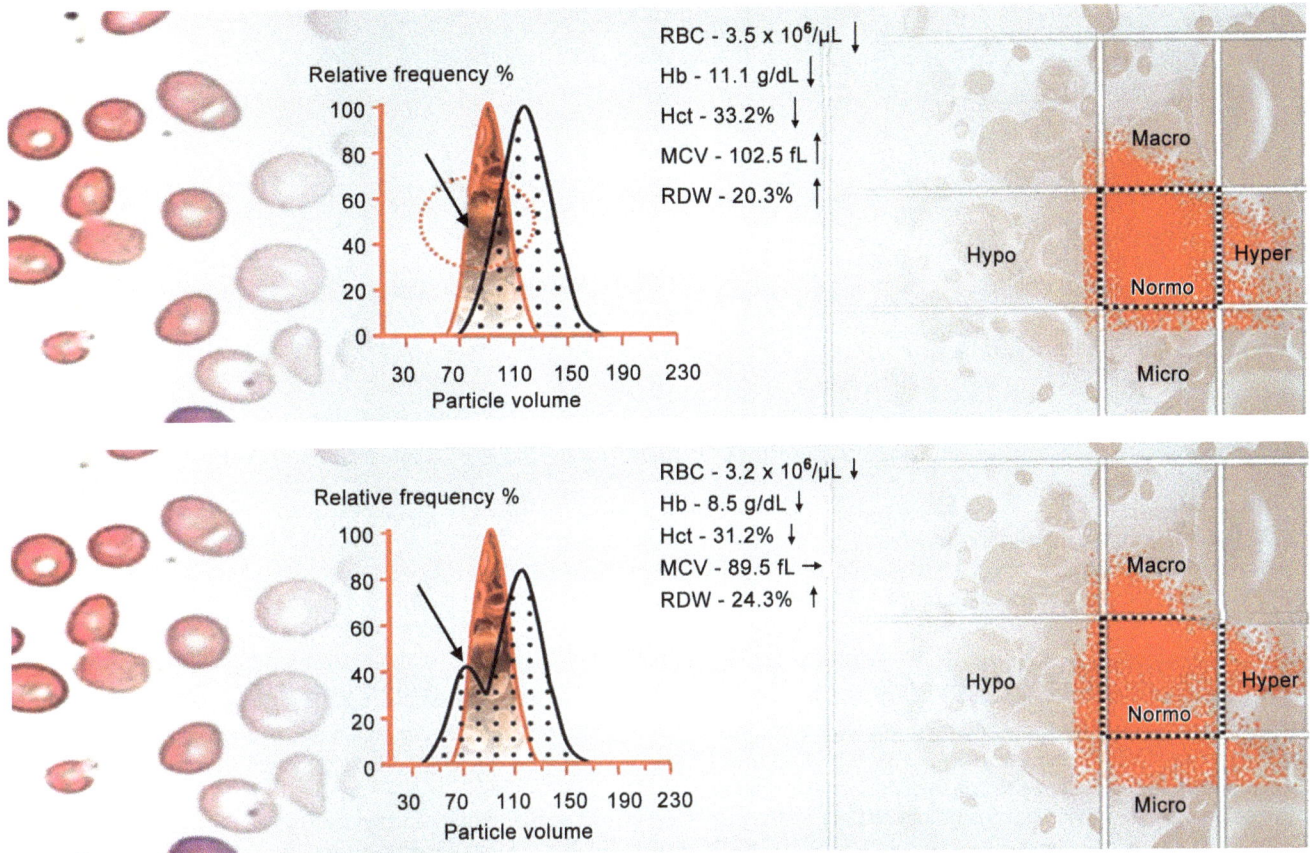

- Double populations of red cells may exist in:
  - Patients on hematinic treatment
  - Following blood transfusion
  - Dual (vitamin B_{12}/folate and iron) deficiency anemia
- Due to their different size and hemoglobin concentration leading to varying scatter properties, these populations can be identified on the RBC cytogram
- Presence of a dual red cell populations may only be visible on the scatter plot and may not always be reflected in the numerical data due to the antagonistic effect of macrocytes and microcytes on the MCV.

Normocytic recovery (circle and arrow)
- A small peak of cells in the normal range.
- RDW is higher than untreated megaloblastic anemia due to two cell population contributing to the heterogeneity.

Microcytic recovery (arrow)
- Two cell populations are seen in this histogram—Old macrocytes and newly produced or surfaced up microcytes.
- Concomitant iron deficiency has been unmasked.
- RDW is markedly increased due to increased heterogeneity.
- MCV is normal only because it reflects the average of two abnormal populations.

Multiple populations of red cells causing significant heterogeneity may exist in patients on vitamin treatment. Due to their different size and hemoglobin concentration leading to varying scatter properties, many populations (Hypo, Normo and Hyper) can be identified on the RBC cytogram. The presence of a such red cell population may only be visible on the scatterplot and may not always be reflected in the numerical data due to the averaging effect of macrocytes and microcytes on the MCV.

RBC Fragmentation in Megaloblastic Anemia

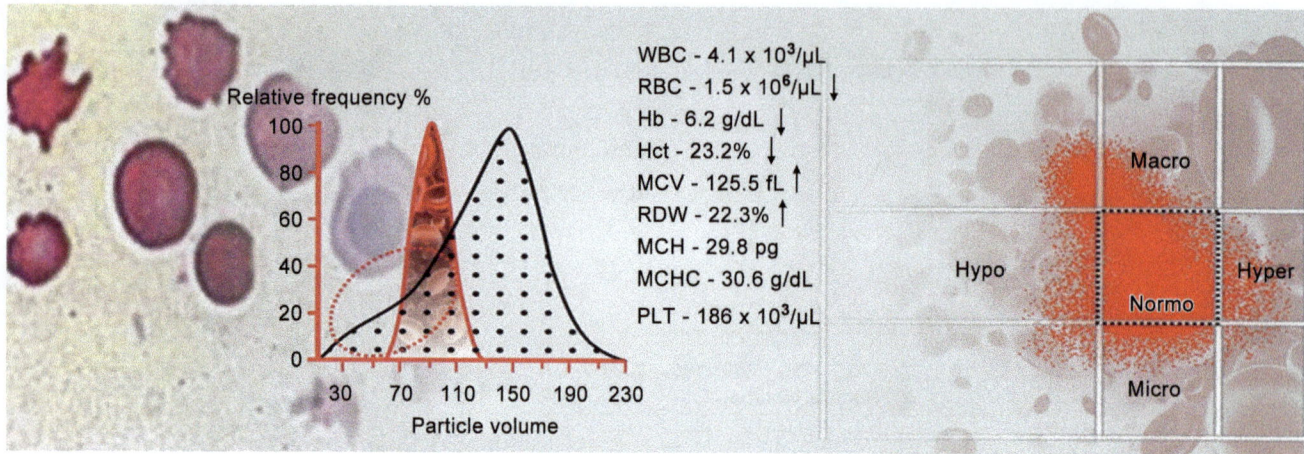

- The fragments form a plateau is of small size.
- Because the fragments are averaged with intact cells, the MCV is less than expected.
- RDW is increased due to heterogeneity of cells (fragmented RBCs).

Megaloblastic Anemia

Erythroid maturation during erythropoiesis involves a progressive condensation of nuclear chromatin (termed nuclear maturation) and finally its extrusion from the cell, followed by the synthesis of hemoglobin in the cytoplasm (termed cytoplasmic maturation), and a concomitant reduction in cell size due to division and water loss.
- Megaloblastic anemia is caused by impaired DNA synthesis, defects in nuclear maturation, and nuclear-cytoplasmic desynchronization due to folate or B12 deficiency, result in ineffective erythropoiesis with large oval erythrocytes (macroovalocytes) with normal hemoglobin content.
- MCV increases much before the onset of anemia or clinical symptoms.
- MCV >95 fL should prompt further study.
- MCV >115 fL is most likely due to megaloblastic anemia.
- MCV may be normal if coexisting iron deficiency, thalassemia trait, inflammatory disease, or chronic renal failure.
- MCH may increase with normal MCHC.
- RDW is often increased due to anisopoikilocytosis.
- Hypersegmented neutrophil (≥5 lobes) is the earliest diagnostic morphologic sign.
- WBC and platelet counts – Low or normal (DD of pancytopenia).
- LDH increases.
- Vitamin B_{12} (<100 pg/mL), folic acid (< 4 ng/mL) levels decrease.
- Bone marrow—hypercellular with megaloblastic erythropoiesis, giant metamyelocytes, and dysplastic megakaryocytes, reduced M:E ratio.

RBC Fragmentation

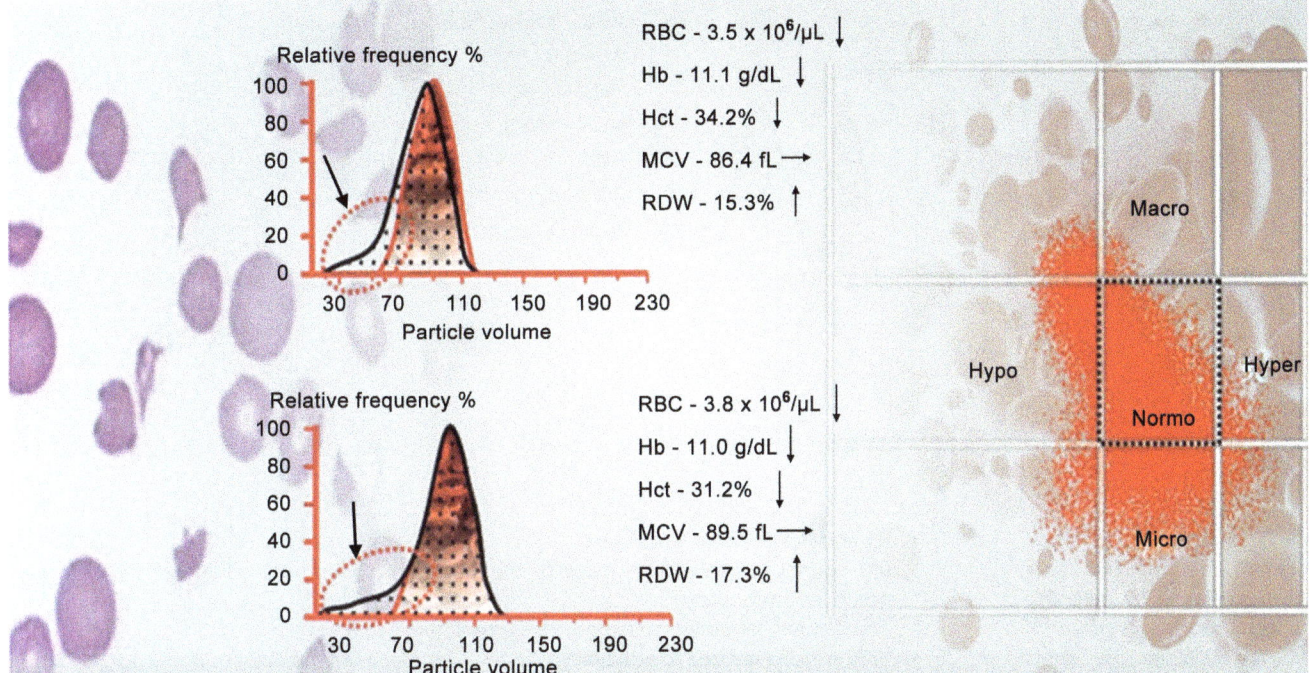

Red Cell Fragmentation may be caused by	
• Malfunctioning of cardiac prosthetic valves • Sickle cell anemia • Thrombotic thrombocytopenic purpura (TTP) • Hemolytic uremic syndrome (HUS)	• DIC • Megaloblastic anemia • Burns • Metastatic tumor • Cytotoxic chemotherapy

- MCV is normal but RDW is increased
- Histogram is pathognomonic of RBC fragmentation
- This is the only direct indicator of fragmentation for the clinician
- Without fragmentation there would be no plateau to the left side of the peak

RBC Fragmentation

- The characteristic features of fragmentation hemolysis are the appearance of the fragments of RBCs, leukoerythroblastic changes, low platelet count, and the presence of intravascular hemolysis.
- Depending on the underlying vascular pathology, there may be a reduction in the platelet count and evidence of DIC.
- Signs of intravascular hemolysis vary from the absence of haptoglobin, ↑LDH, and minimal hemosiderinuria to acute intravascular destruction with hemoglobinemia, and hemoglobinuria.
- With protracted intravascular hemolysis, urinary hemoglobin loss may cause iron deficiency, with hypochromic, microcytic red cells.
- When diseases affecting the small vessels produce fragmented red cells, the term used is microangiopathic hemolytic anemia.
- **RBC cytogram** exhibits Variable population in the hypochromic microcytic zone

Immune Hemolytic Anemia

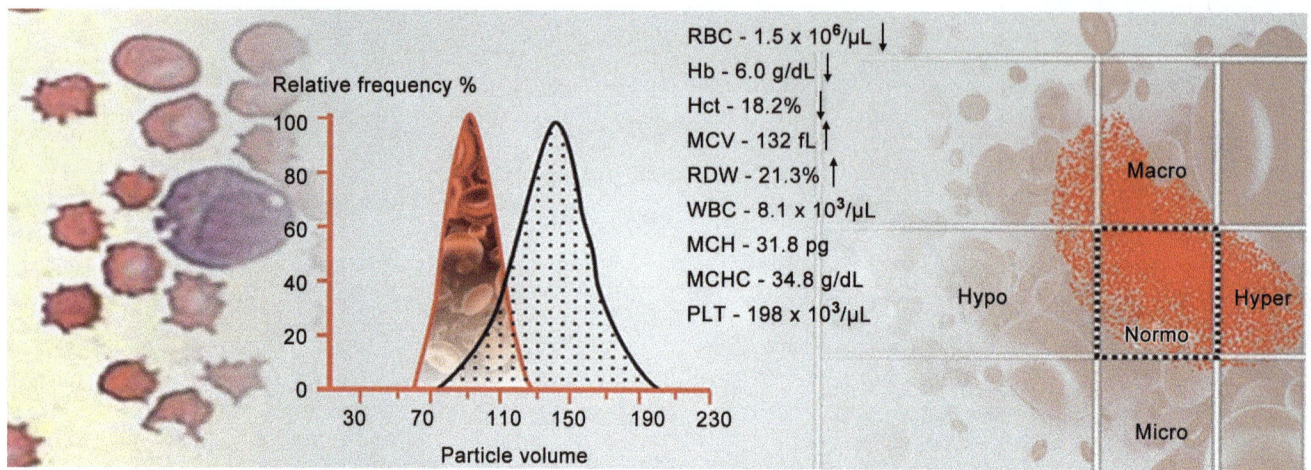

The immune hemolytic anemias are distinguished from the nonimmune by detecting antibody on the surface of the red cells by the direct antiglobulin test (DAT), also known as the Coombs test.	• Hb and Hct levels are decreased. • RBC count decreased, destruction by the mechanism of immune adherence by the patient produced antibodies. • At maximum hemolysis reticulocytosis is profound. • MCV is increased due to reticulocytosis. • RDW also increased to make a macrocytic heterogeneous anemia. • **RBC cytogram** shows the variable population in the hyperchromic and macrocytic zone

Immune Hemolytic Anemia

- Blood smear shows anisocytosis, poikilocytosis, polychromasia and spherocytosis
- MCV reflects immaturity of circulating RBCs
- Reticulocyte count is increased
- Erythroid hyperplasia of bone marrow
- Slight abnormality of osmotic fragility occurs

- Increased indirect serum bilirubin
- Urine urobilinogen is increased
- Hemoglobinemia and hemoglobinuria are present when hemolysis is very rapid
- Haptoglobins are decreased or absent in chronic hemolytic diseases
- WBC count is usually elevated.

Chapter 8: RBC Histogram and Cytogram

Recovery from Immune Hemolytic Anemia

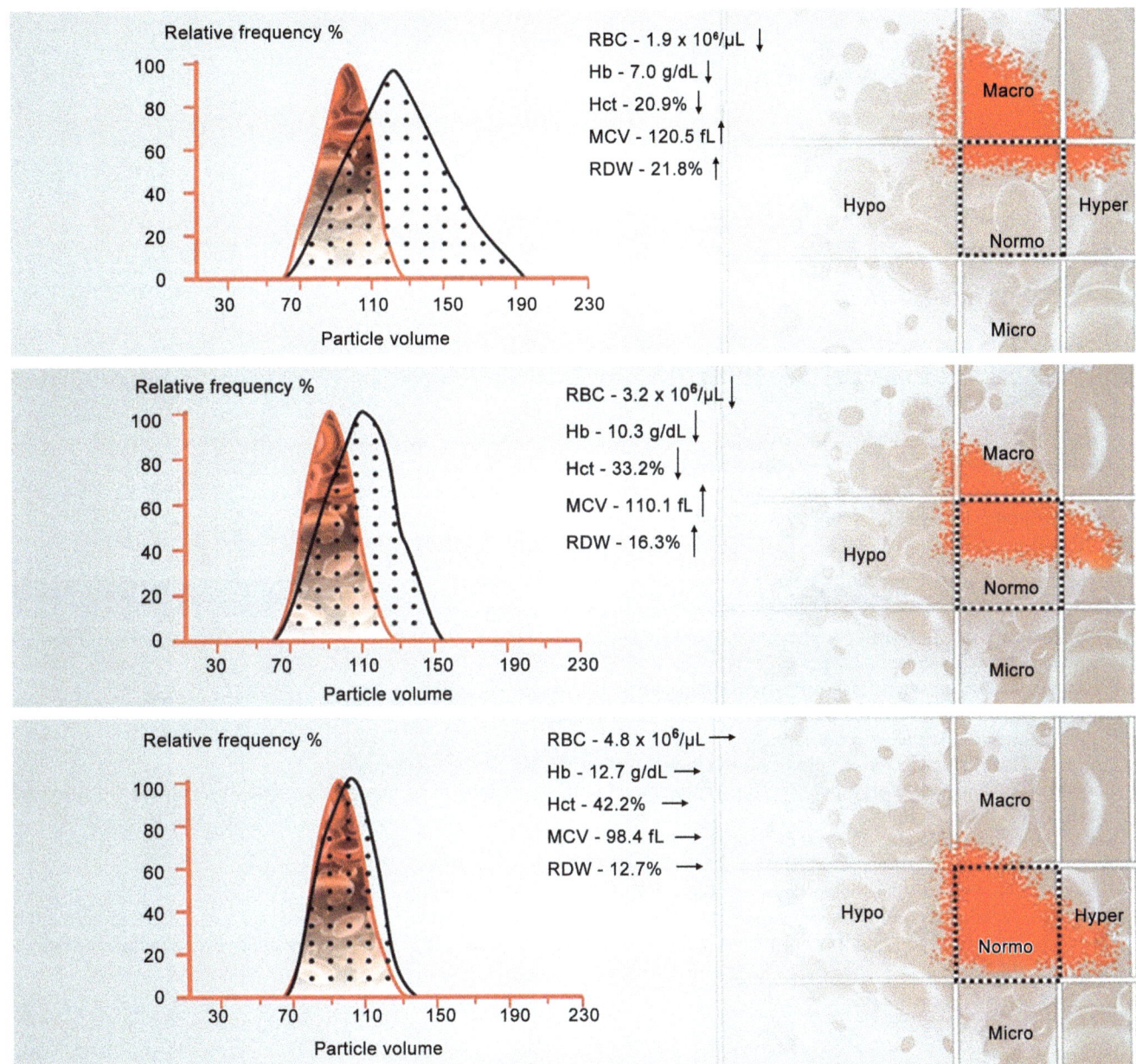

- As the hemoglobin rises the MCV falls.
- In all cases there is only a single peak of cells.
- RDW is directly proportionate to the degree of anemia.
- Red cell heterogeneity parallels anemia.

"Stress" Erythropoiesis is seen exclusively in 'immune hemolytic anemia' resulting in reticulocytosis substantial enough to change MCV and RDW.

Otherwise: Reticulocytes (8% bigger than mature RBC) per se do not change MCV or RDW substantially

Aplastic Anemia Untreated

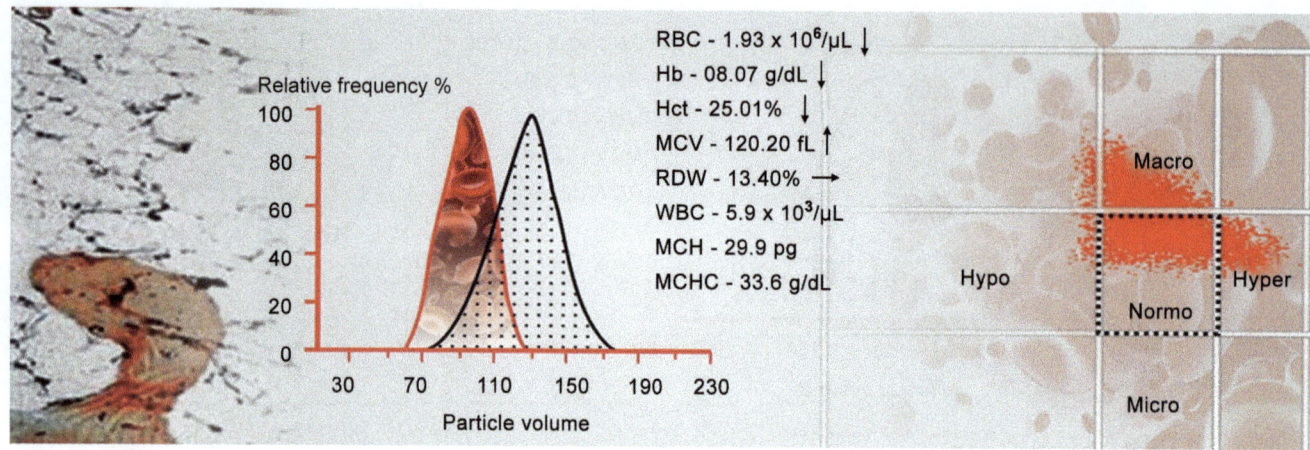

- **The hemoglobin is reduced, MCV increased and RDW is normal.**
- Aplastic anemia is typically macrocytic, homogeneous anemia if there has been no recent transfusion.
- **RBC cytogram** is showing cell condensation in the macrocytic zone also

Aplastic Anemia

Aplastic anemia is characterized by peripheral blood pancytopenia with variable bone marrow hypocellularity in the absence of underlying myeloproliferative or malignant disease.
- Neutropenia (absolute neutrophil count <1,500/μL), often monocytopenia is present.
- Lymphocyte count is normal; reduced helper/inducer: cytotoxic/suppressor ratio.
- Platelet count <150,000/μL; severity varies.
- Anemia is usually normochromic, normocytic but maybe slightly macrocytic; RDW is normal.
- Bone marrow is hypocellular; aspiration and biopsy should both be performed to rule out leukemia, myelodysplastic syndrome, granulomas disease, or tumor.
- Reticulocyte count corrected for Hct is decreased.
- Serum iron is increased.
- Flow cytometry phenotyping shows the virtual absence of CD34 stem cells in blood and marrow.
- Laboratory findings represent the whole spectrum, from the most severe condition of the classic type with marked leukopenia, thrombocytopenia, anemia, and acellular bone marrow, to the cases with pure RBC aplasia or agranulocytosis or amegakaryocytic thrombocytopenia.

Aplastic Transfused

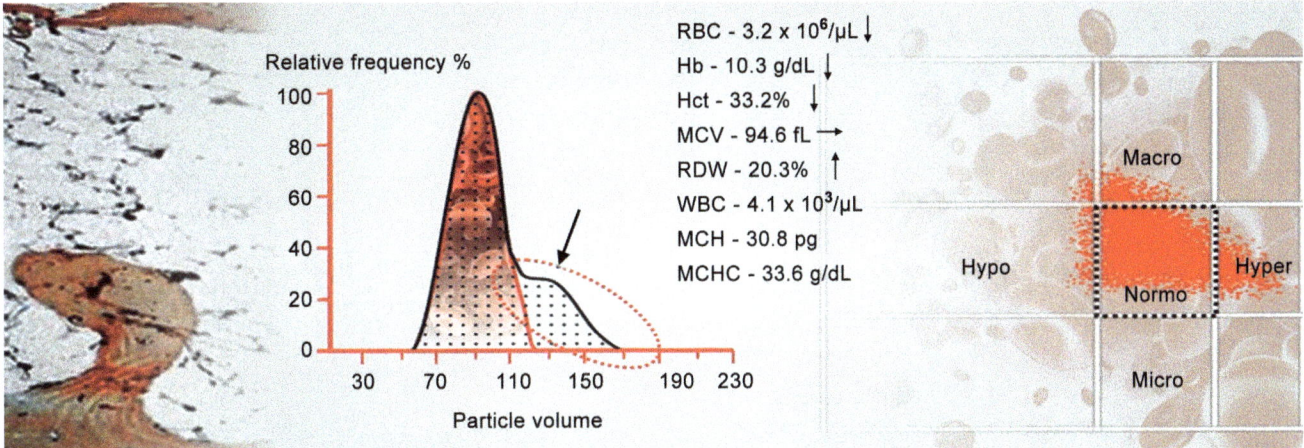

RDW is a very useful parameter to differentiate between megaloblastic anemia and aplastic anemia when MCV >97 fL. Also, iron deficiency anemia and thalassemia minor when MCV < 80 fL. As it is high in megaloblastic and iron deficiency.	• MCV is now normal in contrast to non-transfused. • Two populations of RBCs are seen on histogram-transfused normocytes and patient's macrocytes. • This fact can only be appreciated better on PS after seeing the histogram.

- International aplastic anemia study group criteria for aplastic anemia ≥ 2 peripheral blood criteria plus one of the marrow criterias
  - Peripheral blood criteria:
    - Neutrophils < 500/µL; < 200/µL in very severe aplastic anemia
    - Platelets < 20,000/µL
    - Reticulocyte count ≤ 40 × 10^3/µL or ≤ 60 × 10^3
  - Marrow criteria
    - Severe hypocellularity
    - Moderate hypocellularity with < 30% of residual cells being hematopoietic

Heterozygous Thalassemia

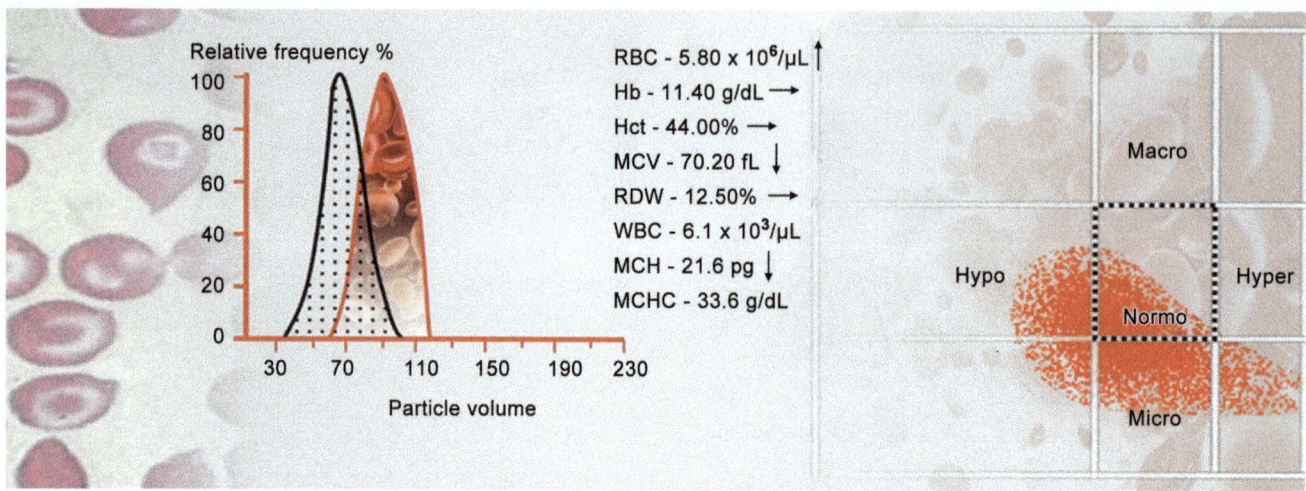

Heterozygous -Thalassemia (Two Locus Deletion)

- Although the peripheral blood may show a slight variation of the size of RBC but it is more reflected as target cells rather than the true anisocytosis or hypochromia.
- Low MCV with normal RDW (microcytosis with normal heterogeneity).
- Coexisting nutritional deficiency with thalassemia carrier may change the values of RDW beyond expected.
- This simple test thus eliminates the need for expensive and time-consuming tests like Hb-electrophoresis and A2 estimation or iron studies to differentiate other causes of microcytosis to a greater extent.
- Thalassemia trait tend to be more microcytic than hypochromic.
- The ratio of microcytic % cells to hypochromic % cells **(MH ratio)** is usually **greater than 1**.
- Red cell distribution width (RDW) and hemoglobin distribution width (HDW) tend to be normal in cases of thalassemia trait whereas both parameters are typically raised in iron deficiency.
- The RBC cytogram show red cell spread with close clustering of the cell plot owing to the uniform microcytosis.
- A characteristic **"comma-shaped cytogram"** is seen in the thalassemia trait.

Heterozygous Thalassemia

- The thalassemia's are imbalance between productions of the α or β globin chains. The imbalance is caused by deletion or abnormality of one or more of the four α or two β alleles.
- Phenotypically, every single α-locus deletion on average reduces MCV approximately 9 fL whereas every single β-locus deletion on an average reduces MCV approximately 18 fL.
- Single β-locus deletion will bring MCV below normal.
- Whereas in more than half of subjects the 9 fL reduction of a single α-locus deletion may not bring MCV below 80 fL, the bottom of the normal range.

So, these α thalassemia subjects are truly silent carriers whereas β thalassemias patients are expressed.

Sickle Cell Anemia

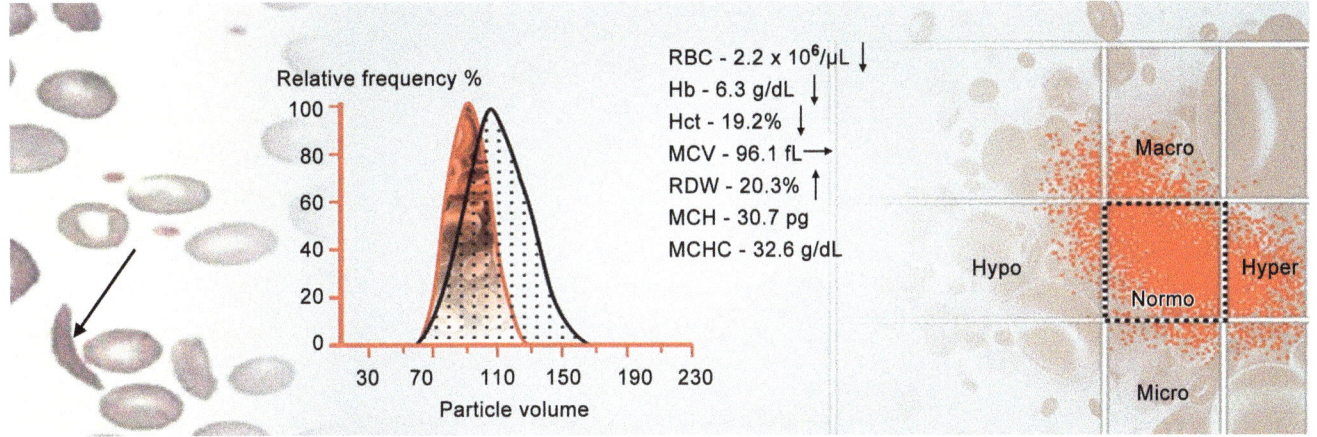

- The RBC count is markedly reduced.
- MCV is high normal.
- RDW is high, due to heterogeneity of RBCs.
- **RBC cytogram** is spreading minimally into hypo, hyper and macrocytic zone.

Sickle Cell Anemia

- Blood smear may show a variable number of RBCs with target cells (especially in HbS/HbC disease), nucleated RBCs, Howell-Jolly bodies, polychromasia.
- Sickle cells in smear are present if RBCs contain >60% HbS.
- Post-autosplenectomy, basophilic stippling, and nucleated RBCs may be seen.
- Reticulocyte count is increased may cause a slight increase in MCV.
- WBC count may rise during sickling crises, with normal differential or shift to the left.
- Infection may be indicated by intracellular bacteria (best seen on buffy coat preparations), Döhle bodies, toxic granules, and vacuoles of WBCs.
- Platelet count may increase (3–5 lac/μL), with abnormal forms.
- Bone marrow shows hyperplasia of all elements, causing bone changes on radiographs.
- Osmotic fragility is decreased (more resistant RBCs).
- Mechanical fragility of RBCs is increased.
- RBC survival time is decreased (17 days in HbSS, 28 days in HbS/HbC).
- Laboratory findings of hemolysis, e.g., increased indirect serum bilirubin (≤6 mg/dL), increased urobilinogen in urine and stool, but urine is negative for bile.

Red cells acquire the sickle or elongated shape upon deoxygenation as a result of intracellular polymerization of HbS that is reversible upon reoxygenation.

Hemoglobin SC Disease

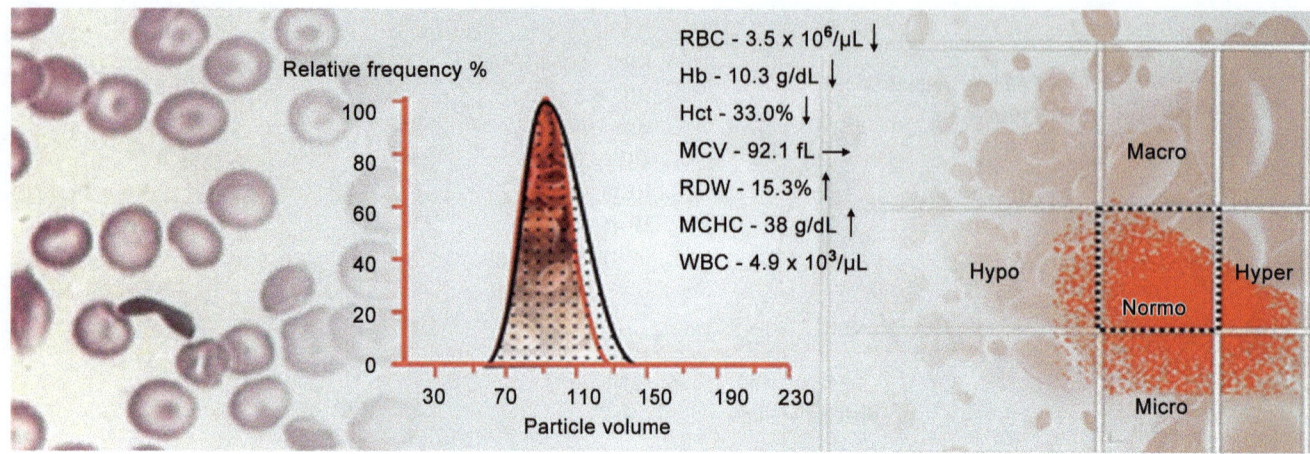

Hemoglobin SC Disease

Hb electrophoresis shows:
- HbA is absent
- HbS and HbC are present in approximately equal amounts (30 to 60%)
- HbF is ≤ 5%

Blood smear: PS shows a wide variation of shape and size, peculiar to hemoglobin SC disease

Tetragonal crystals within RBC
- Plump and angulated rather than typical sickle cells in which Hb is concentrated more in one area of the cell than another; target cell are present
- Sickling test is positive

- This is a severe sickling disease intermediate between sickle cell disease and sickle cell trait.
- The RBC is moderately reduced.
- MCV is normal.
- MCHC is high.
- Histogram shows mild widening.
- RDW is moderately increased, consistent with the moderate degree of anemia.
- **RBC cytogram** is extending to hyperchromic zone.

Sideroblastic Anemia

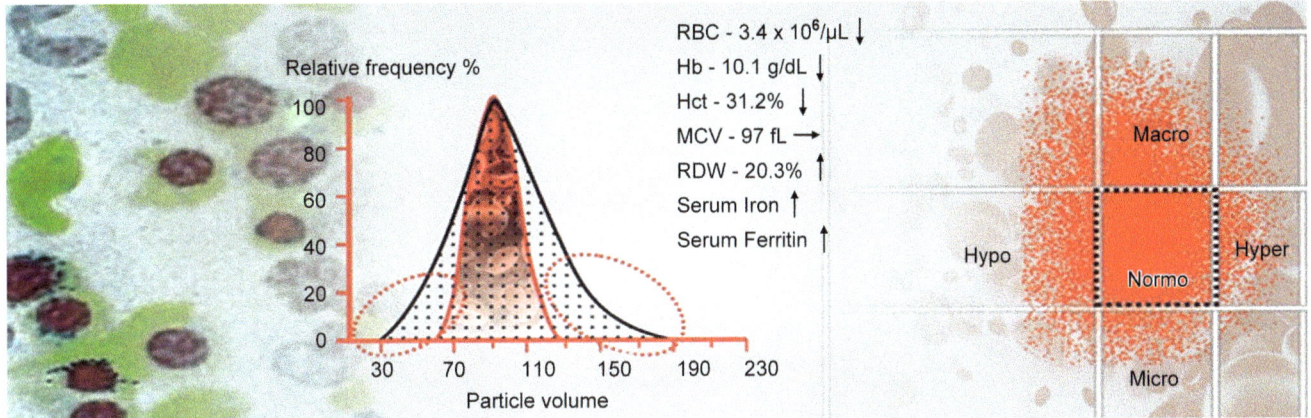

Sideroblastic Anemia

- Two types:
  - Inherited: Either sex-linked or autosomal
  - Acquired: Idiopathic MDS-RARS variant (refractory anemia with ring sideroblast)
- Ringed sideroblasts (abnormal erythroblasts with excessive mitochondrial iron deposition) in the bone marrow.
- The cardinal feature of sideroblastic anemia is mitochondrial iron deposition. In sideroblastic anemia, the iron-containing particles are larger and more numerous than normal.
- Sideroblastic bone marrows often show erythroid hyperplasia, consistent with the ineffective erythropoiesis characteristic of this condition.
- Ineffective erythropoiesis increases gastrointestinal iron absorption. Therefore, patients with even mild sideroblastic anemia can develop substantial iron overload.

- Classically the RBCs in idiopathic sideroblastic **anemia is that of a "Dimorphic population" both macrocytes and microcytes**.
- MCV is +/− normal because of averaging of micro and macro sizes of RBCs.
- Histogram is always markedly widened.
- High RDW with generally a single peak.
- Basophilic stippling and Pappenheimer bodies may be seen.
- Biochemical iron studies show elevated levels.

The presence of microcytic and macrocytic cells in the same sample may result in a normal MCV and may mislead if only observed numerically, but the characteristic RBC cytogram spreading from micro to macro zone is informative.

Dimorphic Anemia

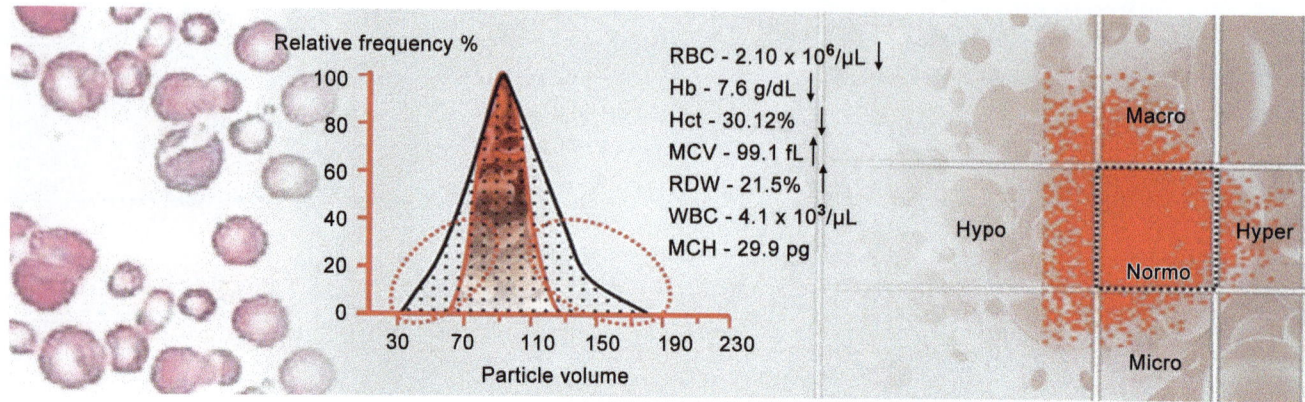

Dimorphism is the presence of two distinct erythrocyte populations of differing sizes.

Causes include:
- Transfusion of normal cells into patients with microcytic or macrocytic anemias.
- Combined iron deficiency and B_{12} or folate deficiency.
- Myelodysplastic syndromes.
- Sideroblastic anemias.
- Treatment of iron deficiency anemia, in which older microcytic cells coexist with younger normocytic cells.

The MCV, since it is an average value can be normal in the presence of two different cell populations, e.g., dimorphic anemias, red cell fragmentation with reticulocyte response. It is, therefore, important to examine the peripheral smear.

In dual deficiency anemia, the **red cell cytogram** is wide and shows 2 distinct red cell populations in the macrocytic and microcytic zones

Low RBC count
High RDW (heterogeneity)
MCV generally is normal
- The diagnosis is missed usually because of consideration of numerically normal MCV which is due to averaging of macro and micro RBCs.

Red Cell Agglutinins (Cold)

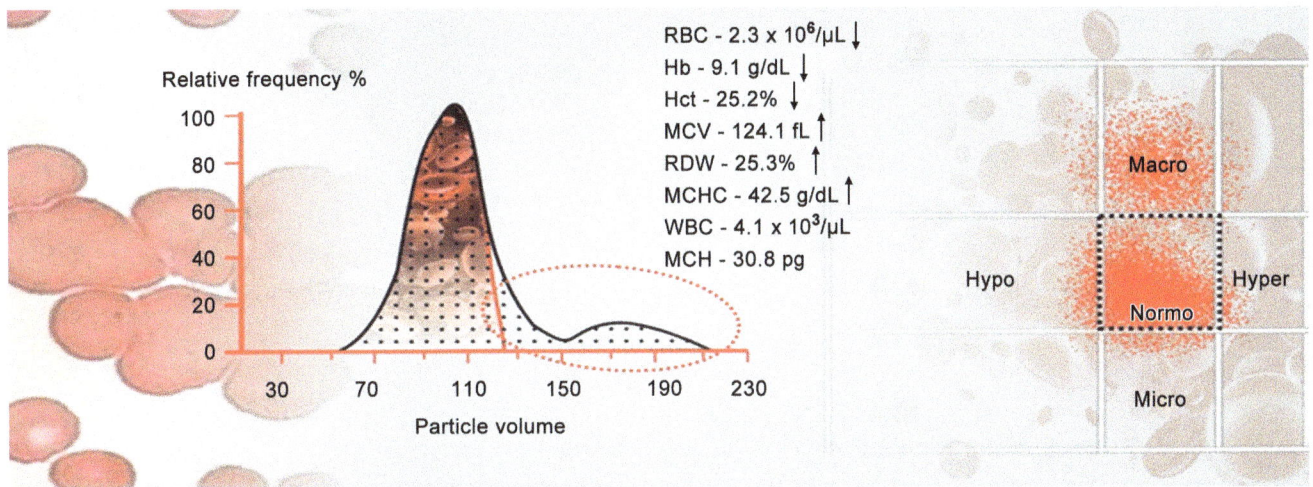

Red Cell Agglutinins
• Hemolysis is usually present and the patient may be mildly icteric.
• The cold agglutinins are monoclonal IgG.
• Automated cell counters detect the agglutinates and record erroneously high MCV and low RBC values.
• In red cell agglutination, doublet erythrocytes are counted as one, and larger clumps are not counted as red blood cells at all. This leads to a "decrease" in red cell count and a falsely elevated MCV. Determination of the hemoglobin value is not affected.
• Prewarming the sample eliminates these spurious values.
• Important fact is—in a warm climate—cold agglutinins are a more common cause for high MCHC than in hereditary spherocytosis.
• Sometimes a set of spurious values may be the first clue to an otherwise unsuspected clinical condition, (e.g., the combination of low hematocrit, normal hemoglobin, and high MCV and MCHC is characteristic of cold agglutinins).
• In the dilute blood suspension used by automated counters agglutination will be as red cell doublets, rather than the large clumps seen on the peripheral smear.
• Fall in the RBC count is caused by clumping therefore is not quite matched by a rise in MCV.
• As a result, the product of, RBC × MCV, i.e., Hct, is artifactually reduced.
• Hb is not affected by agglutination.
• The ratio of Hb/Hct, i.e., MCHC raises.
• The best clue is that the mode of RBC histogram does not match MCV.

- RBC agglutinins show a bizarre spread of the red cell population on the **cytogram**.
- The doublets and triplets of agglutinated RBCs (with volumes over 200 fL or beyond) are plotted in the macrocytic zone on the cytogram.
- Cytogram, histogram, and red cell parameters return to normal after incubating blood sample at 37°C.
- ***Histogram and cytogram is diagnostic in this condition and can help a physician in proper diagnosis and treatment.***

Chronic Lymphocytic Leukemia

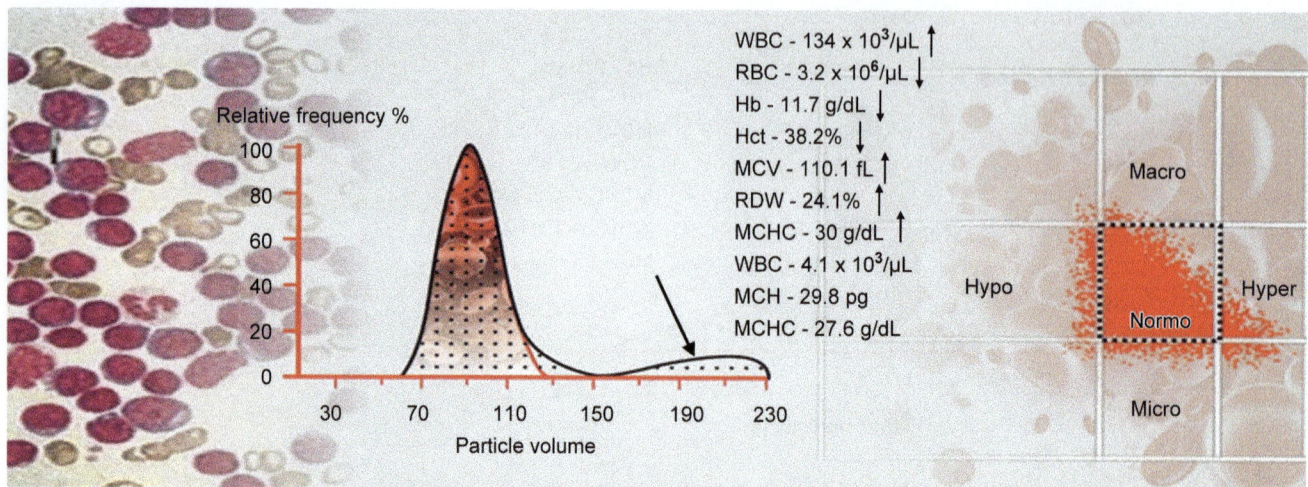

Chronic Lymphocytic Leukemia

- When whole blood is analyzed, RBCs are not defined by criteria of traditional morphology and hemoglobin pigment but by nominal volume.
- If other cells also fall within the criteria defining red cell volume, such cells are counted as red cells.
- Small lymphocytes with 150–180 fL volume may be counted as red cells.
- This mixing is significant when such lymphocytes are high in number like in CLL.
- In such case:
  - Additional peaks on the right side of the RBC histogram may be seen along with spurious low MCHC, high MCV, and high RDW.
  - True RBC macrocytes never exceed 145 fL so any plateau or peak beyond this is due to such lymphocytes.
  - A similar peak is seen in red cell agglutinins, but the high MCHC differentiates it from CLL.

- In CLL, the lymphocytes usually appear normal, but they may be large or have deeply cleft nuclei (Rieder cells).
- They sometimes contain coarse, clumped chromatin, and the cytoplasm may be vacuolated.
- With the preparation of the blood film, lymphocytes commonly disintegrate.
- Smudge cells, the cytoplasm is lost and the nucleus spreads out.
- When autoimmune hemolytic anemia complicates CLL, polychromatophilia, and spherocytosis appear on the smear.

The diagnosis of CLL requires evidence of lymphocytosis, at least 10×10^9/L and lymphocytic infiltration in the bone marrow of at least 40%.

Hemoglobin - H Disease

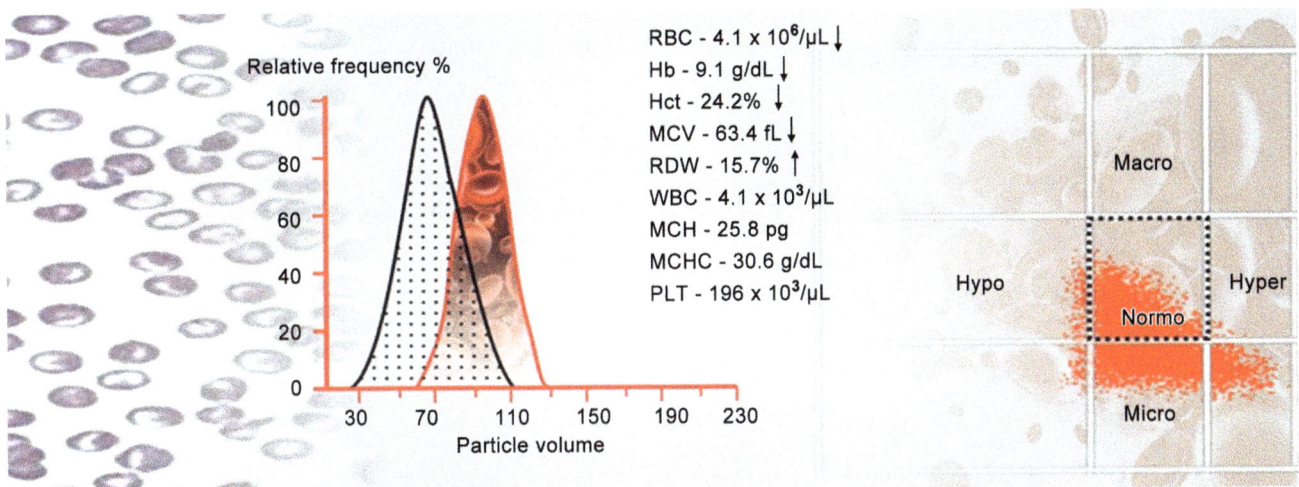

RBC - 4.1 x 10⁶/µL ↓
Hb - 9.1 g/dL ↓
Hct - 24.2% ↓
MCV - 63.4 fL ↓
RDW - 15.7% ↑
WBC - 4.1 x 10³/µL
MCH - 25.8 pg
MCHC - 30.6 g/dL
PLT - 196 x 10³/µL

Peripheral smear includes polychromatophilia, spherocytosis, and sometimes erythrocyte agglutination. Hemoglobin analysis reveals 5–40% HbH, together with HbA, and a normal or reduced level of HbA_2

- HbH disease occurs when three of four α-globin alleles are absent and an excess of β-globins exists.
- Hemoglobinopathy associated with anemia.
- Marked microcytosis.
- Decreased MCV.
- Increased RDW.
- This condition is characterized by a variable degree of anemia and splenomegaly but it is unusual to find severe thalassemic bone changes or growth retardation.
- Patients usually survive into adult life, and the course may be interspersed with severe episodes of hemolysis associated with infection or worsening of the anemia due to progressive hypersplenism.
- Hemoglobin values range from 7–10 g/dL and the blood film show typical thalassemic changes.
- Oxidant drugs may increase the rate of precipitation of HbH and exacerbate the anemia.

Myelofibrosis

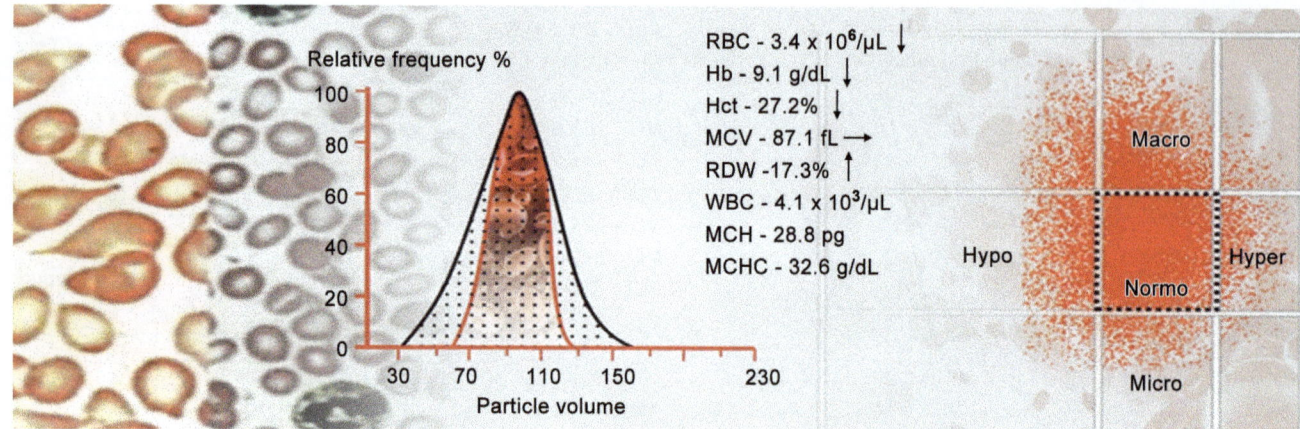

- The peripheral blood smear discloses leukoerythroblastosis (the presence of nucleated red cells and immature myeloid cells) and teardrop erythrocytes in almost all patients.
- Other red cell abnormalities include fragments, numerous polychromatophilic cells, ovalocytes, elliptocyes, and basophilic stippling.
- Increased basophils and eosinophils are common.
- Large platelets and intact or fragmented megakaryocytes are characteristic.

Usually, spleen becomes the site of hematopoiesis with immature granulocytes, nucleated RBC, and increased reticulocytes in the peripheral blood. On examination, splenomegaly is universal and may be massive.
- Low RBC count
- High RDW (heterogeneity)
- MCV generally is normal

In myelodysplasia, due to the diversity of the syndromes MCV, RDW, and Hb range from normal to abnormal—alerting the clinician to the abnormality!

RBC cytogram *is exhibiting wider spread all around the central square due to heterogeneity of cells*

Osmotic Change due to Hyperglycemia

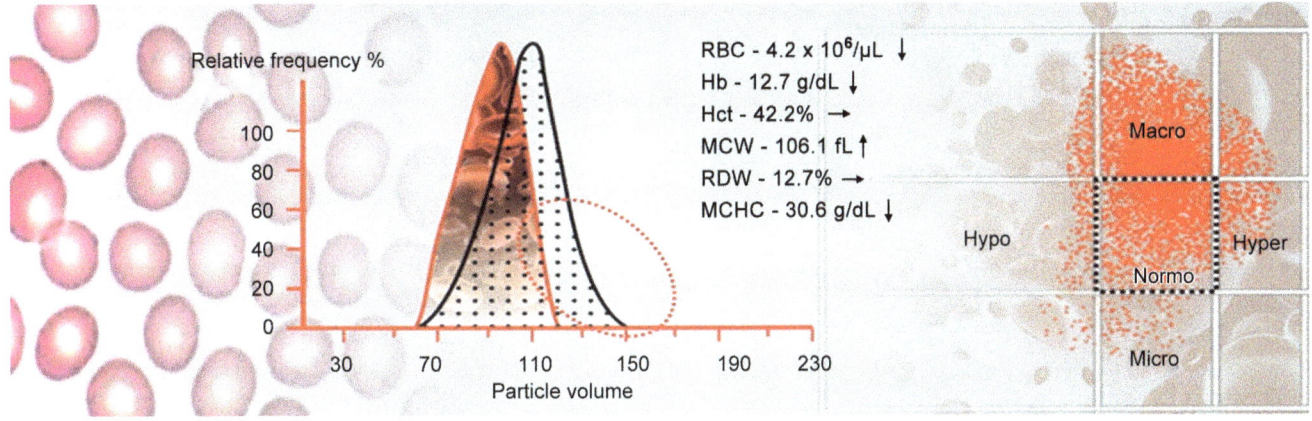

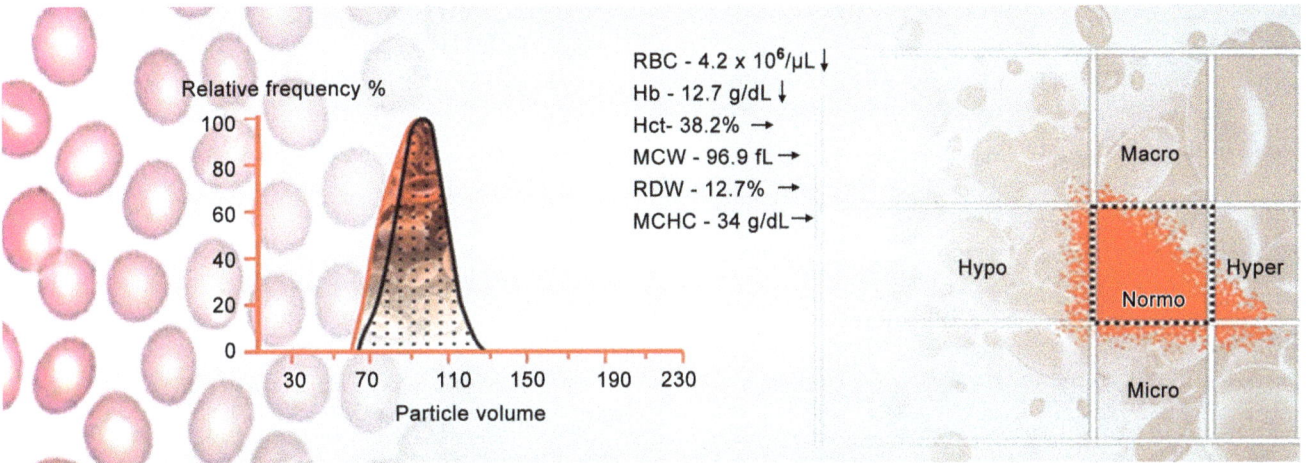

In hyperglycemia, red cells are transiently hypertonic as compared to the isotonic diluting fluid, resulting in swollen cells and an elevated MCV. This can be avoided if some time is allowed for the equilibration after dilution.	• This artifact may cause serious overstatement of the red cell size (MCV). • RBC count and Hb are accurate. Therefore, Hct is spuriously high. • MCH is correct and MCHC is spuriously low in proportion to the amount of spurious macrocytosis because all red cells affected equally. • RDW does not change during hyperglycemia-induced macrocytosis. • Water from diluents flows into the red cells far more rapidly than glucose can flow out, so the red cells initial osmotic equilibration is achieved by net red cell swelling.

Key Diagnostic Features of Various Common Hematological Conditions						
Condition	*Hb*	*MCV*	*MCH*	*MCHC*	*RDW*	*RBC Plots on Cystogram*
Normal	Normal	Normal	Normal	Normal	Normal	In normocytic normochromic zone
Iron deficiency anemia	Low	Low	*Low*	Normal or low	High	Microcytic hypochromic zone (triangular spread)
Beta thalassemia trait (minor)	Normal or low	Low	Low	Normal or low	Normal or near normal	Narrow clustering in the microcytic hypochromic zone (comma-shaped)
Beta thalassemia (major)	Very low	Low	Low	Low	Very high	Widespread in the microcytic hypochromic zone (simulates an exaggerated version of the cystogram seen in iron deficiency)
Nonmegaloblastic macrocytosis	Normal or low	High	Normal	Normal	Normal	Closely clustered in macrocytic zone
Megaloblastic anemia	Low	High	Normal	Normal	High	Widespread in the macrocytic zone
Dual deficiency anemia	Low	Low variable (depends on the type of anemia)	Variable (depends on the type of anemia)	Variable	High	Wide cystogram extending in both macrocytic and microcytic zones
Blood transfusion	Normal or low	Variable (depends on the type of anemia)	Variable (depends on the type of anemia)	Variable	High	Double plot of patient's and transfused cells
Cold agglutinins	Normal or low	Bizarre	Bizarre	Bizarre	Bizarre	Most RBC plots in the high macrocytic zone; cytogram and red cell parameters return to normal after incubating blood sample at 37°C
Spherocytosis	Low	Normal	Normal	Usually high	Normal	Variable population in the hyperchromic zone

WBC and Platelet Histogram and Scatterogram

CHAPTER 9

Interpretation of histograms and scatter plots, in conjunction with the numerical data are clinically useful tools in the diagnosis and follow-up of many hematological conditions and unfortunately graphical representations have been largely ignored in favour of newer parameters, which have been available over the years.

THE VOLUME HISTOGRAM FOR WBCs

The WBC histogram is generated with a size of cells in femtoliters on the X-axis and the relative frequency of the cells on the Y-axis. The automated counter sets a lower discriminator (LD) fluctuating between 30 fL and 60 fL and an upper discriminator (UD) fixed at 300 fL. The number of cells between the UD and the LD is the WBC count. WBC histograms consist of two troughs, T1 between 78 fL and 114 fL and T2 < 150 fL.

There are three groups:
1. The peak between the LD and T1 represents small cells, i.e., lymphocytes. The volume of the cells ranges from 35 to 90 fL.
2. The peak that lies between T1 and T2 represents the mid-cell count which includes the eosinophils, basophils, monocytes, blasts, and promyelocytes. The volume of the cell ranges from 90 to 160 fL.
3. The peak after T2 represents neutrophils. Volume ranging between 160 fL and 300 fL.

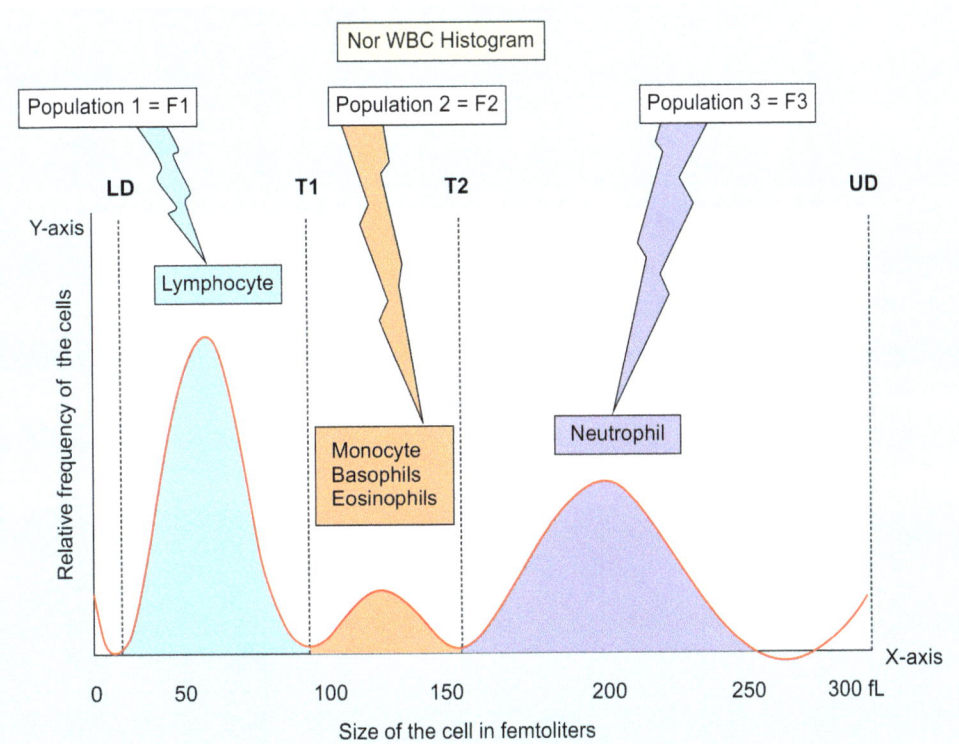

The histogram curve should start within the lower and upper discriminator at the baseline

FLAGGING AND ABNORMAL WBC HISTOGRAM

- Whenever there is any parameter that is abnormal and does not fit into the normal expected graph described above, the analysis system will flag those areas.
- Abnormal curves are flagged with WL, WU, T1, T2, F1, F2, and F3, etc. with some variations depending on the make of the instrument. These situations demand a visual review of the patient's blood smear for confirmation.

1. **Abnormal Curve in Front of the Lower Discriminator**

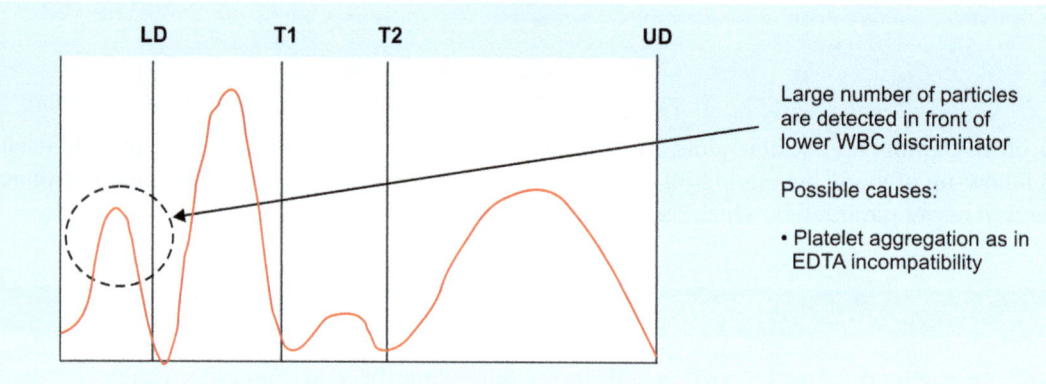

2. **Abnormal Curve at the Lower Discriminator–Wl Flag**

This appears when height of LD is greater than the preset 20% of y-axis. As a result, the WBC count, W-SCR (small cell region), W-MCR (mid cell region) and W-LCR (large cell region) will show a Wl flag.

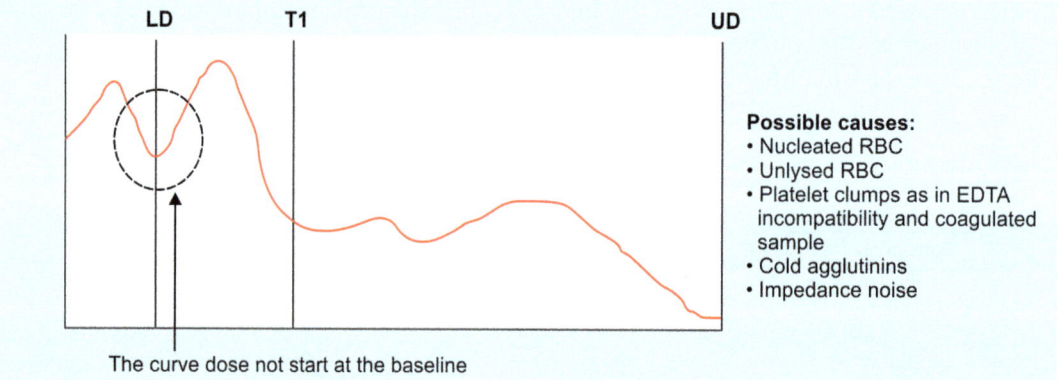

3. **Abnormal Curve at the Upper Discriminator–WU Flag**

This appears when the height of UD is greater than the preset 10% on the y-axis. As a result, the WBC count will show a WU flag. It occurs when there is insufficient WBC lysing.

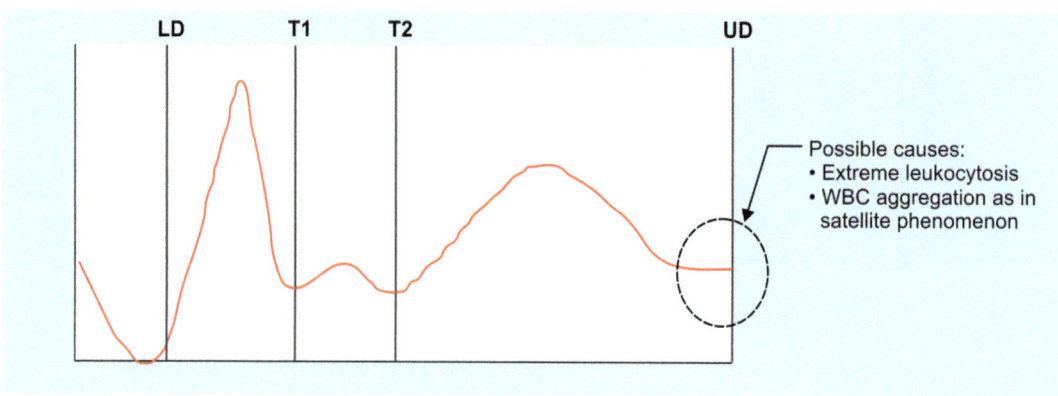

4. Abnormal Curve at T1 Level—T1 Flag

T1 and T2 are valley discriminators defined by the plateau. This discriminator separate leukocyte population into three population. The T1 and T2 discriminators are flexible and will be set automatically according to the sample. In extreme pathological conditions discrimination between 3 populations is not possible. Flag T1 occurs when discrimination between lymphocytes and mid cell population is not done as in abnormal leukocytosis like chronic myeloid leukemia.

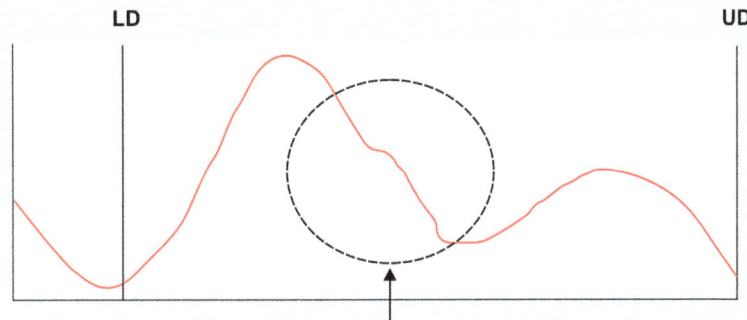

T1 not found here autodiscriminator unable to find first valley

5. Abnormal Curve and Flagging—F1, F2 and F3 Flag

F1 flag appears when the relative height of T1 exceeds the pre-set limit of 40%. F1 flag means that the small cell and middle cell data may be inaccurate. It may occur in acute lymphoblastic leukemia.

F2 flag appears when the relative heights exceed the preset of T1 (40%) or T2 (50%). F2 flag means that the middle cell data is inaccurate. This often occurs in eosinophilia, acute myeloid leukemia, monocytosis, etc.

F3 flag appears when the T2 exceeds the preset limit of 50%. F3 Flag means that the large cell data is inaccurate.

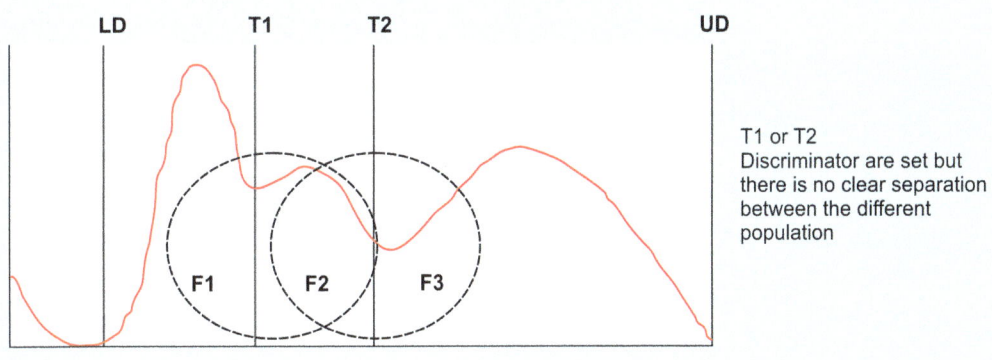

T1 or T2 Discriminator are set but there is no clear separation between the different population

6. Abnormal Curve at T2—T2 Flag

Flag T2 appear when discrimination between mixed cell and neutrophil could not be done, as in chronic lymphocytic leukemia.

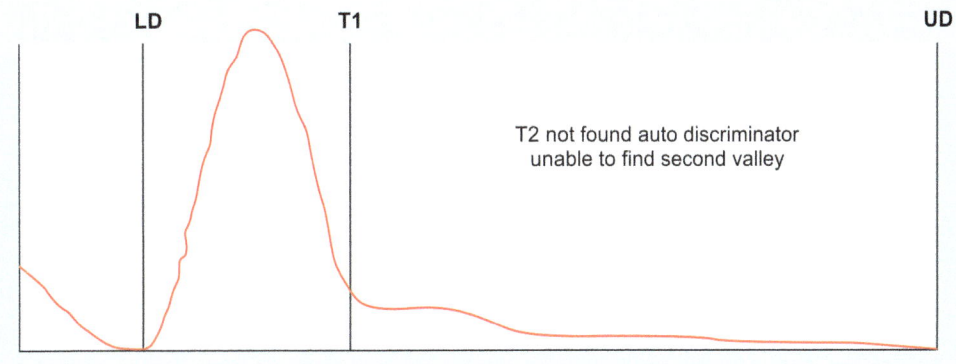

T2 not found auto discriminator unable to find second valley

Some of the examples of flagging and the relevant clues are:

- If there is a leukocytosis due to increased neutrophils, then the peak may occur in the extreme right region of the histogram.
- Cells that fall between the lymphocyte and mononuclear cell region, if flagged the alert signal are due to: increased basophils, increased eosinophils, larger than normal lymphocytes, plasma cells, or certain blast cells.
- If the peak is between the mononuclear and granulocyte region, then the cause could be increased immature granulocytes, certain blast cells, or eosinophils.
- If nucleated red blood cells, giant platelets, or non-lysed erythrocytes make up the particle population being counted, there may be an interference peak formed between 30 and 35 fL or at 35 fL.
- In acute leukemia there may be a peak between T1 and T2 since blasts are larger than small lymphocytes and smaller than neutrophils.
- In chronic lymphocytic leukemia the peak is between LD and T1 since the size of the cell is of lymphocytes.
- In neutrophilia the peak is between T2 and UD.

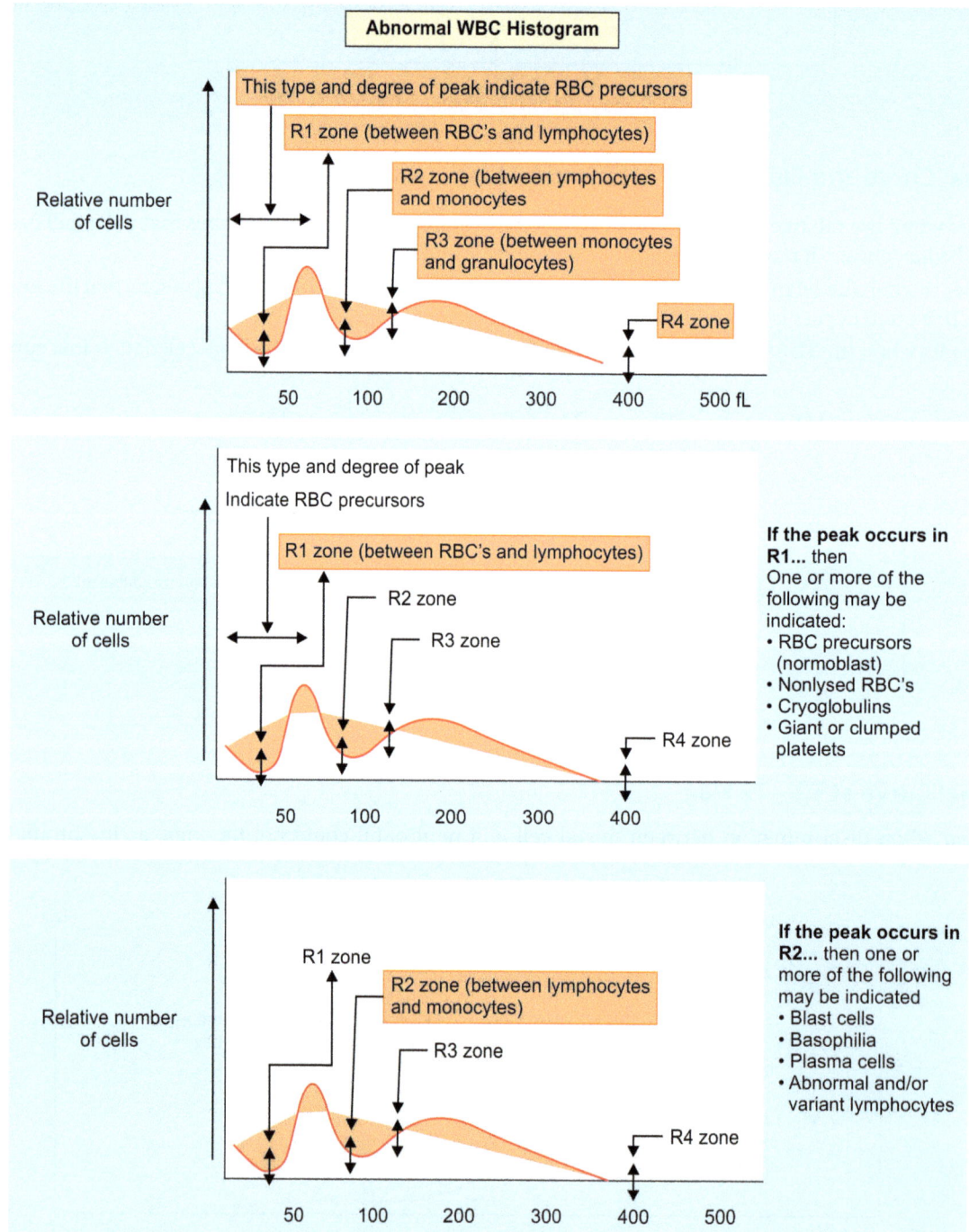

Chapter 9: WBC and Platelet Histogram and Scatterogram

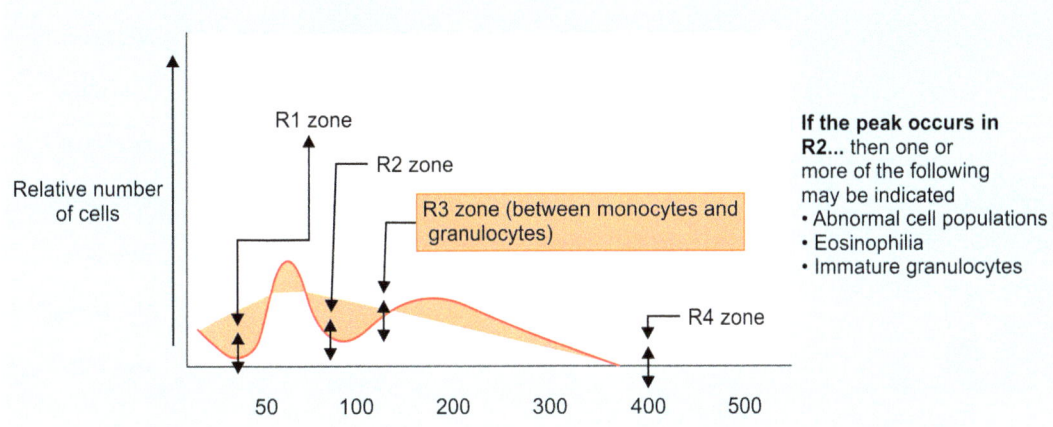

If the peak occurs in R2... then one or more of the following may be indicated
- Abnormal cell populations
- Eosinophilia
- Immature granulocytes

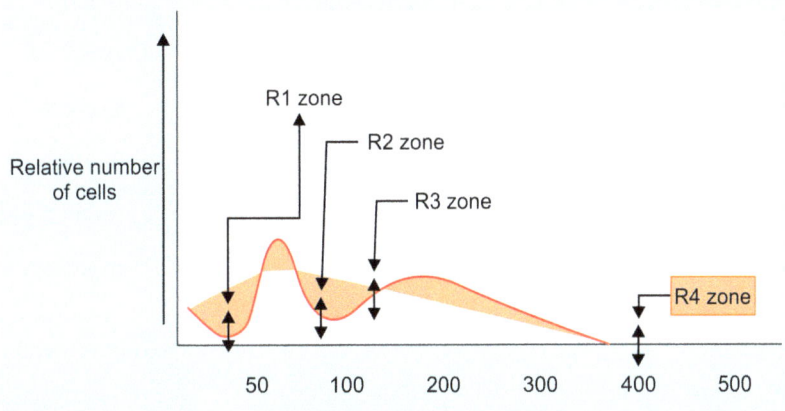

If the peak occurs in R4... then there is most likely an absolute granulocytosis (shift-to-the-right)
- Any abnormal peak display will require a manual

VARIOUS TYPES OF WBC HISTOGRAMS

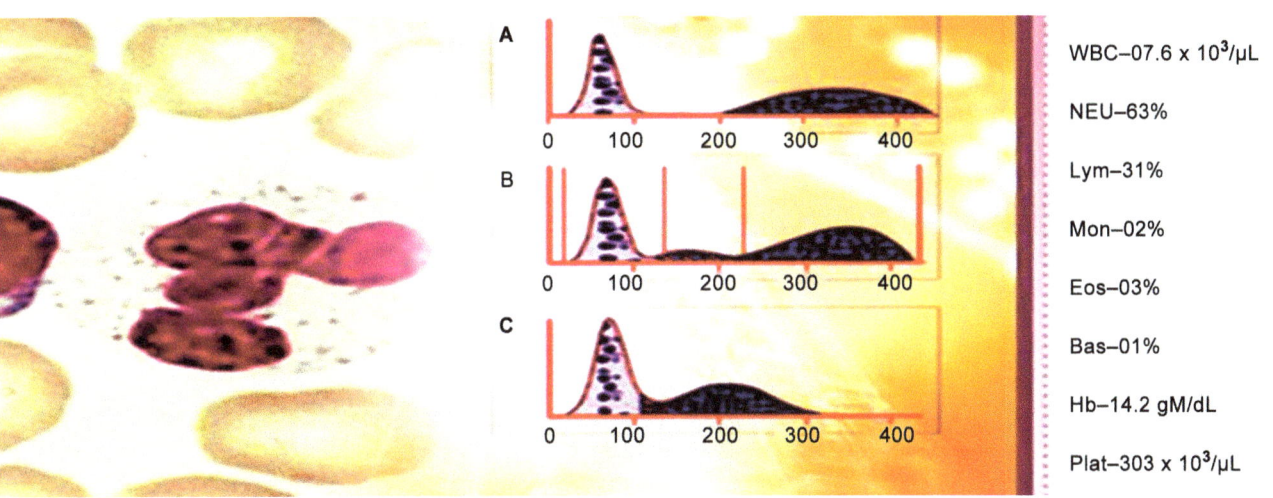

WBC–07.6 x 10³/µL
NEU–63%
Lym–31%
Mon–02%
Eos–03%
Bas–01%
Hb–14.2 gM/dL
Plat–303 x 10³/µL

Normal trimodal curve of WBC presents with many variations depending upon the permutation combinations possible within the reference range.

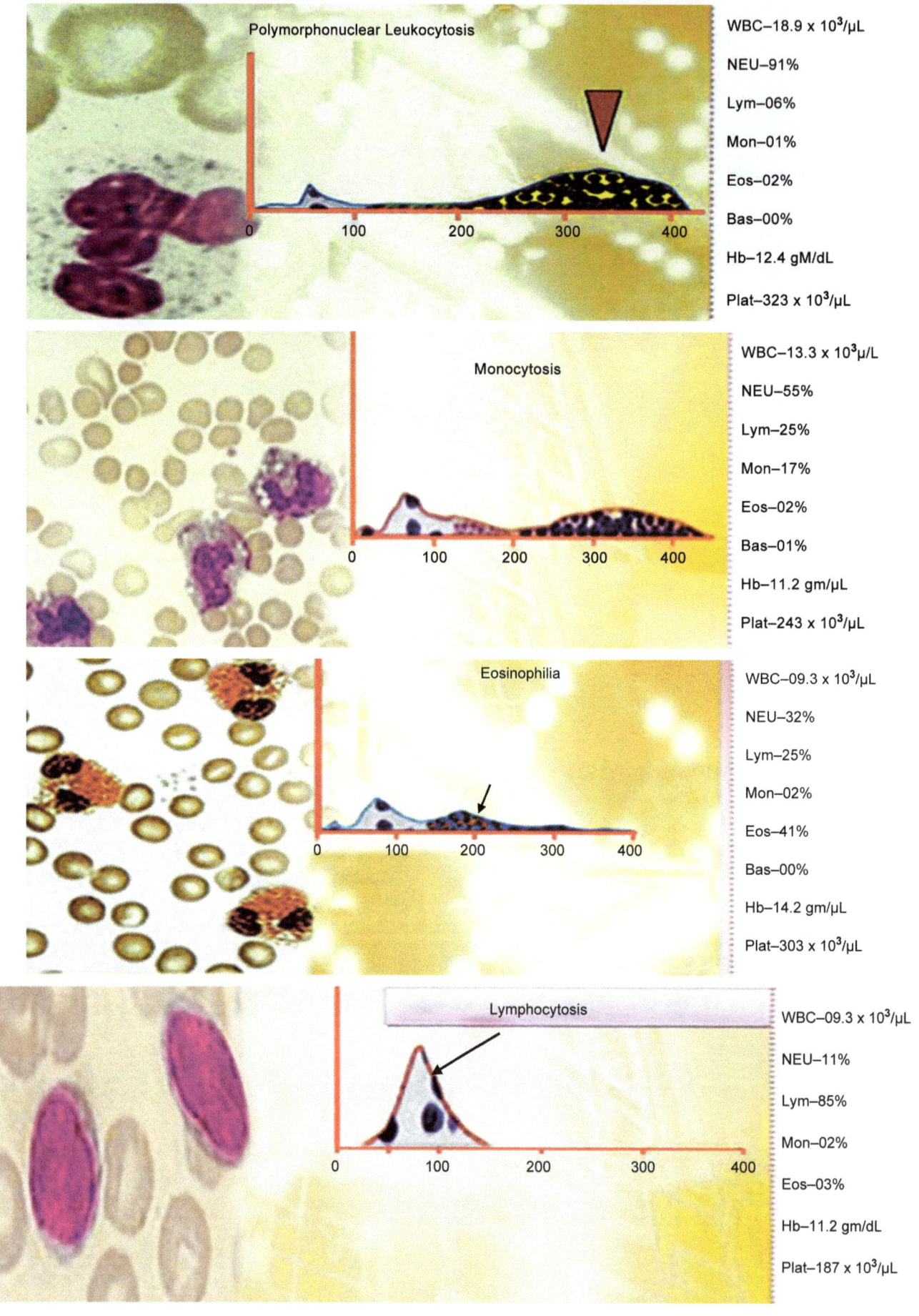

THE VOLUME HISTOGRAM FOR PLATELETS

Platelet-derived histograms are obtained from volume sizes of 2 to 30 fL. Platelet counting and sizing in both the electrical impedance and optical systems reflect the native cell size. The counting of the platelets takes place in the RBC aperture and the instrument is designed to count the particles in a range of 0 to 70 fL.

The actual count against mathematical criteria that eliminates nonplatelet particles is finally derived from the "best-fit" log-normal curve which generally falls in the 2 to 20 fL range.

An alert is generated if the three generated histograms do not agree or if the results are not within the range.

Particles within the platelet size range can interfere with the platelet count and histogram. Small particles, such as bubbles or dust, can overlap at the lower end of the histogram; microcytic erythrocytes can interfere at the upper end.

If the histogram does not return to the baseline at both the right and left of the peak, either there is severe thrombocytopenia or nonplatelets are being counted, either erythrocyte or leukocyte fragments may be responsible.

In such cases, the platelet count and derived parameters of MPV and PDW are not reliable.

With the application of computer technology, two other parameters can be obtained from the platelet histogram:
1. Mean platelet volume (MPV)—This is a mathematical calculation to determine the average size of the platelets. The average MPV range = 7.4 to 10.4 fL.
   If the MPV is >10.4 fL, then this indicates that immature platelets are being released, which may be due to some pathology. The MPV is also known as the platelet index (PI) and is analogous to the MCV. The normal MPV histogram is a right-skewed, single-peak normogram.
2. Platelet distribution width (PDW)—The platelet distribution width (PDW) is the width of the curve of distribution of platelets related to the different sizes produced by these cells (anisocytosis of platelets).
   Like MPV, abnormal PDW indicates the presence of some disorder in the production of platelets.

Platelet (PLT) Histogram

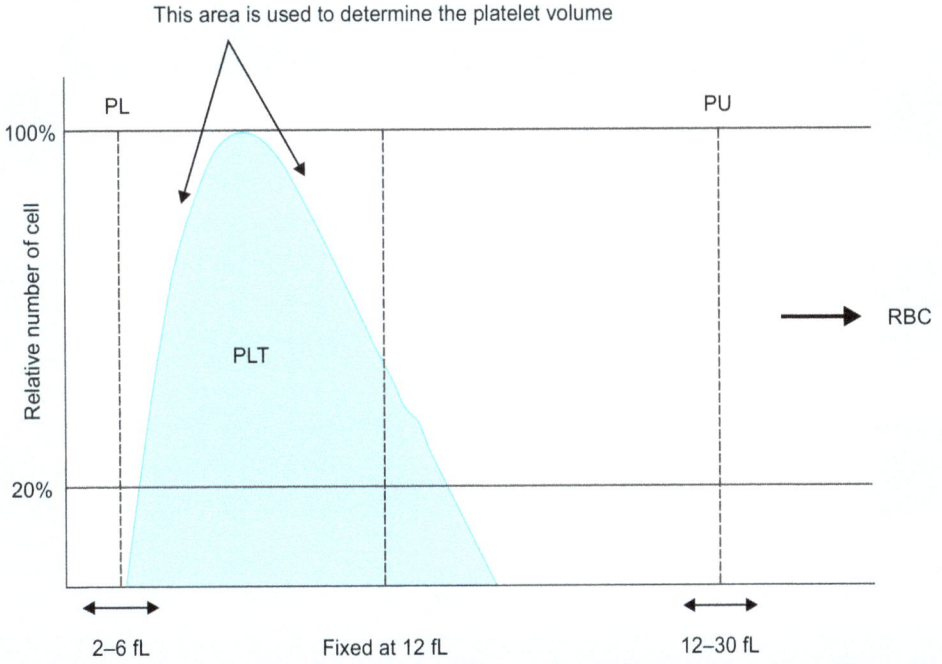

Platelet Distribution Curves

Three discriminators are used in these curves, the LD which is set at 2–6 fL, UD at 12–30 fL, and a fixed discriminator at 12 fL. In case of abnormal histogram, the platelet histogram may show the following flags:
- **PL:** Abnormal height at lower discriminator
- **PU:** Abnormal height at upper discriminator
- **MP:** (Multi peak) Platelet anisocytosis

PL Flag

This occurs when the lower discriminator exceeds the preset height by 10% the platelet count, MPV and P-LCR will show the PL flag.

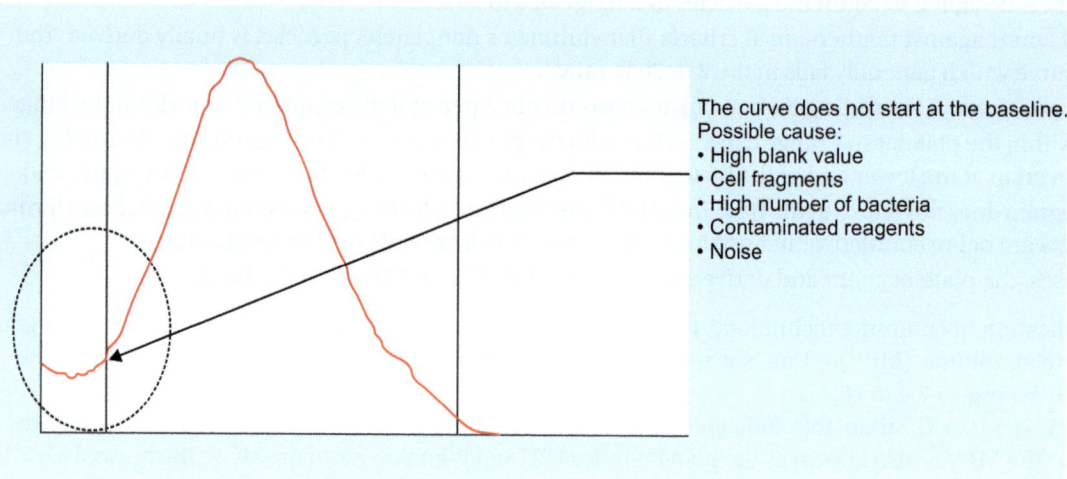

The curve does not start at the baseline.
Possible cause:
- High blank value
- Cell fragments
- High number of bacteria
- Contaminated reagents
- Noise

PU Flag

This occurs when the upper discriminator exceeds the preset height by more than 40%.

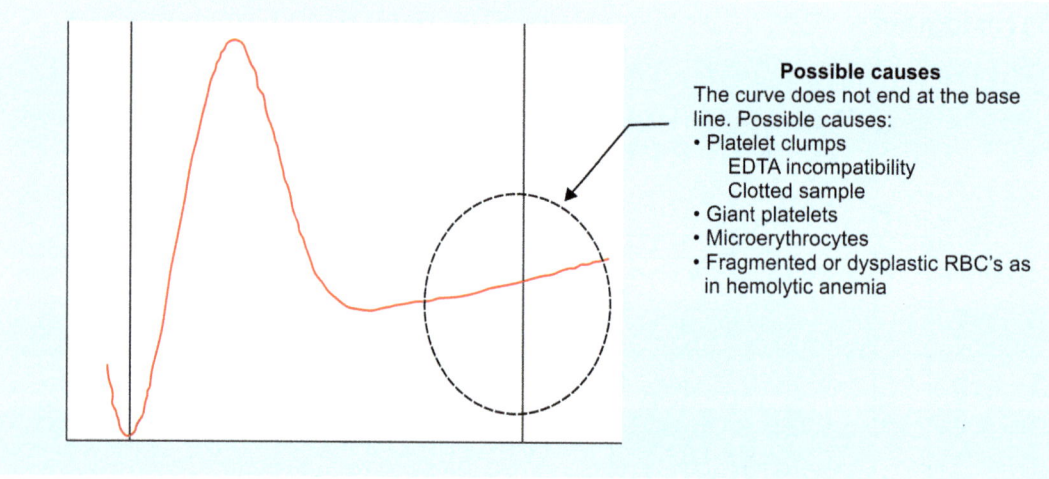

Possible causes
The curve does not end at the base line. Possible causes:
- Platelet clumps
    - EDTA incompatibility
    - Clotted sample
- Giant platelets
- Microerythrocytes
- Fragmented or dysplastic RBC's as in hemolytic anemia

MP Flag (Multipeaks in PLT Histogram)

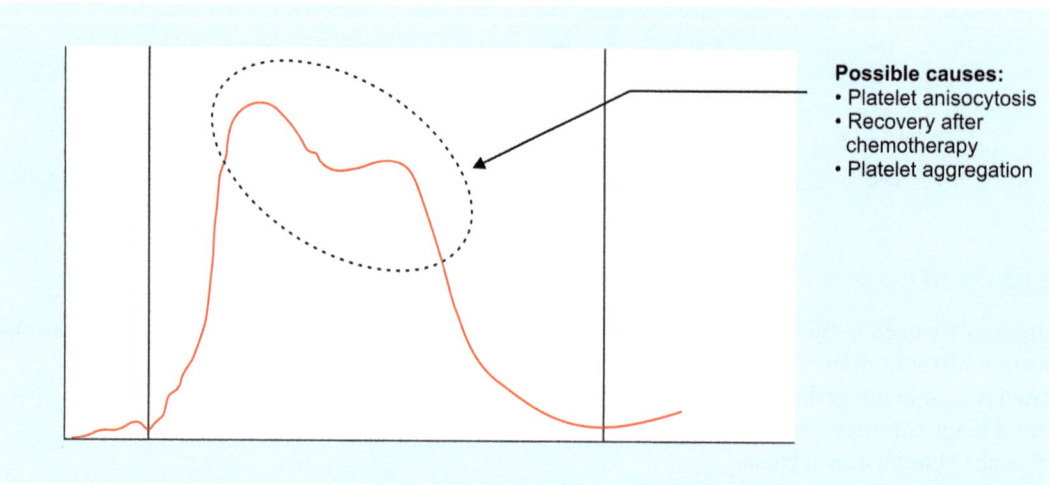

Possible causes:
- Platelet anisocytosis
- Recovery after chemotherapy
- Platelet aggregation

SCATTER PLOTS (SCATTERGRAM)

- Scattergram is a graph representing the distribution of two variables in a sample population.
- One variable is plotted on the vertical axis; the second is plotted on the horizontal axis. The scores or values of each sample unit are usually represented by dots.
- A scattergram demonstrates the degree or tendency with which the variables occur in association with each other.
- Scatter plots or scatter graphs is a type of mathematical diagram using Cartesian coordinates to display values for two variables for a set of data.

Technologies

There are various technologies available which generate scatter plots or scatter graphs which has been discussed in the chapter of manual versus automation, the basic technologies used are:
- The volume conductivity scatter (VCS) technology.
- Peroxidase staining.
- Fluorescence flow cytometry.

The Volume Conductivity Scatter Technology (VCS Technology)

Volume

Volume conductivity scatter (VCS) utilizes the Coulter principle of counting and sizing to measure the volume of the cell by using Direct Current (DC) across the two electrodes in a flow cell to physically measure the volume that the entire cell displaces in an isotonic diluent.

Conductivity

Alternating current in the radiofrequency (RF) range short circuits the bipolar lipid layer of a cell's membrane, allowing the energy to penetrate the cell. It reveals information about the internal structure of the cell, including chemical composition and nuclear volume.

Scatter

As cells are pass in a single-stream (flow cell) they are struck by a laser which gets scattered. The light scatter at angles between 10° and 70° is used by VCS instruments. The scattered light gives information about cell surface and granularity.

Fluorescence Flow Cytometry

Two scattergrams are used for the WBC differential.
1. Different channels for the measurement of lymphocytes, monocytes, neutrophils, and eosinophils. The cell populations are separated by the side scatter based upon the internal structure of the cells and side fluorescence-based upon the RNA and DNA content of the cells.
   The neutrophil population also contains the basophils which are counted in the WBC/BASO channel.
2. WBC/BASO channel for the measurement of the total white blood cells and the basophils. The cells are separated by internal structure (side scatter) and cell size (forward scatter).

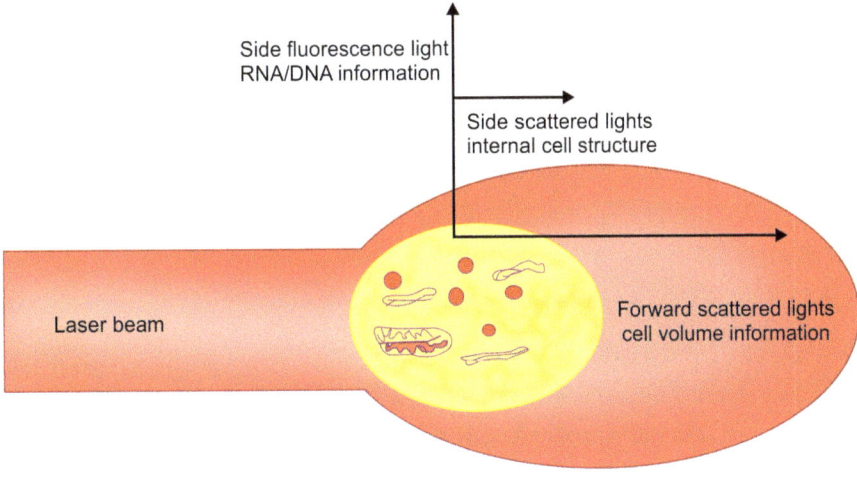

The Basic Cytogram for the Coulter Counter and how to Interpret it

The positions that the dots appear on the cytogram screen are determined by the degree of side scatter (SS). The degree of forward angle light scatter (FALS), absorption of light by each cell, and dyes (if any used). Low FALS and SS are indicative of lymphocytes. As the angle of FALS and SS increases monocytes appear on the cytogram followed by neutrophils. Eosinophils have the highest FALS and SS angles. The basophil requires a special window and detection technology. If a NRBC is present, it will most likely be counted as a WBC.

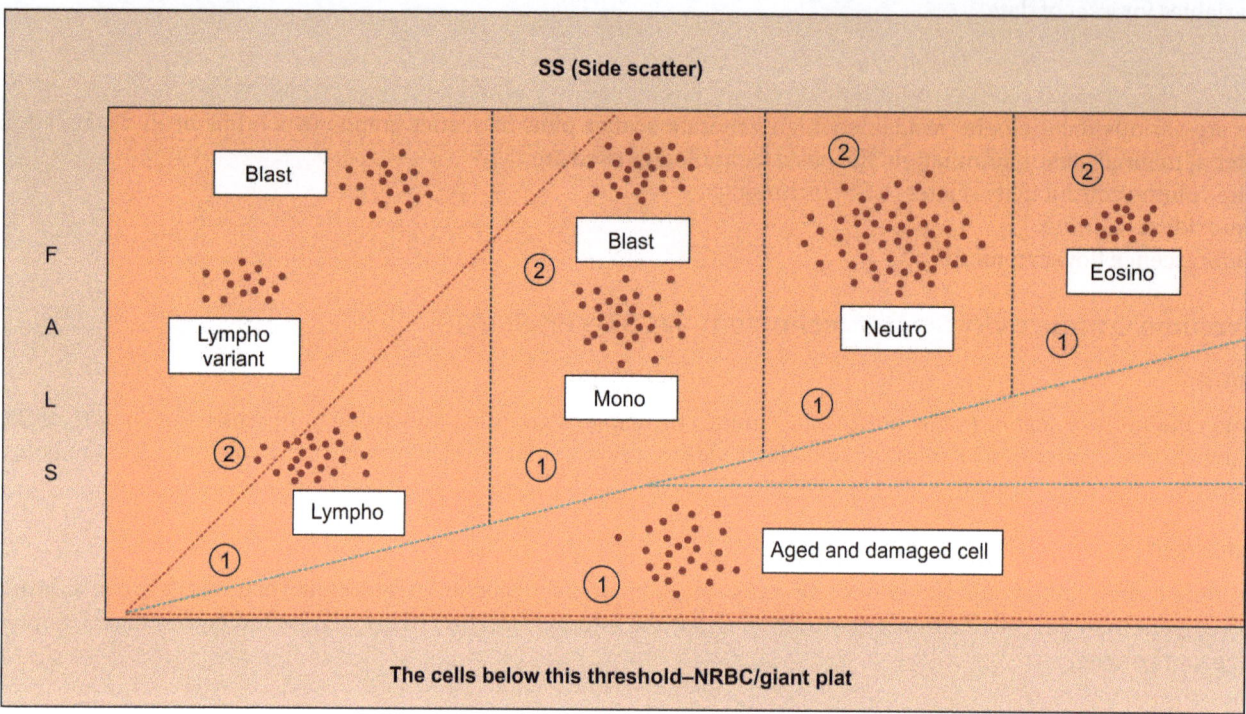

This combination of technologies (VCS) enables the presentation of a **three-dimensional plot (cube display or cytograph)** of the leukocyte population. The general placement of the five types of leukocytes may be noted in the following schematic.

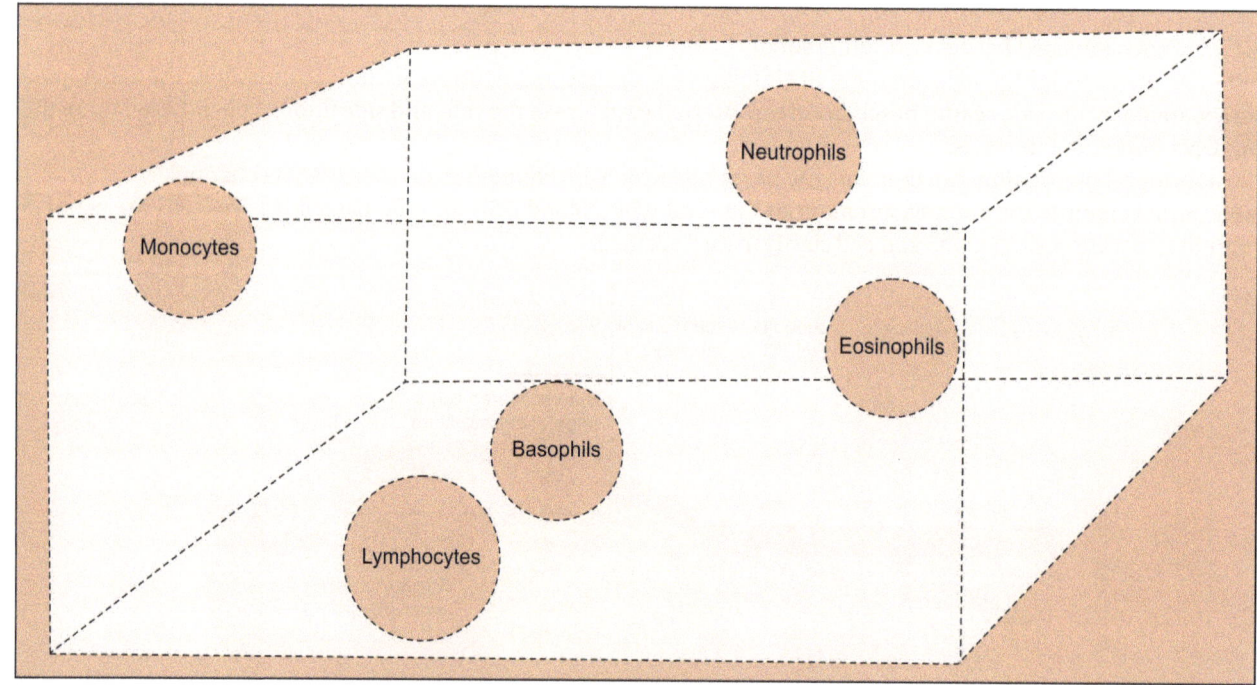

The pattern of cell distribution of the cell cytogram

DUAL WBC - PEROX AND BASOLOBULARITY METHODS

PEROXIDASE STAINING

In this technology, the peroxidase channel of the cell counterstains the cells with peroxidase stain and the cells are measured according to the staining intensity of the cell.
- Cells are stained by peroxidase reagent and analyzed for size and peroxidase stain intensity.
- Cell-specific lysis reagents are used to separate basophils from all other white cells.
- Basophils are subtracted from the lymph/basal cluster in the peroxidase channel to calculate the lymph.

Peroxidase staining intensity of various cells:
- Eosinophils: Strong staining
- Neutrophils: Medium staining
- Monocytes: Weak staining
- Lymphocytes and basophils: No staining
- Large unstained cells (LUC): No staining.

PEROX METHOD

Perox Cytogram Method

- The PEROX channel uses a combination of white light scatter and myeloperoxidase (MPO) cytochemistry to rapidly differentiate lymphocytes, monocytes, neutrophils, and eosinophils.
- Cytochemical reaction is a two-stage chemistry method using the intracellular myeloperoxidase enzyme to differentiate cells using stain and size characteristics.
- This approach makes use of both cell size and the different degrees of MPO positivity shown by different white cell types.
- **Neutrophils are strongly positive and eosinophils are very strongly positive**.
- **Lymphocytes are MPO negative whilst monocytes exhibit an intermediate staining pattern**.
- Large cells that do not stain with MPO, are called **Large unstained cells (LUCs)**.
- LUCs may be reactive lymphocytes (usually viral response), plasma cells, MPO deficient neutrophils, or neoplastic cells.
- LUCs are a unique parameter that allows the user to extend beyond the traditional 5-part differential.

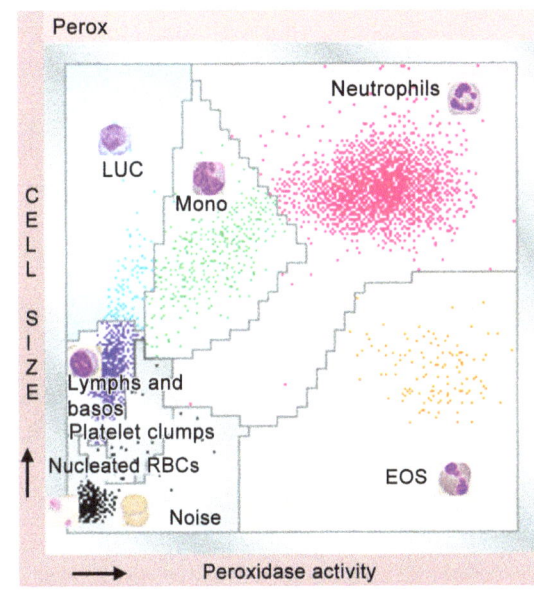

- LUCs are important because their presence quickly highlights cells in the peripheral blood that may be abnormal and warrant further blood film review.
- Use of an MPO based white cell differential is termed as **'cytochemical differential.'**
- MPO positivity is a strong indicator that the cells are likely to be myeloid.

Perox Cytogram

- The cells absorb light proportional to the **amount of peroxidase** stain present, and this is represented on the **x-axis**.
- Cells scatter light proportional to their **size**, and this is represented on the y-axis.
- When the light scatter and absorption data are plotted, distinct populations or clusters are formed.
- Cluster analysis identifies each population based on its **position, area, and density**, and then the number of cells in each population is processed.
- The PEROX cytogram is divided into 100 counting channels on each axis.
- The lines that separate the different cell populations are calculated by the software on a sample-by-sample basis.

A Normal Perox Cytogram showing positions of Neutrophil, Eosinophil, Monocyte, Lymphocyte, Basophil, Large unstained cell, Platelet clump, Nucleated RBCs and Noise (debris, etc).

BASO METHOD

BASO Cytogram Method (BASO Channel)
- The BASO channel, in addition to the WBC and basophil count, provides lobularity and nuclear density information about the white cell nuclei as they pass through the flow cell.
- Acidic reagent mixture strips the cytoplasm from the white cells and the remaining nuclei are counted using laser light scatter.
- Basophils are resistant to the acid stripping process and therefore remain intact. Because the intact basophils are much larger than the bare nuclei of all of the other white cells they can be detected and counted as a separate population.

BASO Cytogram: Cluster Analysis
- When the high-angle light scatter (nuclear configuration) is plotted on the x-axis, and the low-angle light scatter (cell size) is plotted on the y-axis, distinct populations or clusters are formed.
- Cluster analysis identifies each population based on its position, area, and density, and then counts the number of cells/nuclei in each population.
- The BASO cytogram is divided into 50 counting channels on each axis.

The Basophil/Lobularity Method
- Lobularity information allows the cell counter to separate mononuclear cells (lymphocytes and monocytes) from polymorphonuclear cells (neutrophils and eosinophils).
- Provides the primary total white cell count
- BASO reagent lyses the red cells, platelets, and cytoplasm of all white cell types except basophils
- BASO cytogram uses cluster analysis to identify and count cells and nuclei in each population based on position, area, and density **PANDA**
- Information from the PEROX and BASO cytograms can be combined and this forms the basis of '**peroxidase activity and nuclear density analysis**' **(PANDA). PANDA** is a powerful tool to assist in the pre-classification of haematological malignancy.

(Healthcare.siemens.co.uk)

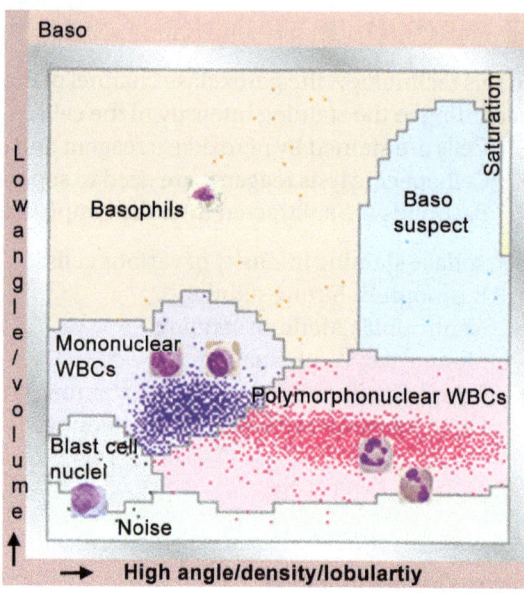

A normal BASO cytogram showing positions of mononuclear cells (MN), polymorphonuclear cells (PMNs), blasts (BLASTS), basophils (BASOPHILLS), Baso suspect (includes unlysed cells other than basophils), and noise (contains Platelets, RBCs, and other cellular debris).

Leukocytosis

Neutrophil left shift/hypolobularity can be seen in cases of:
1. Bacterial infection
2. Sepsis
3. Neutrophil dysplasia

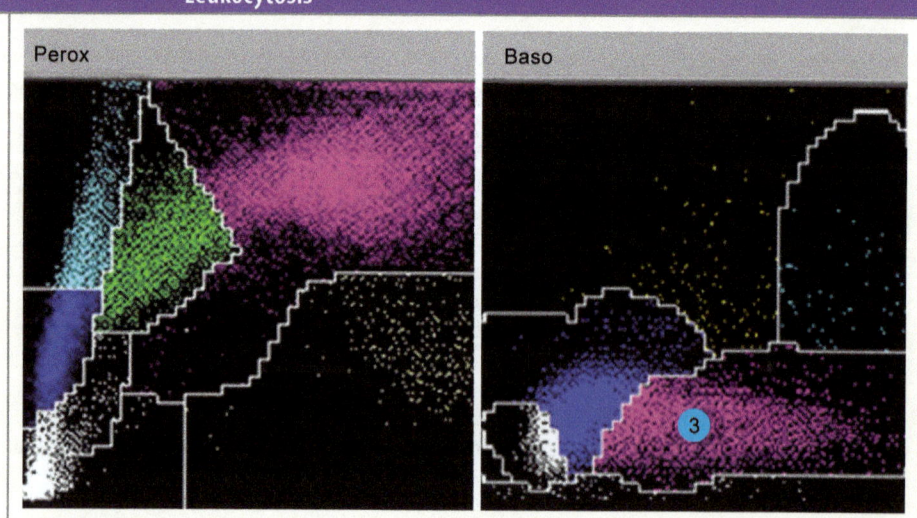

Courtesy: © Siemens Healthcare GmbH 2020

Chapter 9: WBC and Platelet Histogram and Scatterogram   119

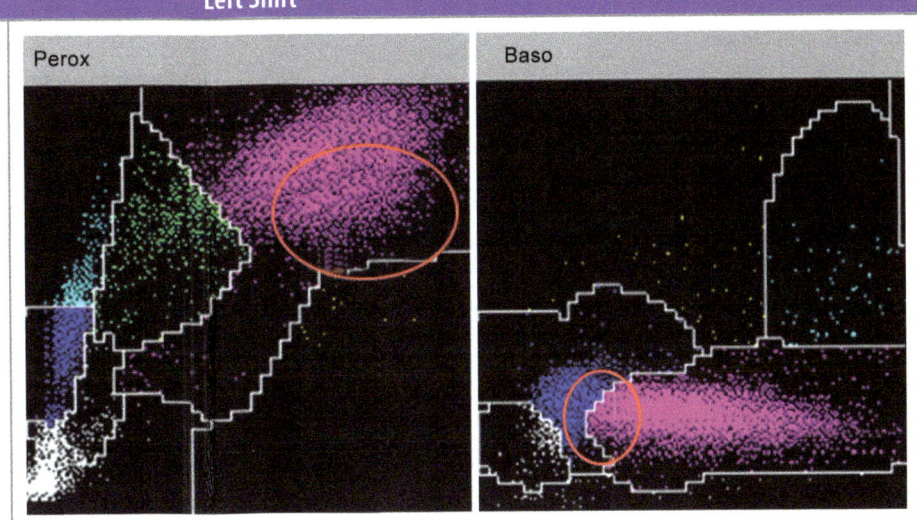

Left Shift

Cytograms from the sample of acute Broncho pneumonia.

The **left shift** flag is triggered by a lobularity index (LI) value less than 1.9 due to increased numbers of immature cell nuclei.

A significant number of band cells observed during a manual differential count on this sample.

Courtesy: © Siemens Healthcare GmbH 2020

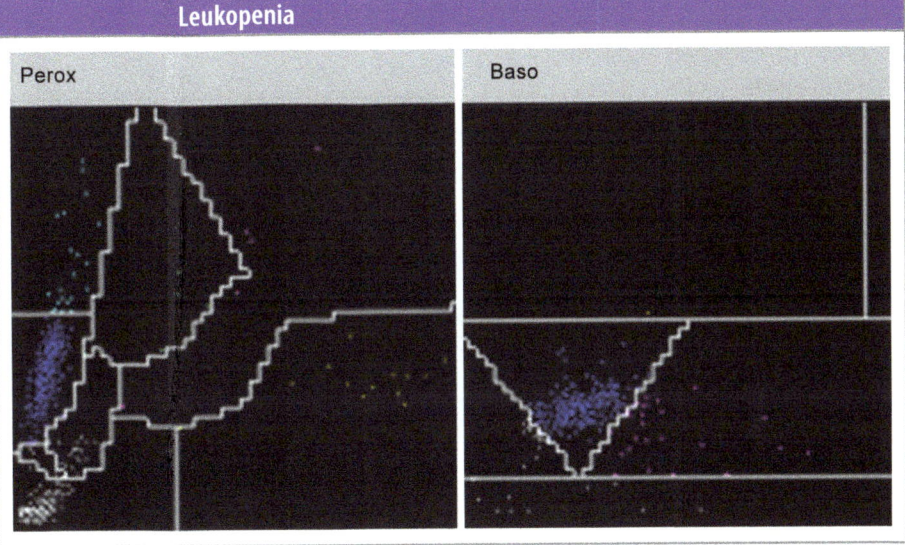

Leukopenia

The significant low WBC count of less than one thousand.

Note: The comparison of the **WBC Perox** and **WBC Baso** on this low count.

Courtesy: © Siemens Healthcare GmbH 2020

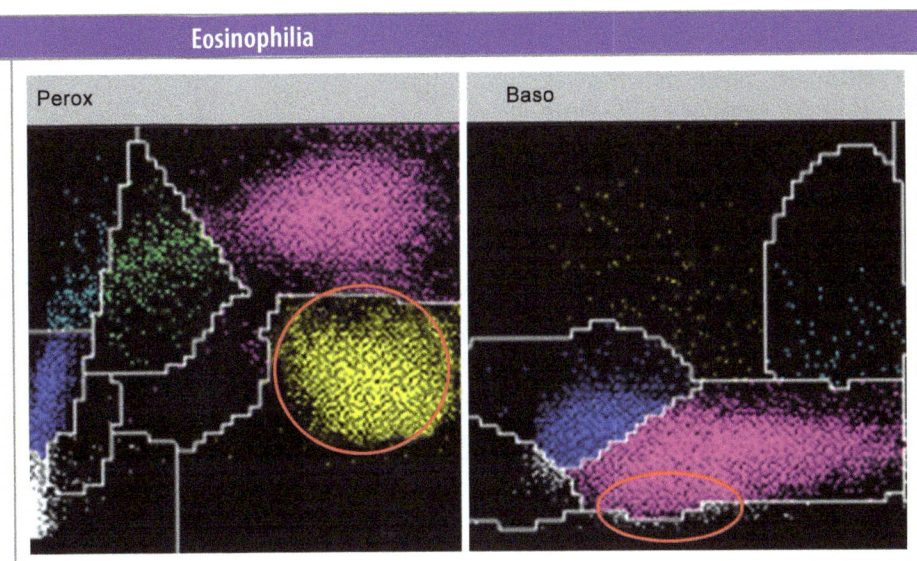

Eosinophilia

- Increased Eosinophils being exhibited in both the Baso and Perox channels.
- The Eosinophils will fall in the **belly of the worm** in the **Baso channel**.
- The Eosinophils will fall in the specific **Eos threshold area** in **Perox channel**.
- Left shift flag is generated as a result of the band form eosinophils, which fill up the valley.

Courtesy: © Siemens Healthcare GmbH 2020

Immature Granulocytes

1. NEUT area (Perox)
2. EOS area (Perox)
3. PMN area (Baso)

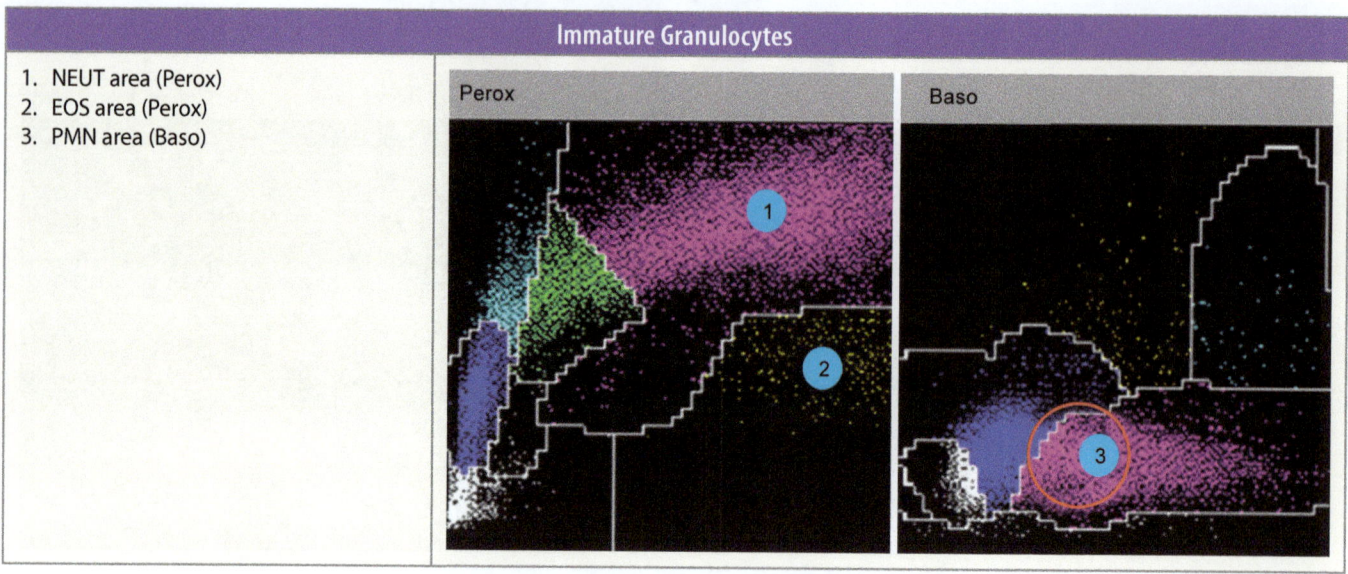

Courtesy: © Siemens Healthcare GmbH 2020

NRBC Location

Location of nucleated RBCs (NRBC) on Baso cytogram.

Location of nucleated RBCs (NRBC) on Perox cytogram.

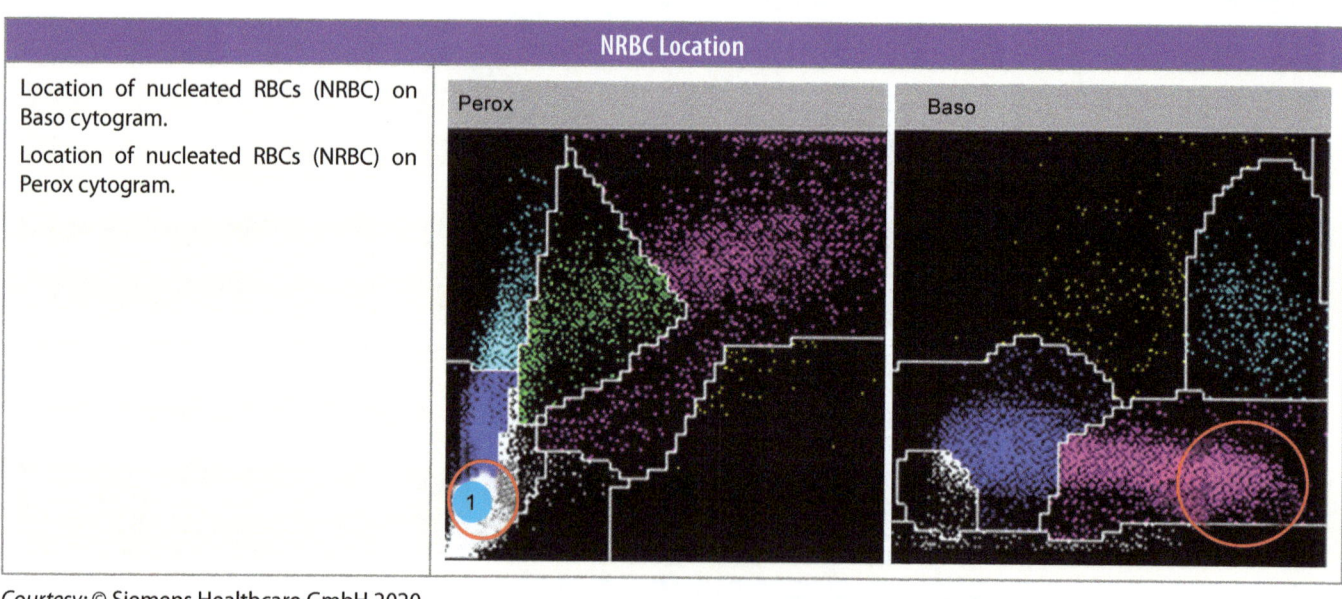

Courtesy: © Siemens Healthcare GmbH 2020

Myelodysplastic Syndrome (MDS)

- **MDS** with neutrophil dysplasia in which the **neutrophils 'dip down'** in the **Perox cytogram** (arrow).
- The **PMN 'tail'** seen in the **Baso cytogram** is significantly shorter than normal (arrow).
- Signifying hypo lobulation and/or pseudo Pelger-Huet neutrophils.

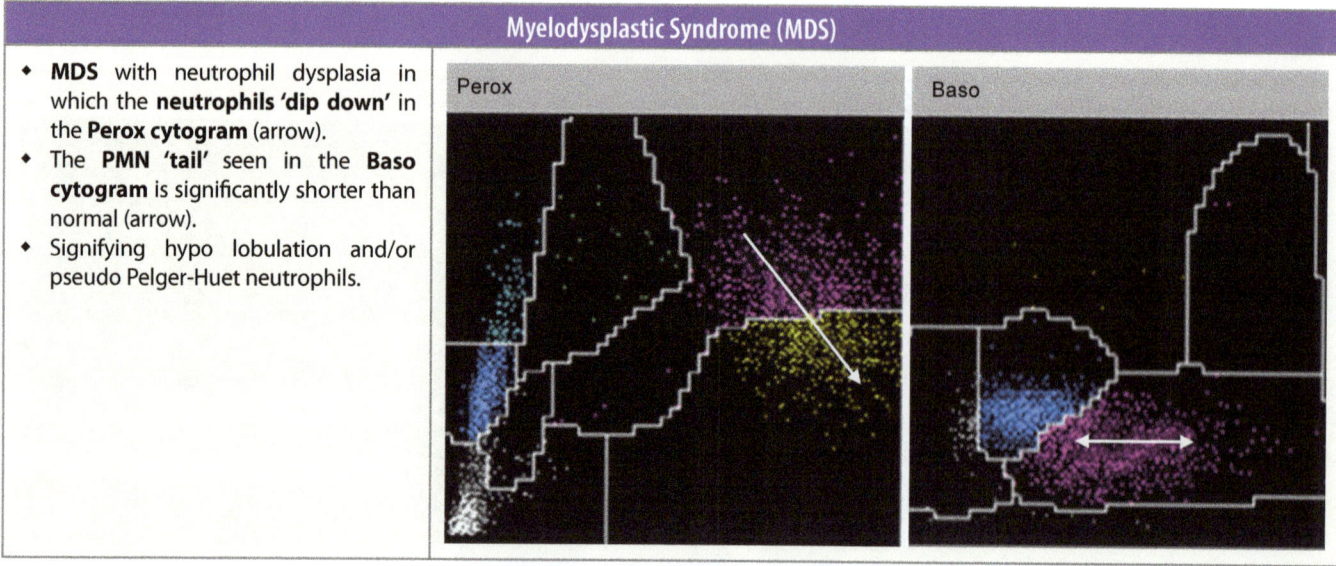

Courtesy: © Siemens Healthcare GmbH 2020

Acute Myelogenous Leukemia

- Acute Myelogenous Leukemia showing presence of **Blast** as identified in the **Baso cytogram**
- Correspondingly in the LUC area of the **Perox cytogram**.
- The cytogram does show that there are mature neutrophils as well as monocytes present.

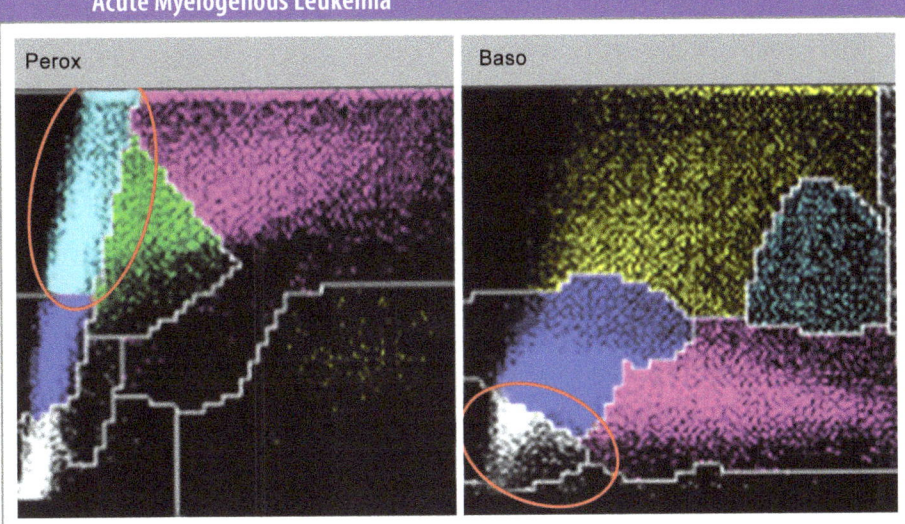

Courtesy: © Siemens Healthcare GmbH 2020

Promyelocytic Leukemia (M3)

- Promyelocytic Leukemia characterized by an increase in pro-myelocytic component of the WBC maturation
- The cells fall in the "neutrophilic" area of **Perox cytogram**, but are seen in the MN area of the **Baso cytogram**.
- Due to high perox positivity, an algorithm is having difficulty in separating the promyelocytes from the eosinophils, in the eosinophil area of the cytogram
- Resulting in false high eosinophilia, whereas these cells are probably promyelocytes.

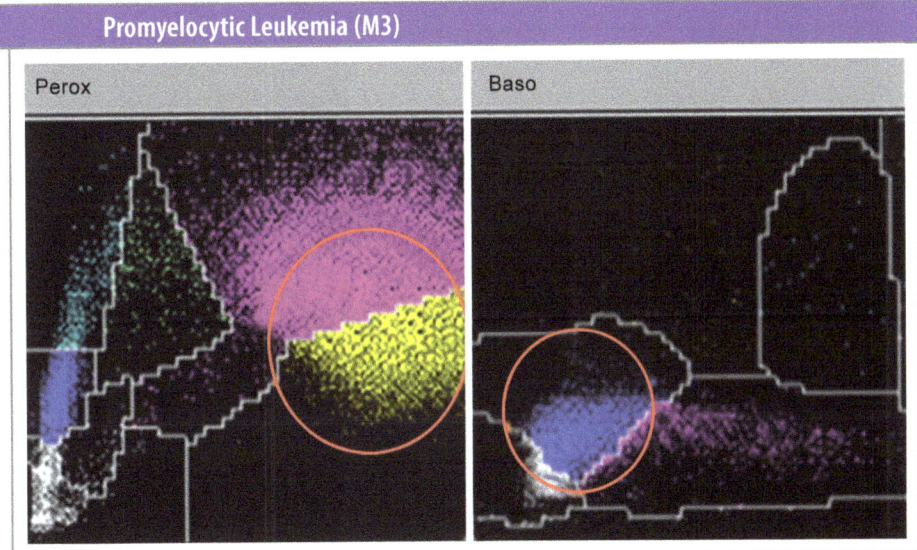

Courtesy: © Siemens Healthcare GmbH 2020

Acute Lymphocytic Leukemia

- Acute Lymphocytic Leukemia showing cell population of **LUC's with the apparent absence of neutrophils**.
- The **Baso channel** shows **blast** indication.
- ALL showing WBC of 194000 with 20% LUC's.
- LUC is evident on Perox cytogram.
- The lab should establish WBC criteria as well as LUC criteria to warn a manual scan in flagging variations.

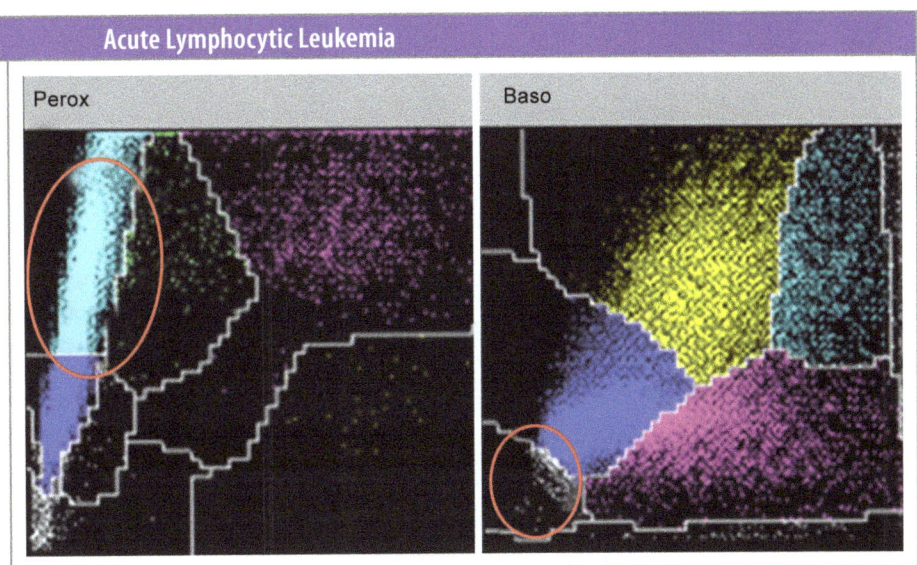

Courtesy: © Siemens Healthcare GmbH 2020

Chronic Lymphocytic Leukemia

Chronic Lymphocytic Leukemia characterized by an increase in atypical lymphocytes with high % **LUC**.

These cells are not blasts.

The cell population in the **Baso cytogram** is to dense and due to the absence of neutrophils, the algorithm is able to find only one population of cells.

The algorithm bisected the lymph and identifies part of the population as mononuclear cells (MN) and the other part as polymorphonuclear cells (PMN).

The **Perox cytogram** and **Baso cytogram** show an inconsistency in the neutrophils plus EOS (Perox) and MN's (Baso).

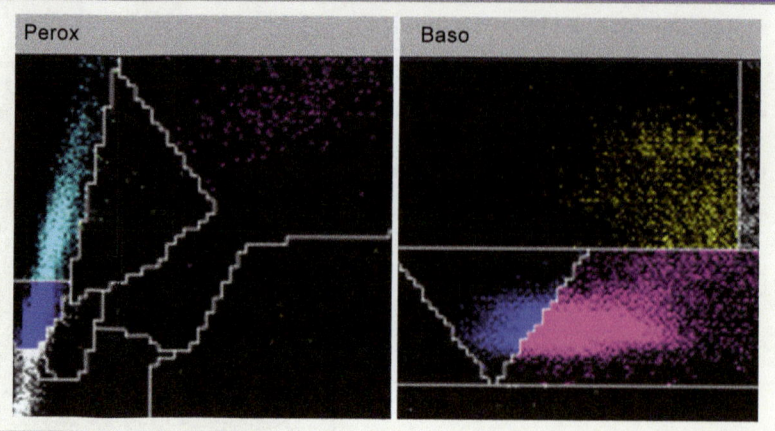

Courtesy: © Siemens Healthcare GmbH 2020

Viral Infections (Dengue)

PEROX cytogram: Reactive lymphocytes/atypical mononuclear cells due to viral infection (like dengue) (yellow cicle).

BASO cytogram: Similar cells seen in the basophill area (yellow circle).

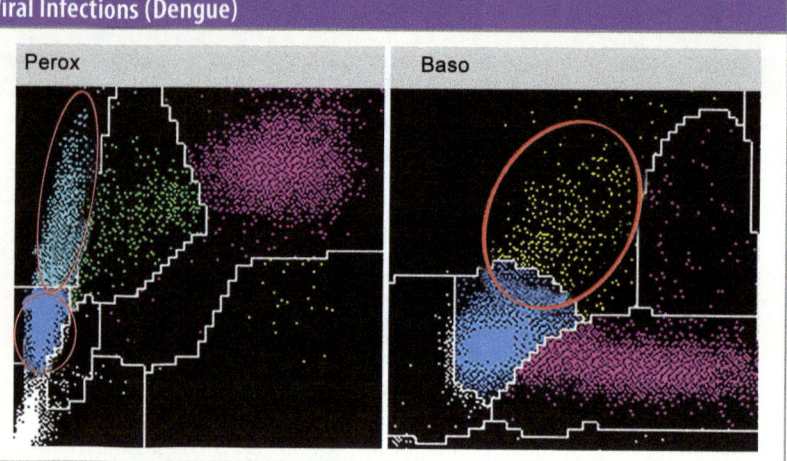

Courtesy: © Siemens Healthcare GmbH 2020

PLATELET SCATTER CYTOGRAM

Using the MIE Theory of light scattering for homogenous spheres, the low-angle, and the high-angle light scatters for each cell are transformed into volume and refractive index values. The vertical axis represents platelet volume (measuring from 0-60 fL), while the horizontal axis shows an increasing refractive index.

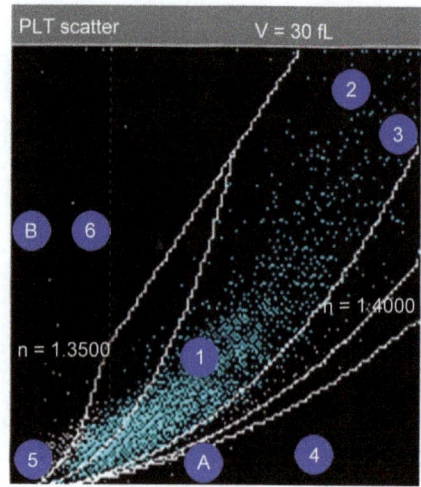

Platelet Scattergram

The Platelet Cytogram is the graphical representation of two light scatter measurements. The high-angle (5°–15°), high-gain light scatter is plotted on the x-axis, while the low-angle (2°–3°), high gain light scatter is plotted on the y-axis.
1. Platelets
2,3. Large platelets
4. RBC fragments
5. Debris
6. RBC Ghost area

Courtesy: © Siemens Healthcare GmbH 2020

Case Studies

CHAPTER 10

This section of the book is for the quick referral and understanding of the comprehensive interpretation of history, physical examination, numerical data, and histogram. The case studies of 30 commonly and uncommonly encountered conditions related to RBC, WBC, and platelet disorder, may not always lead to definitive diagnosis but will narrow the list of differential diagnosis and this will reduce the referral for expensive confirmatory advance investigations.

Abnormalities in the automated counter-generated data will alert the pathologist and technologist to seriously evaluate the peripheral blood smear for confirmation.

The histogram in this section is drawn for a general understanding of different disorders. There will be variation in the drawings of histogram in various makes and brands of the automated cell counters. Each individual laboratory should develop an understanding of the histogram generated by their machine and correlate the data and interpretate it accordingly.

CASE NO. 1 IMPROPER COLLECTION: SPURIOUS RESULTS

HISTORY

A case of a 42-year female receiving chemotherapy for ovarian tumor. She was advised periodic hemograms. On one of the readings, the results were markedly variable from the previous results. This particular sample was collected through intracath.

There was an abnormality in the histogram which had not been apparent on previous histograms. The spurious results were attributed to improper collection and the dilution of the specimen.

A properly collected repeat specimen revealed correct results.

INITIAL SPECIMEN

WBC

The histogram shows lymphocyte zone curve begins at approximately 45% above baseline. The usual causes of such error (fibrin strands, normoblast, or platelet clumps) could not be identified on the peripheral blood smear.

RBC

The histogram shows a broad and slightly shifted curve. The markedly elevated MCV and RDW were corrected in repeat specimen.

Platelet

Unremarkable

	Initial specimen	Repeat specimen
WBC	$9.4 \times 10^3/\mu L$	$9.7 \times 10^3/\mu L$
RBC	$2.6 \times 10^6/\mu L$	$3.9 \times 10^6/\mu L$
Hb	7.9 g/dL	11.9 g/dL
Hct	30%	38%
MCV	118 fL	93 fL
PLT	$183 \times 10^3/\mu L$	$378 \times 10^3/\mu L$
MPV	10.7 fL	8.9 fL
RDW	18.7%	14.8%

Repeat specimen histograms

WBC – unremarkable
RBC – unremarkable
PLT – unremarkable

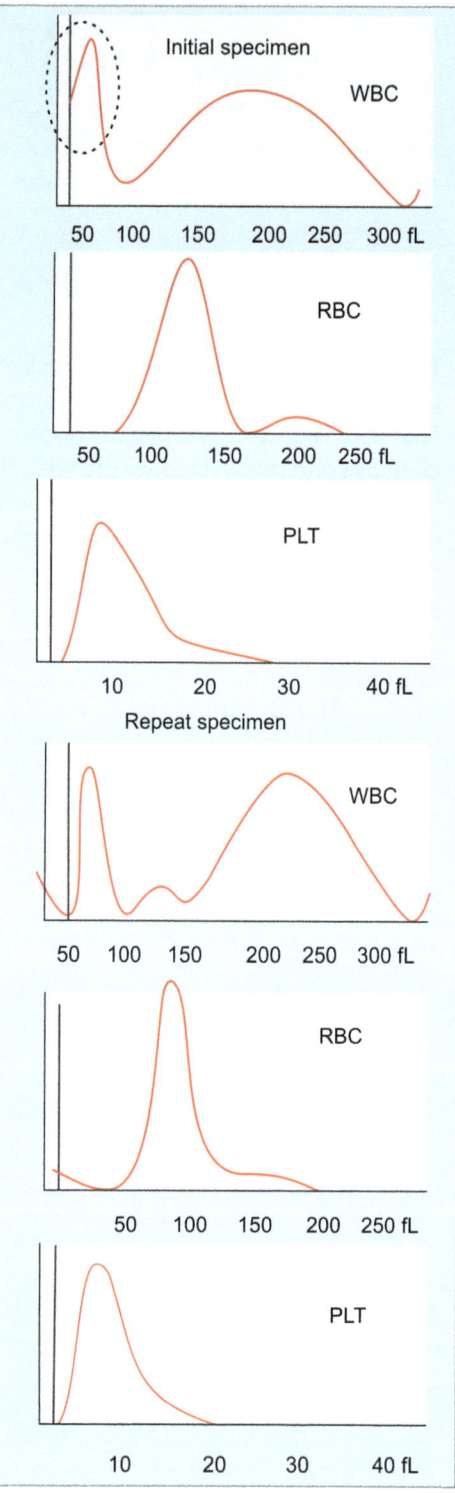

CASE NO. 2 IRON DEFICIENCY ANEMIA

HISTORY
27-year female with pregnancy.

OBSERVATION

RBCs: Numerically normal RBC count shows microcytosis (MCV decreased) and heterogeneity (RDW increased).

RBC histogram: It is shifted to the left and the peak of the curve is falling at 69 fL (microcytic zone). No evidence of fragmentation was seen.

RBC cytogram: It appears characteristically a distinct 'wedge' or 'right-angled triangle' shape, that differs from other causes of microcytosis and hypochromia. The RBC cytogram shows the majority of the red cell population to be in the microcytic hypochromic zone, appearing with a shift to the left and lower region of the cytogram. Hypochromia is more than microcytosis, and the ratio of microcytic % cells to hypochromic % cells (M/H ratio) is usually less than 1.

WBC
Within normal limits.

Platelet
Within normal limits.

DISCUSSION

The differential diagnosis in such observation can be:
- Iron deficiency anemia
- Thalassemia minor (trait)
- Thalassemia intermedia
- Hemoglobin H disease
- Sickle–thalassemia disease
- Red cell fragmentation.

Thalassemia trait can be excluded due to high RDW, unless there is concomitant iron deficiency anemia.

Fragmentation of RBC is excluded as an additional bump is not seen on the left arm of the RBC histogram in this case.

The age of the patient without past history excludes the diagnosis of hemoglobinopathies.

Anemia with low MCV and high RDW is a typical presentation of iron deficiency anemia.

Sometimes false low RBC count is due to non-counting of the microcytic RBCs which are less than 35 fL.

DIAGNOSIS
Iron deficiency anemia.

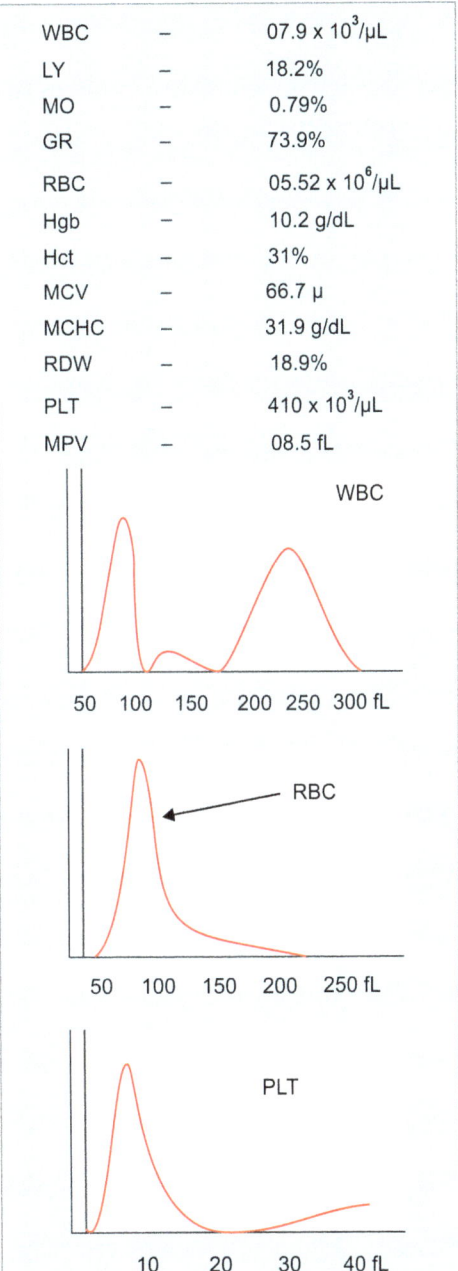

WBC	–	$07.9 \times 10^3/\mu L$
LY	–	18.2%
MO	–	0.79%
GR	–	73.9%
RBC	–	$05.52 \times 10^6/\mu L$
Hgb	–	10.2 g/dL
Hct	–	31%
MCV	–	66.7 µ
MCHC	–	31.9 g/dL
RDW	–	18.9%
PLT	–	$410 \times 10^3/\mu L$
MPV	–	08.5 fL

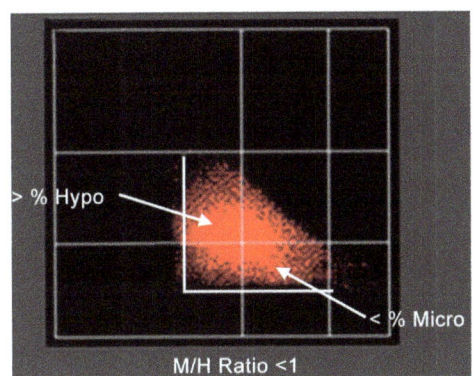

Courtesy: © Siemens Healthcare GmbH 2020

CASE NO. 3 BETA THALASSEMIA MAJOR

HISTORY

A case of a 16-year male of Gujarati Lohana Community referred to the hematology clinic. The patient had been diagnosed with beta thalassemia major in childhood and receives red cell transfusion at short intervals. The hemogram revealed a markedly abnormal WBC histogram along with anemia.

OBSERVATION

WBC

Histogram shows a small cell curve that begins approximately 40% above the normal baseline indicating that the small cell population is not solely lymphocytes but is due to the presence of NRBC in a significant number.

The mixed cell and neutrophil curves appear significantly depressed due to the preponderance of cells in the small cell area. The presence of NRBCs warranted the need for correcting the manual count for NRBCs interference.

RBC

The **histogram** shows an obviously skewed curve. This is due to the excessive number of NRBCs present and extremely heterogeneous morphology associated with this disease-causing raised RDW also.

Cytogram: In this case, red cells are markedly microcytic, hypochromic, and show severe anisopoikilocytosis.

Red cell cytogram due to these cells show a much wider spread compared to iron deficiency anemia.

Platelet

The histogram shows an unremarkable curve with visual evidence of microcytic red cell invasion on the right side of the histogram. The floating upper discriminator is automatically set at 20 fL to eliminate this interference.

DIAGNOSIS

Overall picture with raised Retic count guides towards the diagnosis of beta thalassemia major.

WBC	–	$56.5 \times 10^3/\mu L$
NRBC	–	680/100 WBC
RETIC	–	6.8%
Hgb	–	8.9 g/dL
PLT	–	467×10^3
MCH	–	23.9 pg
MPV	–	11.6 fL
RBC	–	$3.84 \times 10^6/\mu L$
RDW	–	21.9%
MCV	–	80.0 fL

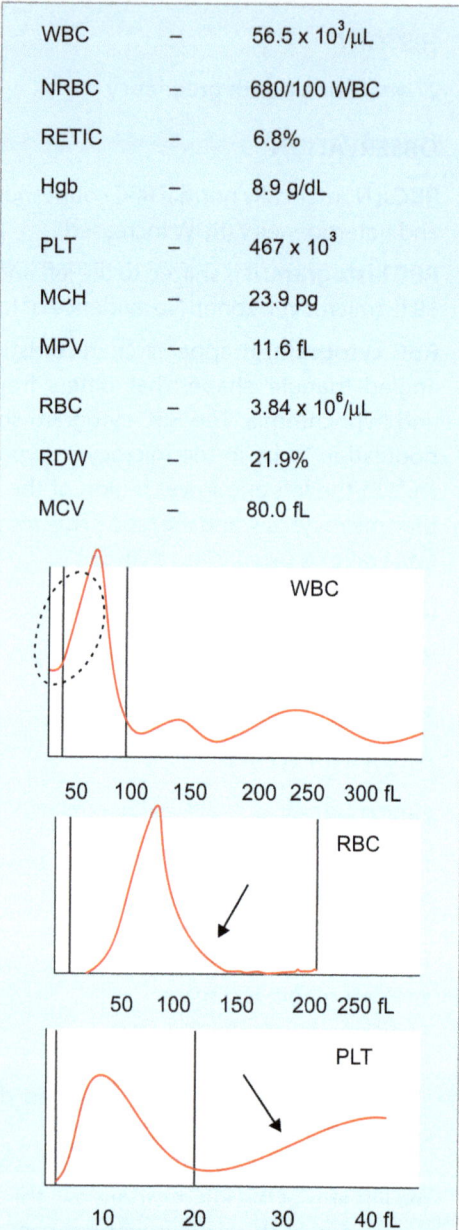

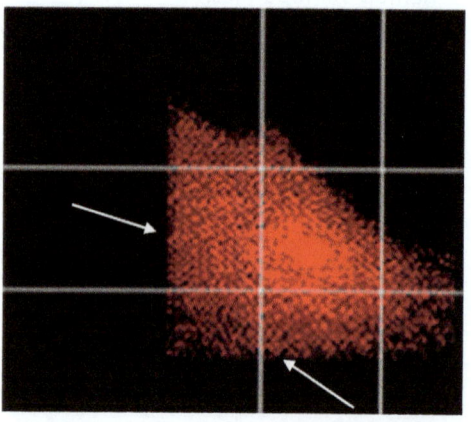

Courtesy: © Siemens Healthcare GmbH 2020

CASE NO. 4 BETA THALASSEMIA MINOR

HISTORY
An 18-year-old female admitted for abortion.

OBSERVATION

WBC
Unremarkable.

RBC
CBC reveals raised RBC count. Significant microcytosis, hypochromia with normal RDW (no significant heterogeneity of red cells).

Histogram: The histogram shows a narrow microcytic curve that peaks at approximately 55 fL.

Cytogram: Thalassemia trait tends to be more microcytic than hypochromic. The ratio of microcytic % cells to hypochromic % cells **(MH ratio)** is usually **greater than 1**. Red cell distribution width (RDW) and hemoglobin distribution width (HDW) tend to be normal in cases of thalassemia trait whereas both parameters are typically raised in iron deficiency. The RBC cytogram show red cell spread with close clustering of the cell plot owing to the uniform microcytosis. A characteristic **"comma-shaped cytogram"** is seen in the thalassemia trait.

Platelet
Histogram shows interference with microcytic red cells on the right side. The MPV was not determined due to the error code.

DISCUSSION
Considering the patients family history, normal red cell distribution width with microcytosis, she was advised hemoglobin electrophoresis which revealed:
Hb A1 – 93.4%, and Hb A2 – 6.6%.

DIAGNOSIS
Beta thalassemia minor.

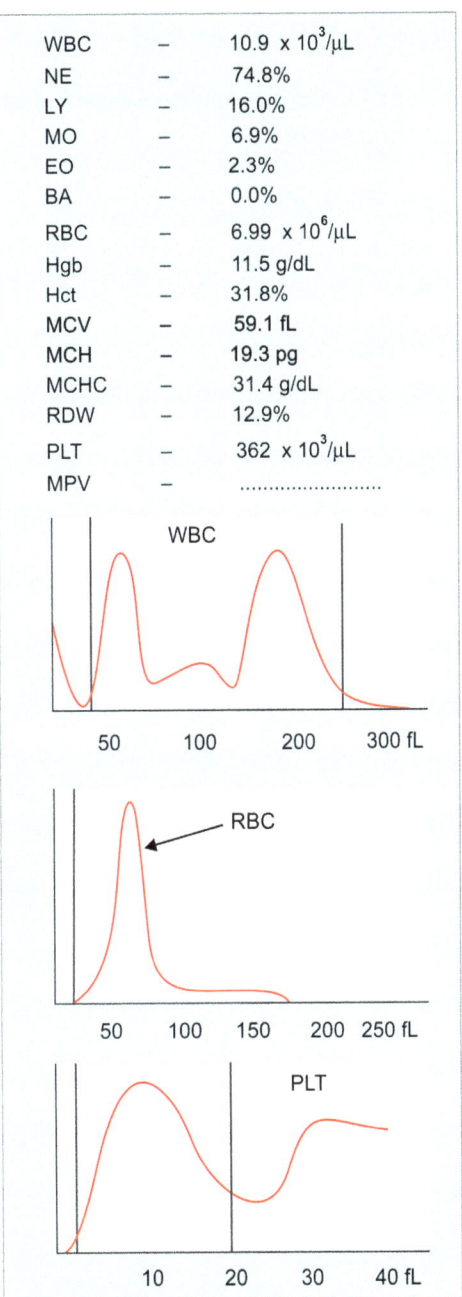

WBC	–	$10.9 \times 10^3/\mu L$
NE	–	74.8%
LY	–	16.0%
MO	–	6.9%
EO	–	2.3%
BA	–	0.0%
RBC	–	$6.99 \times 10^6/\mu L$
Hgb	–	11.5 g/dL
Hct	–	31.8%
MCV	–	59.1 fL
MCH	–	19.3 pg
MCHC	–	31.4 g/dL
RDW	–	12.9%
PLT	–	$362 \times 10^3/\mu L$
MPV	–	....

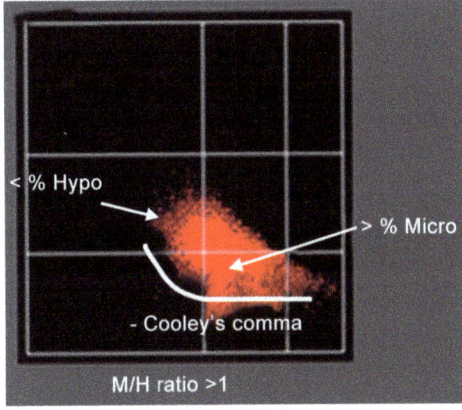

Courtesy: © Siemens Healthcare GmbH 2020

CASE NO. 5 HETEROZYGOUS ALPHA THALASSEMIA

HISTORY

A 27-year-old male with borderline anemia treated with iron without improvement.

OBSERVATION

RBCs–Count upper normal value, MCV reduced and RDW normal.
WBC–Within normal limits.

Platelet
Normal count with higher MPV.

DISCUSSION

Microcytosis with normal heterogeneity includes possibilities of:
* Iron deficiency anemia
* Anemia of chronic disease
* Heterozygous thalassemia.
  – Absence of significant anemia and normal RDW excludes the possibility of first choice diagnosis of microcytosis that is iron deficiency.
  – Anemia of chronic disease is usually normocytic with normal RDW.
  – Increased MPV with normal platelet count also supports the diagnosis.

DIAGNOSIS

Thalassemia trait.

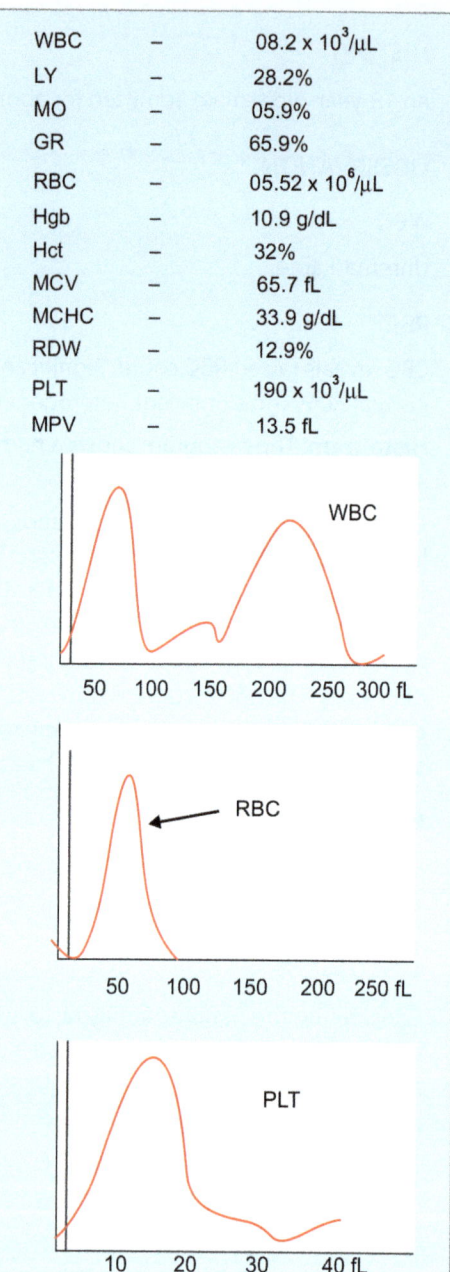

WBC	–	$08.2 \times 10^3/\mu L$
LY	–	28.2%
MO	–	05.9%
GR	–	65.9%
RBC	–	$05.52 \times 10^6/\mu L$
Hgb	–	10.9 g/dL
Hct	–	32%
MCV	–	65.7 fL
MCHC	–	33.9 g/dL
RDW	–	12.9%
PLT	–	$190 \times 10^3/\mu L$
MPV	–	13.5 fL

CASE NO. 6 SICKLE CELL ANEMIA

HISTORY

22-year-old male with severe pain in abdomen.

OBSERVATION

RBC

Count decreased, hemoglobin low, MCV high, RDW elevated.
RBC cytogram is spreading into hypo, hyper and macrocytic zone.

WBC

TLC is high, neutrophil upper normal range.
Histogram–lymphocyte peak shoulder seen.

Platelet

Count increased with high MPV.

DISCUSSION

The macrocytic (MCV increased), and heterogenous (RDW increased) anemia is seen in:
- Chronic liver disease
- Immune hemolytic anemia
- Cytotoxic chemotherapy
- Newborn
- Vitamin B_{12}/folate deficiency anemia
- Sickle cell anemia

Raised WBC count with a shoulder on the small end in the peak of lymphocytic histogram is in the nucleated red cell range, this indicates the presence of normoblasts in peripheral blood, which in turn indicates hemolysis.

A very high RDW again leads to the possibility of anisocytosis may be due to poikilocytosis (sickle cell), thrombocytosis with high MPV also supports the diagnosis.

DIAGNOSIS

Sickle cell anemia (sickle crisis).

WBC	–	$12.2 \times 10^3/\mu L$
LY	–	18.2%
MO	–	09.9%
GR	–	71.9%
RBC	–	$02.02 \times 10^6/\mu L$
Hgb	–	07.9 g/dL
HCl	–	23%
MCV	–	105.7 fL
MCHC	–	33.9 g/dL
RDW	–	19.9%
PLT	–	$619 \times 10^3/\mu L$
MPV	–	10.8 fL

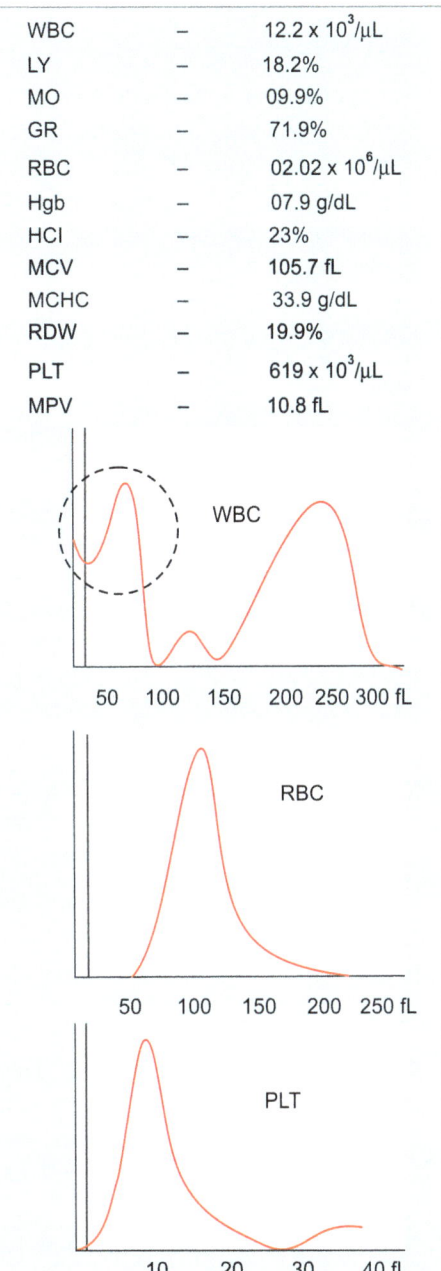

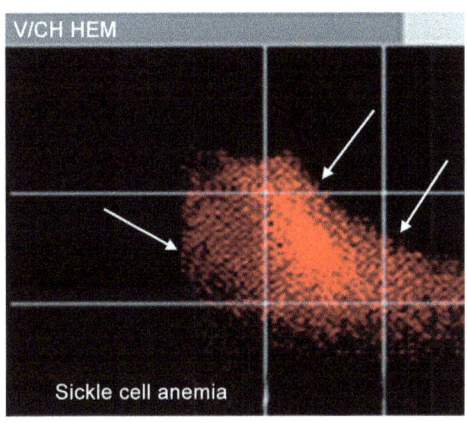

Courtesy: © Siemens Healthcare GmbH 2020

CASE NO. 7 MEGALOBLASTIC ANEMIA–VITAMIN B$_{12}$ DEFICIENCY

HISTORY

A case of a 69-year male suffering from anemia.

Hemogram revealed an Hgb of 3.3 g/dL, macrocytosis (MCV increased), and thrombocytopenia.

The serum vitamin B$_{12}$ was significantly decreased.

The bone marrow aspirate and biopsy revealed megaloblastic erythropoiesis.

OBSERVATION

WBC

The histogram shows a neutrophil population curve that is broader than normal.

The right descending slope is extended, possibly due to the hyper-segmented-neutrophils. (Seg…66%…Hyperseg…13%).

RBC

The histogram shows an extremely broad symmetrical curve with a marked elevation of RDW. The curve is shifted to the right of normal and peaks at approximately 122 fL which correlates with marked macrocytosis. The symmetrical curve indicates the presence of microcytes as well as macrocytes.

Most red cells have a larger volume (>100 fL) and show significant poikilocytosis (macro-ovalocytes).

The red cell cytogram, therefore, shows most cell plots in the macrocytic zone with a wider spread as compared to that seen in non-megaloblastic macrocytosis

Platelet

The histogram shows a slightly depressed curve due to the thrombocytopenia which accentuates the presence of microcytic red cells. The curve does not return to baseline and shows the typical interference caused by microcytes. The MPV was not reported.

DIAGNOSIS

Megaloblastic (pernicious) anemia.

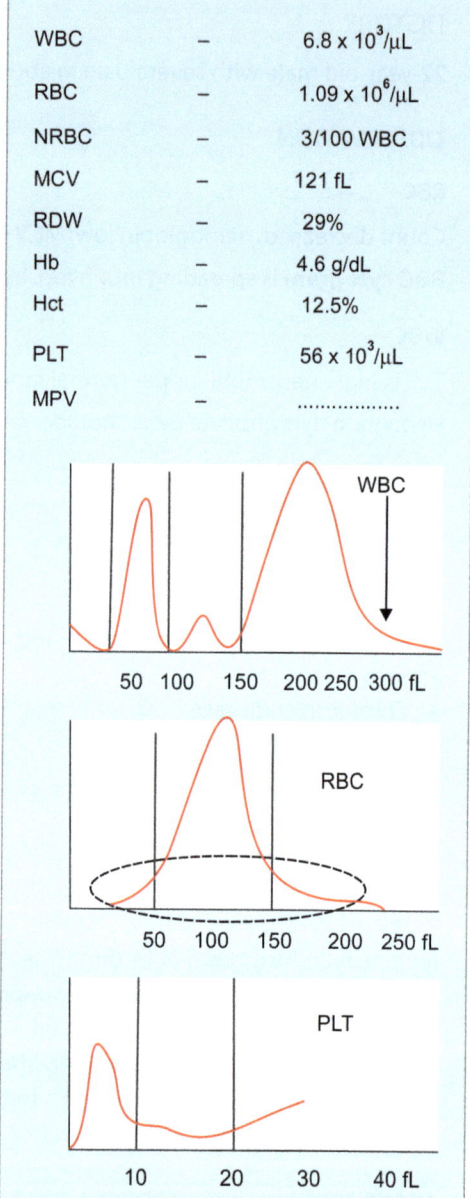

WBC	–	6.8 x 10^3/µL
RBC	–	1.09 x 10^6/µL
NRBC	–	3/100 WBC
MCV	–	121 fL
RDW	–	29%
Hb	–	4.6 g/dL
Hct	–	12.5%
PLT	–	56 x 10^3/µL
MPV	–	…………………

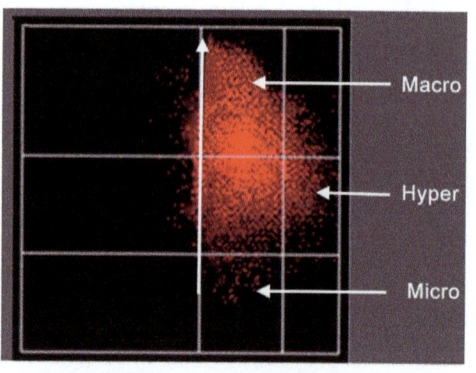

Courtesy: © Siemens Healthcare GmbH 2020

CASE NO. 8 MEGALOBLASTIC ANEMIA–VITAMIN B_{12} DEFICIENCY (POST-THERAPY)

HISTORY

The patient with pernicious anemia (Case no. 7) was treated with transfusion of packed cells and intramuscular vitamin B_{12} therapy.

The post-therapy CBC revealed:

WBC

The histogram curve shifted slightly to the right may be due to the presence of hypersegmented neutrophils.

RBC

The RDW is still elevated.

The histogram reveals a bimodal curve—one tall and one small curve.

Data for the smaller-sized population can be obtained by manually moving the upper discriminator to the valley between the two red-cell populations (black line-arrow).

The RBC population on the left side curve (tall curve) includes RBCs of normocytic size (MCV 83), in response to therapy.

The smaller curve on the histogram has an MCV of 135 fL. These results are determined by moving the upper discriminator to its original position and the lower discriminator to the valley between the two red-cell populations (black dotted line).

RBC population on the right side of the histogram (small curve) includes the patient's original macrocytes and an increased number of reticulocytes produced in response to therapy.

Cytogram: Multiple populations of red cells may exist. Due to different sizes of red cells and hemoglobin concentration, leading to scatter plotting predominantly in normocytic zone, and minimally in hypochromic, macrocytic, and hyperchromic zones.

Platelet

The histogram is unremarkable considering the moderate thrombocytopenia. There is evidence of increased platelet production shown by the presence of a bump on the descending slope of the curve.

DIAGNOSIS

Post-therapy megaloblastic anemia.

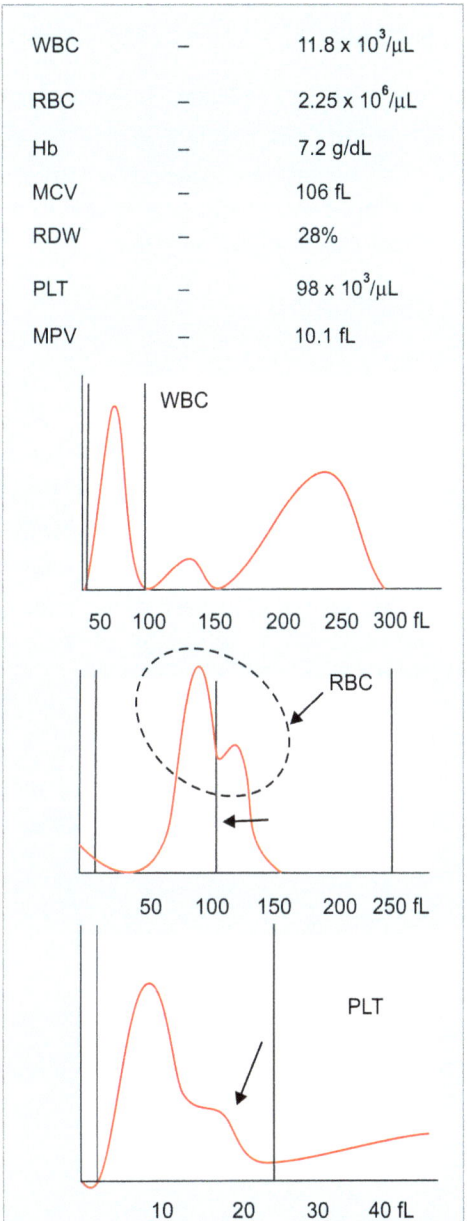

WBC	–	$11.8 \times 10^3/\mu L$
RBC	–	$2.25 \times 10^6/\mu L$
Hb	–	7.2 g/dL
MCV	–	106 fL
RDW	–	28%
PLT	–	$98 \times 10^3/\mu L$
MPV	–	10.1 fL

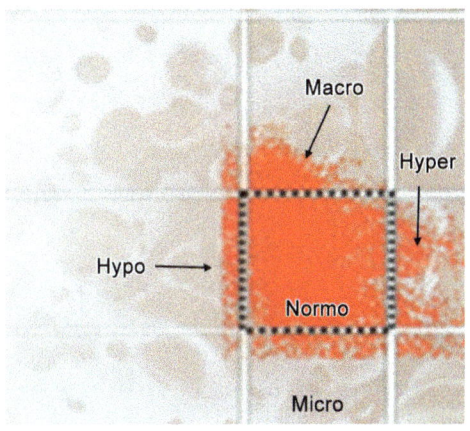

Courtesy: © Siemens Healthcare GmbH 2020

CASE NO. 9 CHRONIC MACROCYTIC ANEMIA—DRUG INDUCED

HISTORY

This case is a 47-year-old male, postrenal transplant, receiving an immunosuppressive drug, to prevent rejection of the transplanted kidney.

The hemogram revealed a marked macrocytosis. The patient has developed macrocytic anemia due to the drug which is known to cause megaloblastic erythropoiesis.

OBSERVATION

WBC

The histogram shows the small cell population curve beginning at approximately 35% above the baseline due to the presence of NRBCs that are interfering with the accuracy of total WBC count and trimodal data.

A manual WBC count with differential correction formula for NRBCs is advised to obtain an accurate total WBC count.

The red cell cytogram shows most cell plots in the macrocytic zone without a wider spread as compared to that seen in megaloblastic macrocytosis.

RBC

The histogram shows an extremely broad curve that has shifted to the right due to the marked macrocytosis.

The RDW is markedly elevated.

Platelet

Unremarkable.

Peripheral smear: Revealed ovoid macrocytes with the presence of Howell-Jolly bodies at places.

DIAGNOSIS

Drug-induced chronic macrocytic anemia.

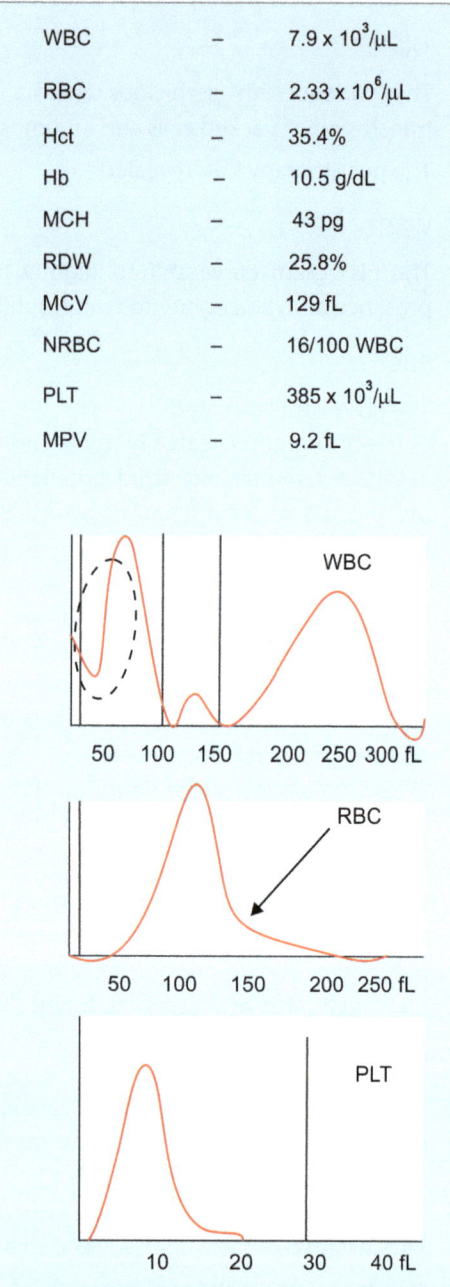

WBC	–	7.9 × 10^3/μL
RBC	–	2.33 × 10^6/μL
Hct	–	35.4%
Hb	–	10.5 g/dL
MCH	–	43 pg
RDW	–	25.8%
MCV	–	129 fL
NRBC	–	16/100 WBC
PLT	–	385 × 10^3/μL
MPV	–	9.2 fL

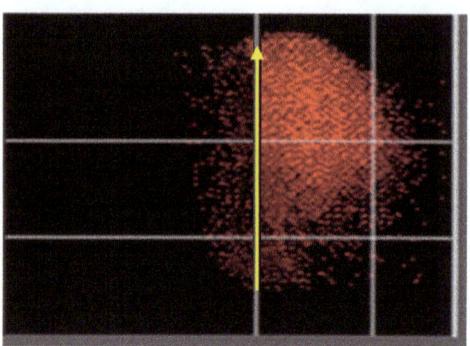

Courtesy: © Siemens Healthcare GmbH 2020

CASE NO. 10 RED CELL FRAGMENTATIONS

HISTORY

59-year male presented in a cardiosurgical clinic for follow-up.

OBSERVATION

RBCs

Count reduced, MCV normal, RDW increased and histogram shows left arm low plateau.

Cytogram exhibits variable population of fragmented RBCs plotted in the microcytic hypochromic zone.

WBC

Within normal limits.

Platelet

Within normal limits.

DISCUSSION

The differential diagnosis for normocytic heterogeneous anemia include:
- Mixed nutritional deficiency anemia
- Myelofibrosis
- Myelodysplasia
- Sideroblastic anemia
- Hemolytic anemia.

The red cell histogram with left arm low plateau in RBC histogram is pathognomonic of red cell fragmentation due to hemolysis. The RBCs are expressed in the zone of < 25 fL. But they are not over numbered to cause a significant increase in platelet count or reduction in total RBC count.

DIAGNOSIS

Red cell fragmentation.

WBC	–	$08.2 \times 10^3/\mu L$
LY	–	30.2%
MO	–	05.9%
GR	–	63.9%
RBC	–	$04.52 \times 10^6/\mu L$
Hgb	–	12.9 g/dL
Hct	–	35%
MCV	–	82.7 fL
MCHC	–	33.9 g/dL
RDW	–	17.9%
PLT	–	$259 \times 10^3/\mu L$
MPV	–	05.5 fL

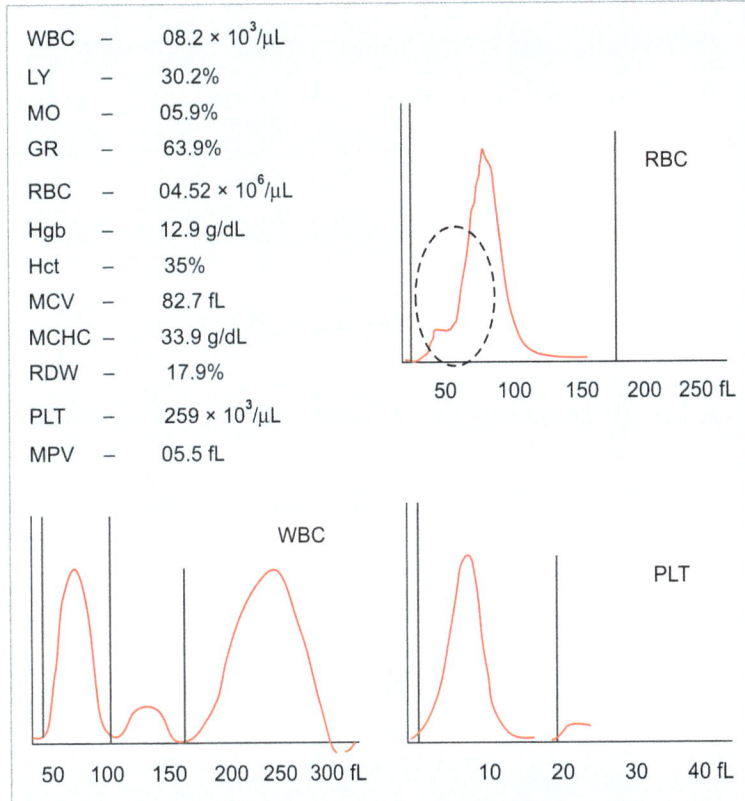

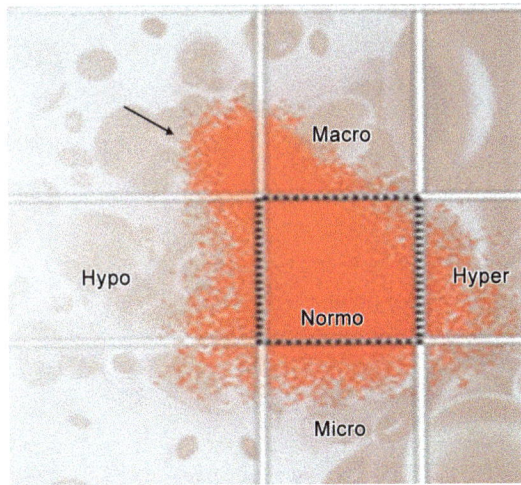

Courtesy: © Siemens Healthcare GmbH 2020

CASE NO. 11 HEMOLYTIC DISEASE OF NEWBORN

HISTORY

This case is a neonate delivered during the 38th week of gestation with signs of fetal distress.

The evaluation revealed a low Apgar score, a positive Coombs test, and raised total bilirubin. It was diagnosed to be a case of Rh incompatibility.

OBSERVATION

WBC

The histogram shows a predominant lymphocytic population that begins at approximately 45% above baseline.

This is classical presentation when normoblasts (nucleated red cell) are present.

The NRBCs interference is significant and obvious because neonatal NRBCs are usually large and the same size as the lymphocytes.

Both mixed cell population and neutrophil are relatively suppressed.

RBC

The histogram shows a very broad curve that peaks at 102 fL. The increased RDW indicates RBC heterogeneity. The histogram shows an increased incidence of cells in the region at 150–250 fL due to numerous nucleated red cells.

Platelet

The histogram shows the presence of large platelets as well as red cell fragments. The upper discriminator was automatically set at 22 fL to eliminate the fragments.

DIAGNOSIS

Hemolytic disease of newborn.

WBC	–	43.8 × 10³/μL
LY	–	39%
MO	–	6%
GR	–	55%
RBC	–	5.2 × 10⁶/μL
Hgb	–	16.7 g/dL
Hct	–	53%
MCV	–	106 fL
MCHC	–	30 g/dL
RDW	–	22%
PLT	–	149 × 10³/μL

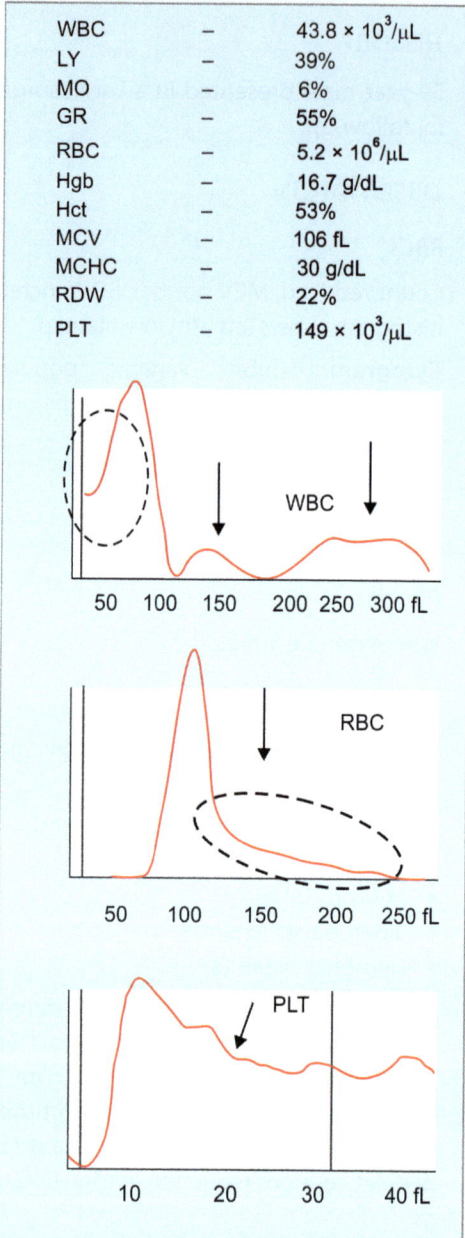

CASE NO. 12 COLD AGGLUTININS

HISTORY

A 25-year-old male with fever, cough, and chest pain.

OBSERVATION

RBC

- RBC count is low
- Hematocrit is within the accepted range
- MCV is too high
- MCHC is also high
- RDW is elevated
- Histogram: Bimodal RBC histogram peaks at a wide apart distance of 90 fL and 150 fL.

Cytogram shows a bizarre spread of the red cell population. The doublets and triplets of agglutinated RBCs are plotted in the macrocytic zone of the cytogram.

WBC

Polymorphonuclear leukocytosis.

Platelet

Within normal limits.

DISCUSSION

High MCHC has limited diagnostic possibilities; diseases with high MCHC like Hereditary spherocytosis can be excluded in this case due to high RDW and unusual RBC vs hemoglobin.

Low RBCs disproportionate to the level of hemoglobin with normal Hct and very high MCV, MCHC, and markedly increased RDW along with bimodal RBC histogram peaks at wide apart a distance of 90 fL and 150 fL is pathognomonic of red cells agglutinins.

Polymorphonuclear leukocytosis is due to infective pathology.

DIAGNOSIS

Cold agglutinins.

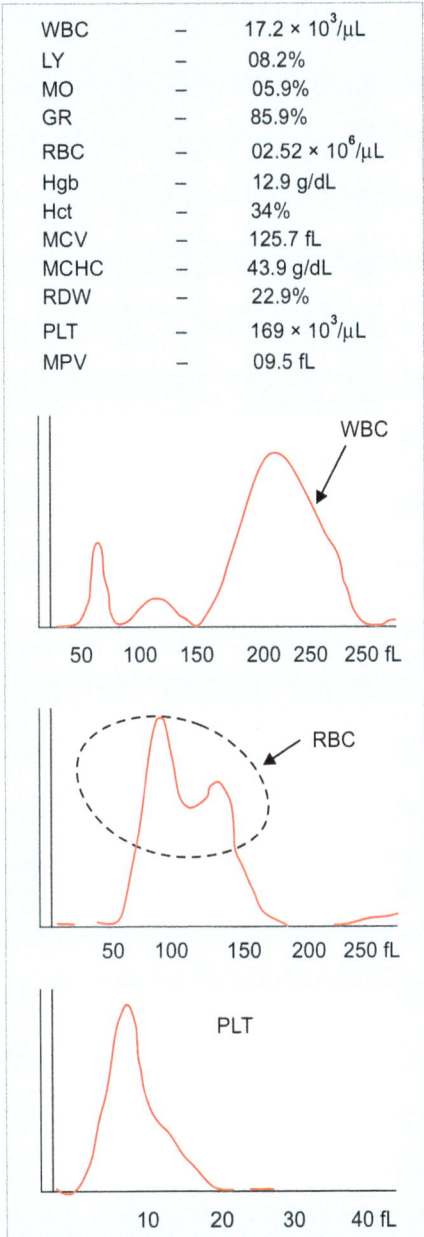

WBC	–	$17.2 \times 10^3/\mu L$
LY	–	08.2%
MO	–	05.9%
GR	–	85.9%
RBC	–	$02.52 \times 10^6/\mu L$
Hgb	–	12.9 g/dL
Hct	–	34%
MCV	–	125.7 fL
MCHC	–	43.9 g/dL
RDW	–	22.9%
PLT	–	$169 \times 10^3/\mu L$
MPV	–	09.5 fL

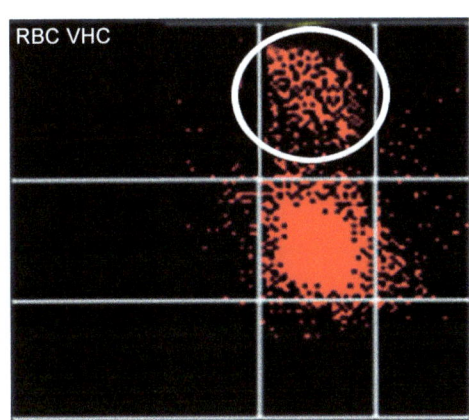

Courtesy: © Siemens Healthcare GmbH 2020

CASE NO. 13 APLASTIC ANEMIA

HISTORY

A case of a 68-year-old male presented with petechial hemorrhage and anemia.

OBSERVATION

- RBC count decreased
- WBC count decreased
- Platelet count decreased
- RDW within normal limits.

HISTOGRAMS

WBC

The histogram shows a predominant lymphocyte curve. The increased lymphocyte population is relative to neutropenia (Relative lymphocytosis).

RBC

The histogram is unremarkable except for an incidence of a shoulder (bump) on the curve from approximately 105–125 fL, which may be due to a small number of neocytes (macrocytes) produced by the patient's own.

RBC cytogram is showing cell condensation in the macrocytic zone also.

Platelet

The histogram shows a severely depressed curve due to a markedly decreased platelet count.

The floating upper discriminator is automatically set at 10 fL to produce a platelet count of $7 \times 10^3/\mu L$.

The MPV was not determined due to the depressed curve.

Bone marrow biopsy confirmed hypoplasia of all myeloid cell lines characteristic of severe aplastic anemia.

DIAGNOSIS

Aplastic anemia.

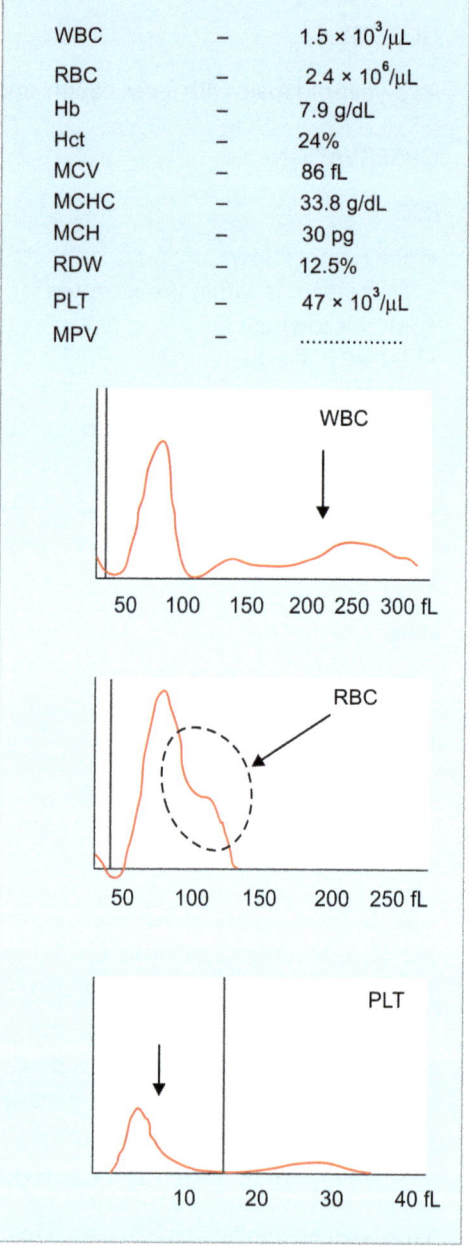

WBC	–	$1.5 \times 10^3/\mu L$
RBC	–	$2.4 \times 10^6/\mu L$
Hb	–	7.9 g/dL
Hct	–	24%
MCV	–	86 fL
MCHC	–	33.8 g/dL
MCH	–	30 pg
RDW	–	12.5%
PLT	–	$47 \times 10^3/\mu L$
MPV	–	....

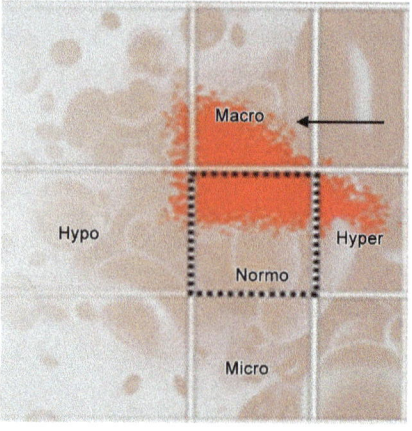

CASE NO. 14 RECOVERY FROM APLASTIC ANEMIA

HISTORY

A 75-year-old male with the history of anemia treated with repeated transfusions and medication. Counts done on recovery and follow-up visits to the physicians.

OBSERVATION

RBCs

Mild reduction in number of RBCs with macrocytosis (increased MCV) with normal heterogeneity (normal RDW).

WBCs

Counts are normal with normal differential count.

Platelet

Reduced platelets with lower normal MPV.

DISCUSSION

Homogeneous macrocytosis (normal RDW and increased MCV) is seen in the cases of:
- Preleukemia
- Early vitamin B_{12} deficiency
- Recovery from aplastic anemia.

Mild thrombocytopenia with borderline lower MPV also favors the above differential diagnosis. With high MCV the most important differential diagnosis is vitamin B_{12} and folate deficiency. But in absence of the past history with homogeneous macrocytosis (normal RDW and increased MCV) the data leads to the diagnosis of recovery from aplastic anemia.

DIAGNOSIS

Aplastic anemia.

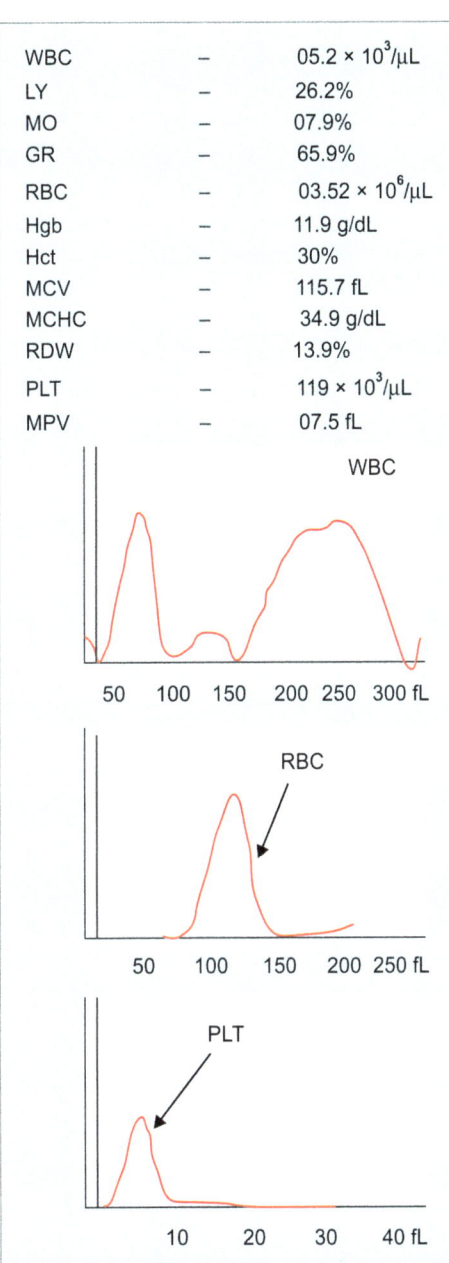

WBC	–	$05.2 \times 10^3/\mu L$
LY	–	26.2%
MO	–	07.9%
GR	–	65.9%
RBC	–	$03.52 \times 10^6/\mu L$
Hgb	–	11.9 g/dL
Hct	–	30%
MCV	–	115.7 fL
MCHC	–	34.9 g/dL
RDW	–	13.9%
PLT	–	$119 \times 10^3/\mu L$
MPV	–	07.5 fL

CASE NO. 15 BIMODAL RBC CURVE-TRANSFUSION RELATED

HISTORY

An 88-year-old patient was admitted with anemia secondary to GI bleed.

Anemia profile and coagulation testing supported a diagnosis of anemia due to blood loss.

The post-transfusion hemogram revealed:

OBSERVATION

WBC

The histogram shows an increase in neutrophil population of (88%) otherwise normal.

RBC

The histogram shows a bimodal curve of almost two equal portions.

The peak to the left is composed primarily of the transfused cells; the peak to the right consists of the patient's original cells.

The RDW on the histogram was not reported due to the multiple peak error.

By manually moving the discriminators (line between RBC histogram shown with an arrow), it is possible to identify and measure these two populations of red cells separately.

The patient's original red cell population shows a microcytosis due to chronic blood loss with a moderate reticulocyte response whereas transfused cells are in the normocytic zone.

Cytogram: Red cell cytogram is wide and shows two distinct red cell populations in the microcytic and normocytic zone.

Platelet

Unremarkable.

DIAGNOSIS

Post-transfusion sample.

WBC	–	9.3×10^3
RBC	–	2.8×10^6
Hb	–	8.9 g/dL
Hct	–	25%
MCV	–	103 fL
MCH	–	31.8 pg
MCHC	–	30.6 g/dL
RDW	–	....
PLT	–	188×10^3
MPV	–	10.9 fL

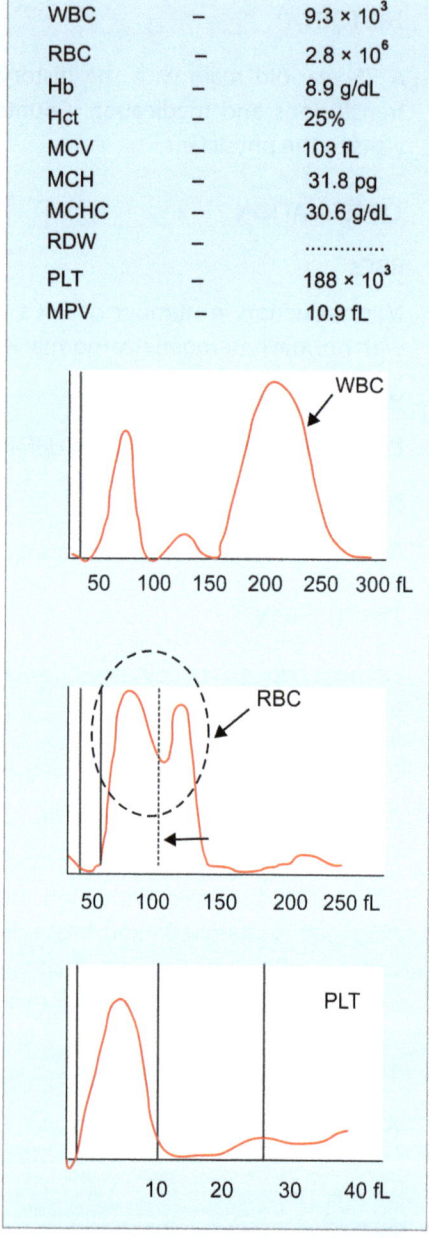

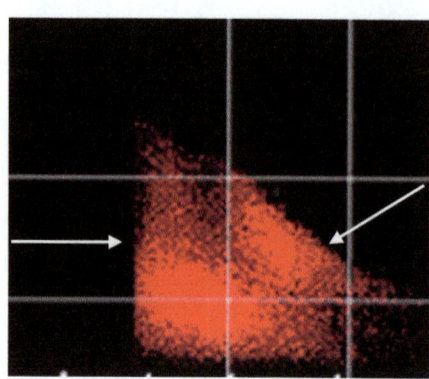

Courtesy: © Siemens Healthcare GmbH 2020

CASE NO. 16 ACUTE LYMPHOCYTIC LEUKEMIA

HISTORY

An 11-year-old male with complaints of fever. CBC was done but the histogram could not be interpreted because of an extremely high WBC count.

HISTOGRAM INTERPRETATION UNDILUTED SPECIMEN

WBC

The histogram shows a curve which neither starts nor ends at the baseline. This is due to an extremely high WBC count.

RBC

The histogram shows evidence of WBC interference especially from 125 to 250 fL. The upper discriminator automatically set at 200 fL attempting to eliminate some of these interferences.

Platelet

The histogram shows a decreased MPV and evidence of particles approaching the size of platelets. The floating upper discriminator is automatically set at 20 fL these particles are probably WBC cytoplasmic fragments.

The blood sample was diluted by 1:4 dilutions and CBC was performed again to obtain results within linearity specifications.

HISTOGRAM OF DILUTED SPECIMEN

WBC

The **histogram** shows a predominantly lymphocytic curve which begins approximately 20% above the normal baseline. This is due to the presence of microblasts and a rare NRBC. Both mixed cell and neutrophil data are suppressed with the lack of a neutrophil peak.

Scatterogram showing cell population of **LUC's with the apparent absence of neutrophils**. The **Baso channel** shows a **blast** indication (red circle). LUC is evident on the perox cytogram (red circle).

RBC

Histogram normal.

Platelet

The histogram is depressed due to the low count of the diluted sample. The MPV is not determined.

Bone marrow aspirate smear shows almost total infiltration with lymphoblasts typical of acute lymphoblastic leukemia.

DIAGNOSIS

Acute lymphoblastic leukemia.

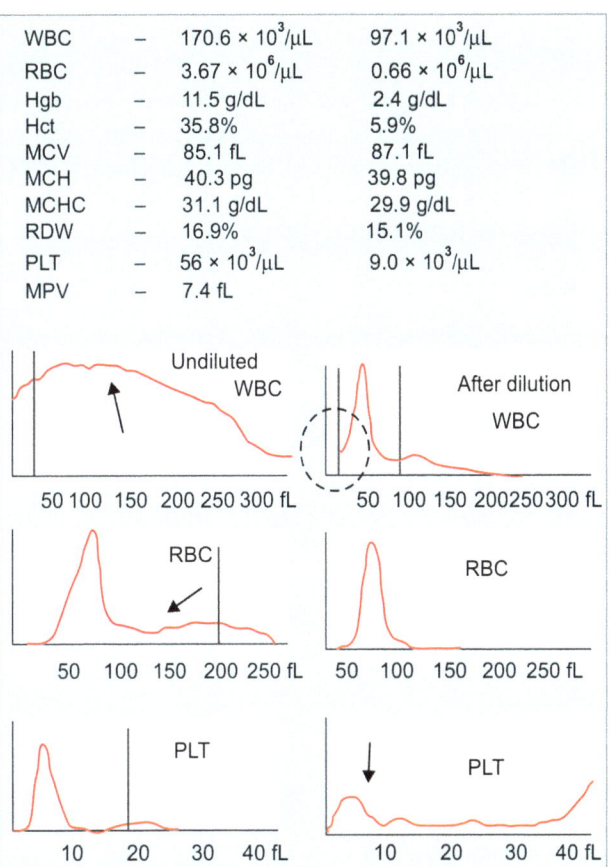

WBC	—	170.6 × 10³/µL	97.1 × 10³/µL
RBC	—	3.67 × 10⁶/µL	0.66 × 10⁶/µL
Hgb	—	11.5 g/dL	2.4 g/dL
Hct	—	35.8%	5.9%
MCV	—	85.1 fL	87.1 fL
MCH	—	40.3 pg	39.8 pg
MCHC	—	31.1 g/dL	29.9 g/dL
RDW	—	16.9%	15.1%
PLT	—	56 × 10³/µL	9.0 × 10³/µL
MPV	—	7.4 fL	

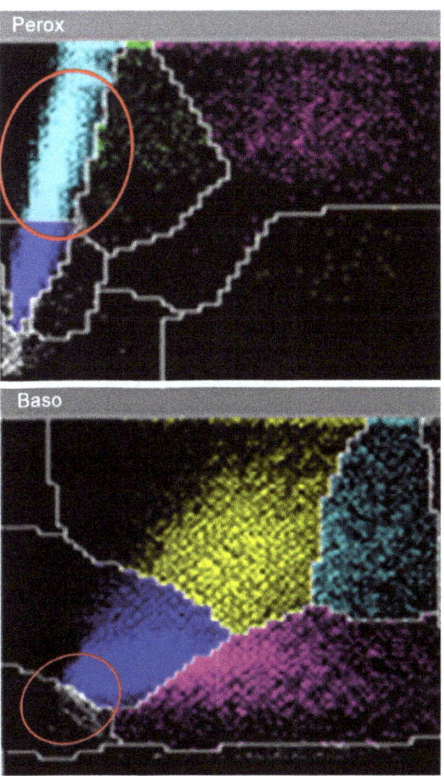

Courtesy: © Siemens Healthcare GmbH 2020

CASE NO. 17 SEPTICEMIA

HISTORY

This case is a 52-year-old male, who underwent GI surgery.

Postoperative sepsis was documented with positive blood cultures. The accompanying hemogram demonstrates the left shift of granulocytes.

OBSERVATION—HISTOGRAM

WBC

The histogram shows very little delineation or valley between the mixed cells and neutrophil populations.

This is due to the presence of immature neutrophils that lie on the ascending neutrophilic slope.

The trimodal histogram demonstrates an increased neutrophil population and a decreased lymphocyte population.

Scattergrams are showing LEFT SHIFT (increased band cells).

RBC

Unremarkable.

Platelet

Unremarkable
Other findings
Band cells present ++
Toxic granulation ++
Blood culture positive for staph.

DIAGNOSIS

Postoperative sepsis.

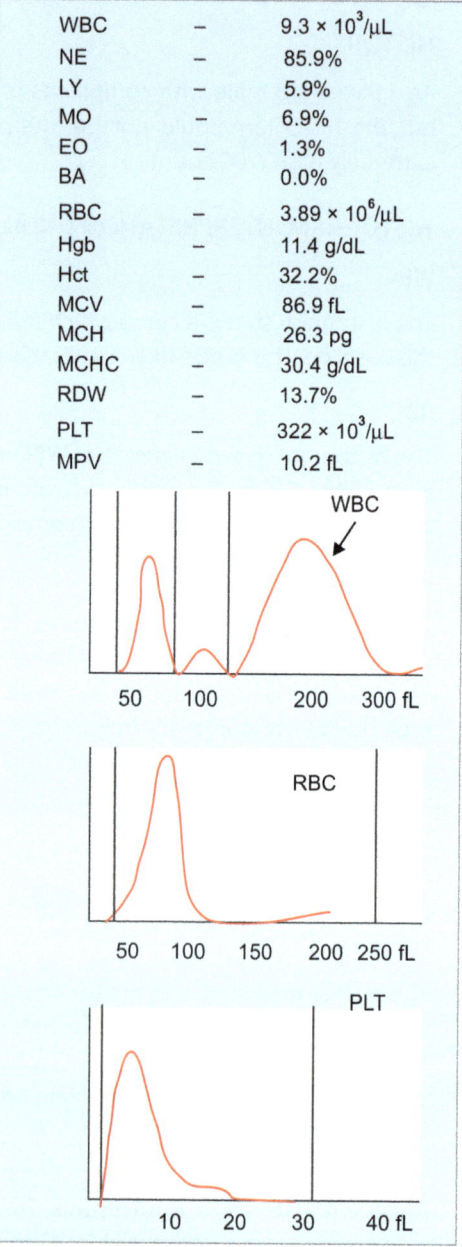

WBC	–	$9.3 \times 10^3/\mu L$
NE	–	85.9%
LY	–	5.9%
MO	–	6.9%
EO	–	1.3%
BA	–	0.0%
RBC	–	$3.89 \times 10^6/\mu L$
Hgb	–	11.4 g/dL
Hct	–	32.2%
MCV	–	86.9 fL
MCH	–	26.3 pg
MCHC	–	30.4 g/dL
RDW	–	13.7%
PLT	–	$322 \times 10^3/\mu L$
MPV	–	10.2 fL

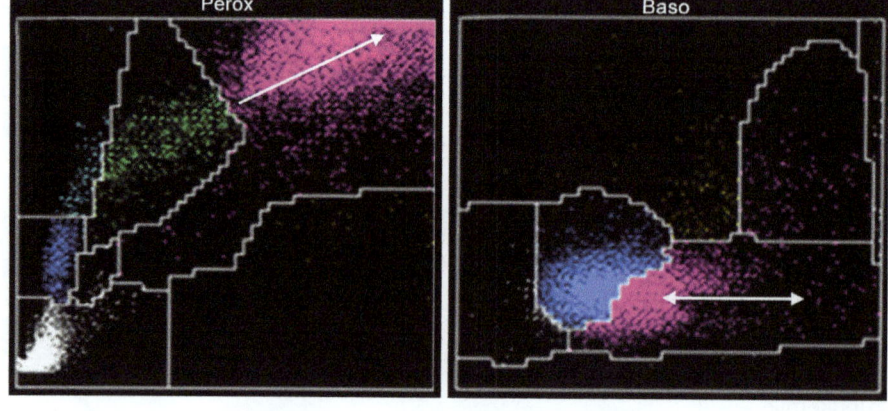

Courtesy: © Siemens Healthcare GmbH 2020

CASE NO. 18 MULTIPLE MYELOMA

HISTORY

A 70-year-old male admitted for evaluation of severe back pain and increased fatigue.

Hemogram revealed anemia.

The RDW is slightly elevated.

A moderate degree of rouleaux formation was noted on the peripheral blood smear.

The bone marrow biopsy and aspirate disclosed a marked increase in plasma cells.

Serum immunoglobulin electrophoresis indicated a monoclonal gammopathy of IgG origin.

HISTOGRAM

WBC

Unremarkable.

RBC

The histogram shows a subtle change to the angle of the ascending slope which is probably due to the presence of abnormal proteins.

Platelet

Unremarkable.

DISCUSSION

Peripheral blood smear: Rouleaux formation – moderate, anisocytosis.

Bone marrow aspirate: Smear shows clusters of pleomorphic plasma cells with occasional binucleated forms.

Serum immunoglobulin electrophoresis: Indicated a monoclonal gammopathy.

DIAGNOSIS

All the above features are suggestive of the multiple myeloma.

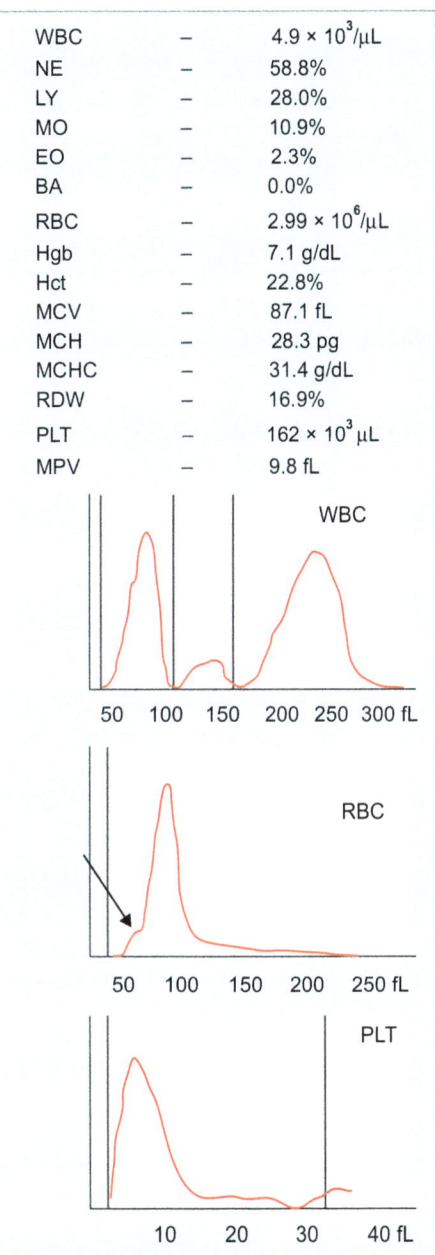

WBC	–	$4.9 \times 10^3/\mu L$
NE	–	58.8%
LY	–	28.0%
MO	–	10.9%
EO	–	2.3%
BA	–	0.0%
RBC	–	$2.99 \times 10^6/\mu L$
Hgb	–	7.1 g/dL
Hct	–	22.8%
MCV	–	87.1 fL
MCH	–	28.3 pg
MCHC	–	31.4 g/dL
RDW	–	16.9%
PLT	–	$162 \times 10^3 \mu L$
MPV	–	9.8 fL

CASE NO. 19 ACUTE MYELOID LEUKEMIA (FAB – M1)

HISTORY

A 65-year-old female with bleeding tendency, clinical findings:
Gingival hyperplasia, multiple hematomas.

WBC

The histogram shows a single curve that peaks in the mixed cell area at approximately 90 fL this is consistent with the location of myeloblasts on the trimodal WBC distribution.

Scattergram: Perox cytogram shows an increased number of undifferentiated cells in the LUC area. Baso cytogram shows plotting of blasts population in the designated blast area.

RBC

Unremarkable.

Platelet

The histogram shows a depressed curve due to the severe thrombocytopenia and the MPV data is not determined by the analyzer.

The peripheral blood smear and bone marrow aspirate smear show a predominance of myeloblast. There is presence of Auer rods in some of the myeloblasts.

Most of the blasts stain positive for the myeloperoxidase.

Cell marker studies were compatible with the diagnosis of acute myeloid leukemia.

DIAGNOSIS

Acute myeloid leukemia.

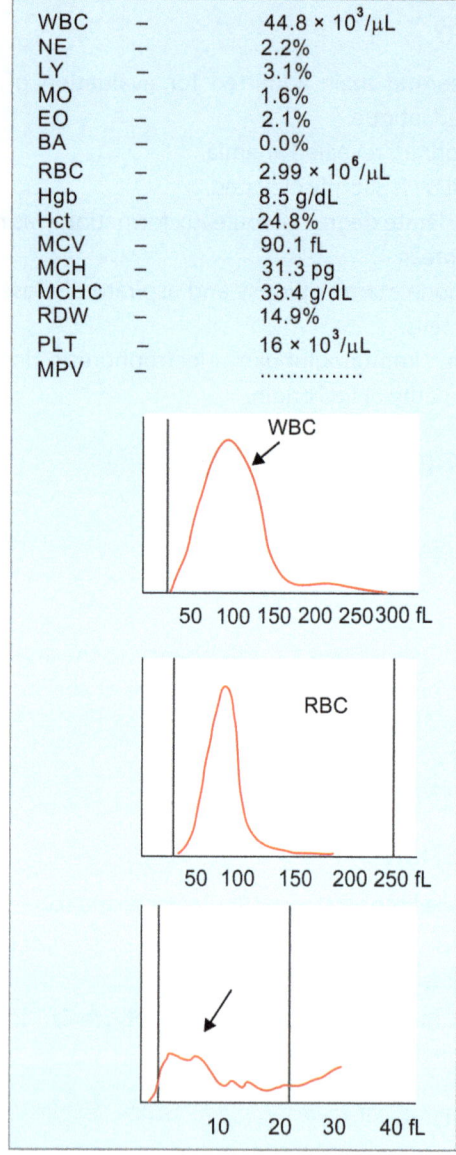

WBC	–	44.8 × 10³/μL
NE	–	2.2%
LY	–	3.1%
MO	–	1.6%
EO	–	2.1%
BA	–	0.0%
RBC	–	2.99 × 10⁶/μL
Hgb	–	8.5 g/dL
Hct	–	24.8%
MCV	–	90.1 fL
MCH	–	31.3 pg
MCHC	–	33.4 g/dL
RDW	–	14.9%
PLT	–	16 × 10³/μL
MPV	–	....

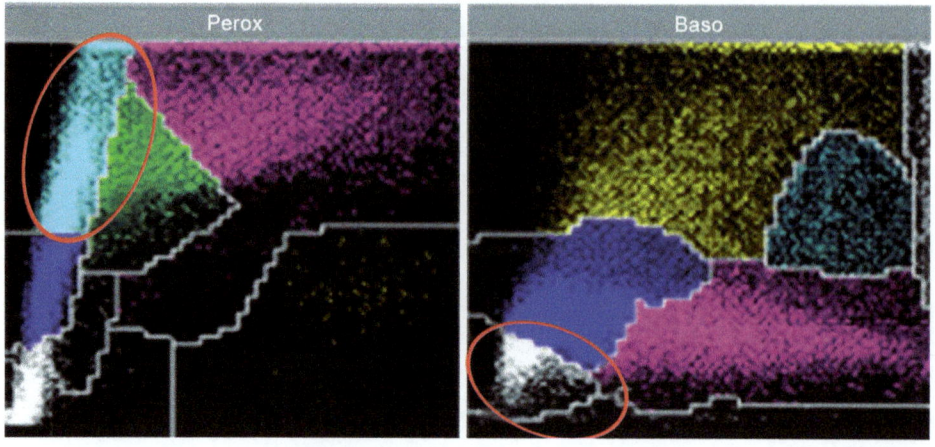

Courtesy: © Siemens Healthcare GmbH 2020

CASE NO. 20 CHRONIC LYMPHOCYTIC LEUKEMIA

HISTORY

A case of a 68-year-old male was admitted for weakness.

The hemogram revealed leukocytosis with a marked lymphocytosis and mild thrombocytopenia.

A bone marrow biopsy and aspiration evaluation confirmed the diagnosis of chronic lymphocytic leukemia (CLL).

WBC

The histogram shows a predominant lymphocyte population curve.

There appears to be little or no discernible neutrophil peak. Both mixed cell and neutrophil data were suppressed.

Scattergram: A large number of atypical lymphocytes with high % LUC. These cells are not blasts.

The cell population in the **Baso cytogram** is too dense due to the absence of neutrophils. The algorithm bisected the lymph and identifies part of the population as mononuclear (MN's) and the other part as polymorphonuclear (PMN's).

The perox cytogram and baso cytogram show an inconsistency in the neutrophils plus eos (perox) and PMN's (baso).

Peripheral Smear

Smudge cells. 15/100 WBCs

SEG—07%
L—91 %
M—01%
E—01%

RBC

Unremarkable.

Platelet

Unremarkable with slight thrombocytopenia.

DIAGNOSIS

Chronic lymphocytic leukemia

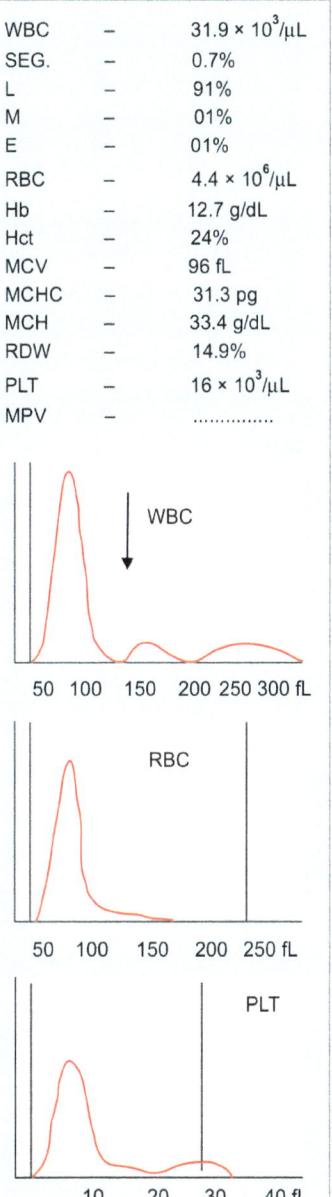

WBC	–	$31.9 \times 10^3/\mu L$
SEG.	–	0.7%
L	–	91%
M	–	01%
E	–	01%
RBC	–	$4.4 \times 10^6/\mu L$
Hb	–	12.7 g/dL
Hct	–	24%
MCV	–	96 fL
MCHC	–	31.3 pg
MCH	–	33.4 g/dL
RDW	–	14.9%
PLT	–	$16 \times 10^3/\mu L$
MPV	–	....

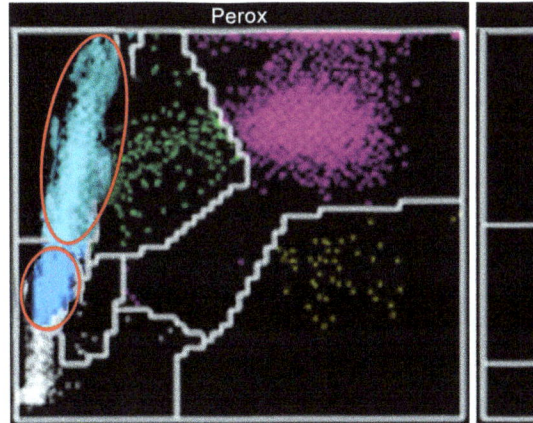
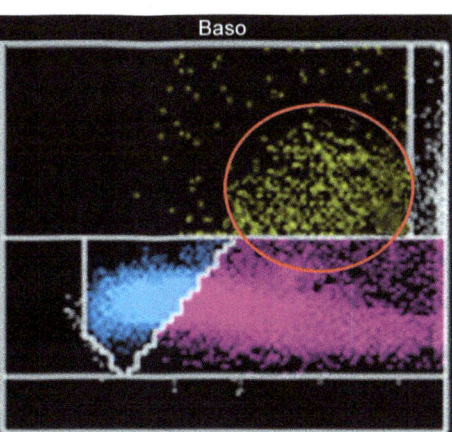

Courtesy: © Siemens Healthcare GmbH 2020

CASE NO. 21 ACUTE MYELOID LEUKEMIA (FAB – M4)

HISTORY

A 65-year-old female with bleeding tendency, clinical findings: Gingival hyperplasia, multiple hematomas.

WBC

The histogram shows a single broad but irregular curve in the mixed cell area which peaks at approximately 90 fL. This is consistent with the predominant population of monocytes and/or blast cells.
   The bump on the ascending slope is probably the lymphocytes population.
   Perox cytogram showing a population of immature myelomonocytoid cells.
   Baso cytogram showing the presence of blasts.

RBC

The curve is shifted into the microcytic region and the MCV is decreased. On the right-hand side, it is atypically-shaped and widened (RDW increased).
   The slightly atypical-shape of the left-hand side of the curve in the histogram. The reason is the presence of microcytic and fragmented cells.

Platelet

The count is markedly decreased.

SPECIAL OBSERVATIONS

Atypical monocytes and monocytoid blast.

Additional Tests

Bone Marrow
Cellularity markedly increased, megakaryocytes decreased, granulopoiesis markedly shifted to the left with 75% blasts.
Cytochemistry: The leukemic blasts are peroxidase positive, nonspecific-esterase positive.

DIAGNOSIS

Acute myelomonocytic leukemia (AML M4 by FAB classification).

WBC	–	56 × 10³/µL
NE	–	24%
LY	–	7%
MO	–	69%
EO	–	0%
BA	–	00%
RBC	–	3.92 × 10⁶/µL
Hgb	–	9.8 g/dL
Hct	–	30.2%
MCV	–	76 fL
MCH	–	24.8 pg
MCHC	–	32.2 g/dL
RDW	–	19.6%
PLT	–	28 × 10³/µL
MPV	–	8.6 fL

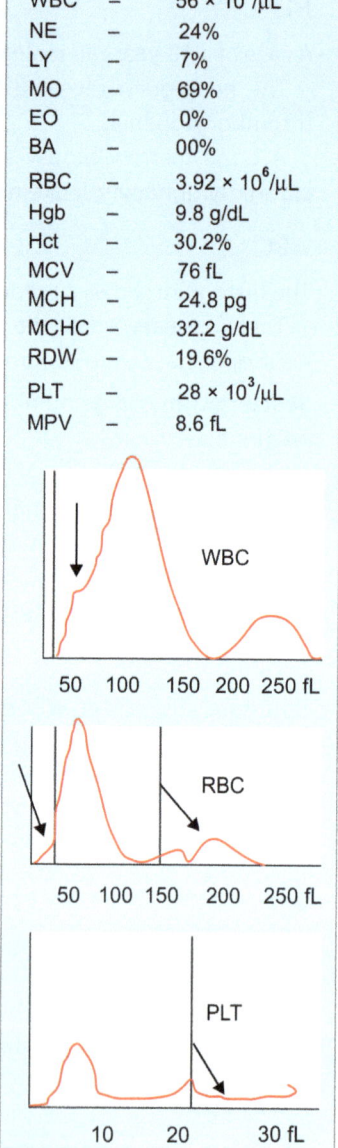

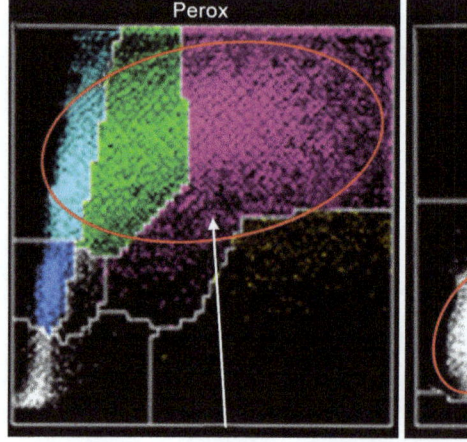
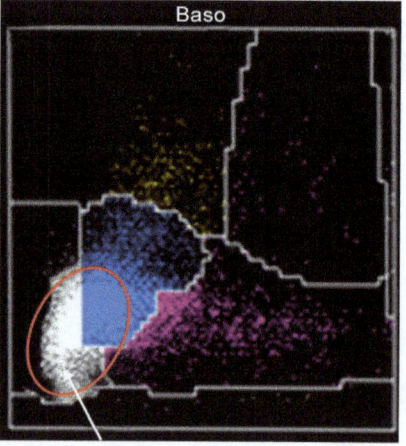

Courtesy: © Siemens Healthcare GmbH 2020

CASE NO. 22 CML IN BLAST CRISIS

HISTORY

A 62-year-old man with CML for 3 years. Presented with general deterioration and splenomegaly.

WBC

The histogram shows a broad curve with a predominant population that peaks at approximately 100 fL which is consistent with a blast population. The descending slope is greatly extended and does not return to the normal baseline at 250 fL.

Baso cytogram shows presence of blasts in the blast designated area and immature cells in the baso designated area.

RBC

The histogram shows a broad asymmetrical curve that peaks at approximately 100 fL. The descending slope is extended which suggests that macrocytes are present and account for the difference between the MCV 107 fL and the peak of the curve at 100 fL.

Platelet

The histogram is unremarkable.

MICROSCOPIC DIFFERENTIAL (%)

Blasts-55, promyelocytes-4, myelocyte-2, metamyelocyte-3, bands-9, segmented-15, lymphocytes-1, monocytes-9, eos-1, baso-1.

RBC MORPHOLOGY

Anisocytosis ++, Toxic granulation +.

CYTOCHEMISTRY

Blasts: Peroxidase negative.

FLOW CYTOMETRY

CD19 positive, CD10 positive, CyCD22 positive, CD34 mostly positive.

DISCUSSION

Although histogram findings resemble those of acute lymphatic leukemia (ALL), recognizing the present episode as part of the course of CML with predominance of lymphatic blasts is possible only with knowledge of the past history.

Blast crises in CML are myeloid 60% of the time, lymphatic (almost always B cell) 30%, and erythroid and megakaryocytic about 5% each.

DIAGNOSIS

CML in blast crisis (lymphatic variant).

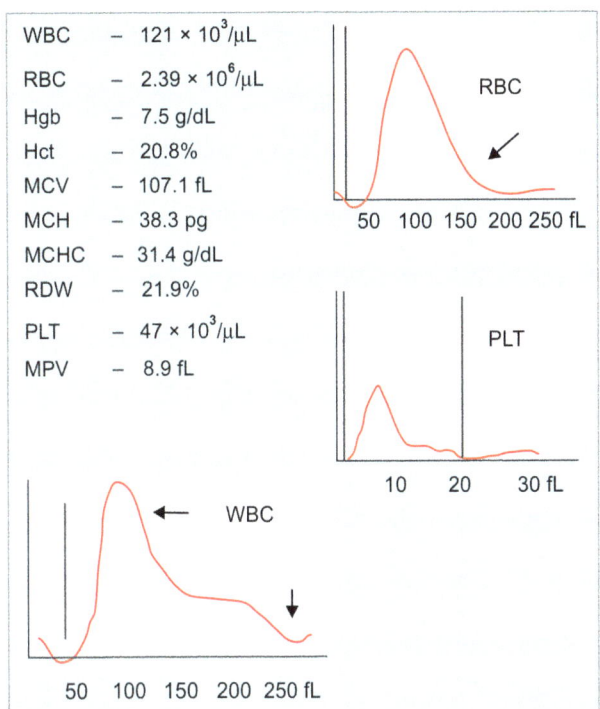

WBC	$121 \times 10^3/\mu L$
RBC	$2.39 \times 10^6/\mu L$
Hgb	7.5 g/dL
Hct	20.8%
MCV	107.1 fL
MCH	38.3 pg
MCHC	31.4 g/dL
RDW	21.9%
PLT	$47 \times 10^3/\mu L$
MPV	8.9 fL

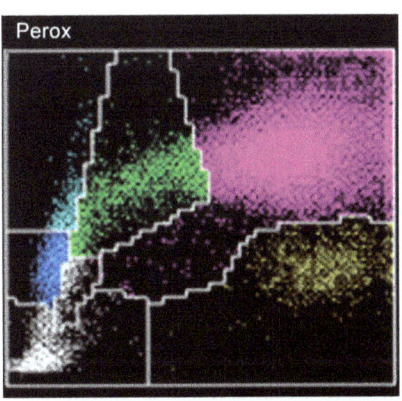

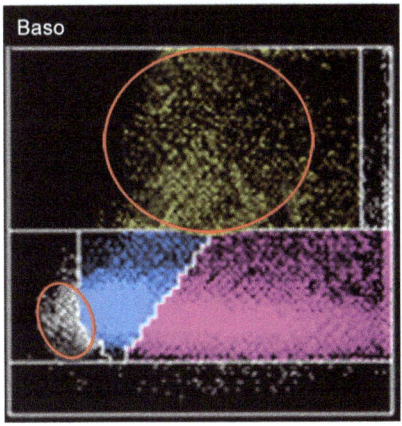

Courtesy: © Siemens Healthcare GmbH 2020

CASE NO. 23 INFECTIOUS MONONUCLEOSIS

HISTORY

A 28-year-old male presented with headache, fever, chills, and night sweats for one week.

Laboratory findings include relative and absolute lymphocytosis and abnormal liver function studies.

HISTOGRAM INTERPRETATION

WBC

The histogram shows a lymphocyte population that is unusually broad at the base of the curve.

The lymphocytes peak lies at approximately 75 fL and to the right of the normal position. This is due to the presence of a large number of reactive lymphocytes.

Manual discrimination was performed to obtain mixed cell and neutrophil data.

Cytogram: Reactive lymphocytes/Atypical mononuclear cells plotted in Lympho and LUC area of **perox** and basophil area in the **baso cytogram**.

This plotting is similar in other viral diseases as well.

RBC

Unremarkable.

Platelet

Unremarkable.

OTHER INVESTIGATIONS

Peripheral smear shows an increase in the large reactive lymphocytes typically seen in infectious mononucleosis.

Serologic tests for infectious mononucleosis were positive.

AST – 654 U/L

ALT – 689 U/L

LDH – 867 U/L

Alk. phosphatase—234 U/L.

DIAGNOSIS

Infectious mononucleosis.

WBC	–	$28.4 \times 10^3/\mu L$
NE	–	21.8%
LY	–	72.6%
MO	–	4.4%
EO	–	1.2%
BA	–	0.0%
RBC	–	$4.10 \times 10^6/\mu L$
Hgb	–	13.1 g/dL
Hct	–	37.5%
MCV	–	86.6 fL
MCH	–	31.0 pg
MCHC	–	34.9 g/dL
RDW	–	13.1%
PLT	–	$147 \times 10^3/\mu L$
MPV	–	9.8 fL

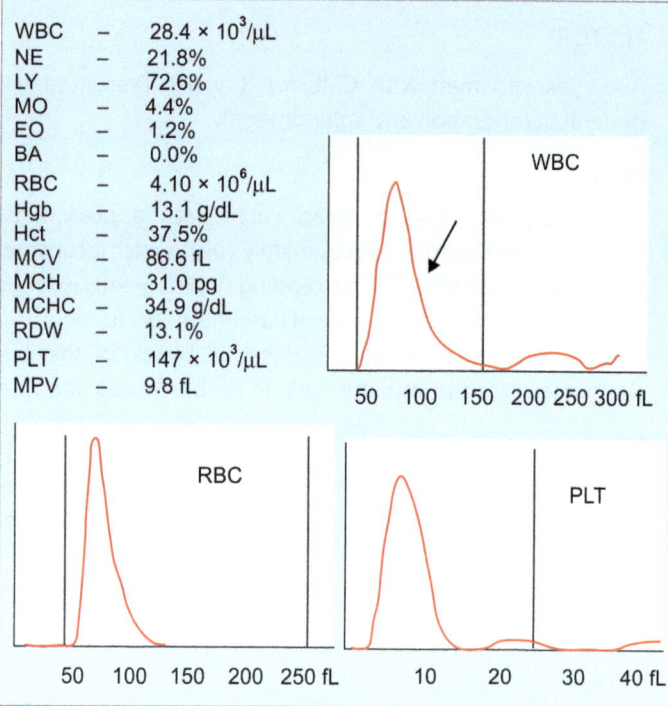

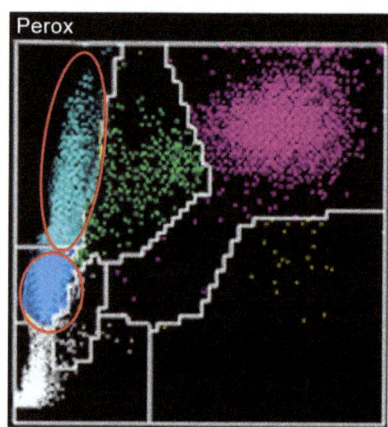

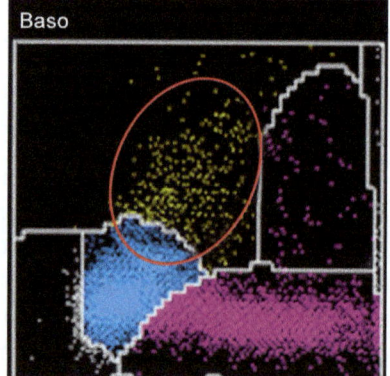

Courtesy: © Siemens Healthcare GmbH 2020

CASE NO. 24 MYELODYSPLASIA

HISTORY

A 65-year-old male was admitted for evaluation of progressing anemia.

CBC revealed pancytopenia with RDW significantly elevated to the marked heterogeneity of size of red cells.

HISTOGRAM INTERPRETATION

WBC

The histogram shows a predominant lymphocyte population that begins approximately 75% above the normal baseline.

This is consistent with the presence of an elevated number of nucleated red blood cells (NRBCs), causing the shift of graph to right and change in numerical values of the lymphocytic population.

The mixed cell and neutrophil data were suppressed due to the abnormal distribution of the cells and the inability of the T2 discriminator to set.

Scatterogram: MDS with neutrophil dysplasia in which the **neutrophils 'dip down'** in the **Perox cytogram** (arrow).

The **PMN 'tail'** seen in the **Baso cytogram** is significantly shorter than normal (arrow).

Signifying hypo lobulation and/or Pseudo Pelger–Huet neutrophils.

RBC

The histogram shows a broad asymmetrical curve with an additional peak on the left side, owing to the presence of microcytes and an extended descending slope (due to the presence of numerous large numbers of NRBCs).

Platelet

The histogram shows a ragged appearance on the descending slope possibly due to large platelets or microcytic red cells.

The MPV could not be determined by the analyzer because the platelet curve does not return to the baseline.

PERIPHERAL SMEAR

Reveals a significant number of NRBCs (87/100 WBCs), anisocytosis, poikilocytosis, target cells, schistocytes and, polychromasia.

A battery of investigations including bone marrow performed revealed the—diagnosis of myelodysplasia.

DIAGNOSIS

Myelodysplasia.

WBC	–	$4.8 \times 10^3/\mu L$
NE	–	38.8%
LY	–	55.0%
MO	–	4.9%
EO	–	1.3%
BA	–	0.0%
RBC	–	$1.99 \times 10^6/\mu L$
Hgb	–	7.5 g/dL
Hct	–	20.8%
MCV	–	107.1 fL
MCH	–	38.3 pg
MCHC	–	31.4 g/dL
RDW	–	24.9%
PLT	–	$189 \times 10^3/\mu L$
MPV	–	....

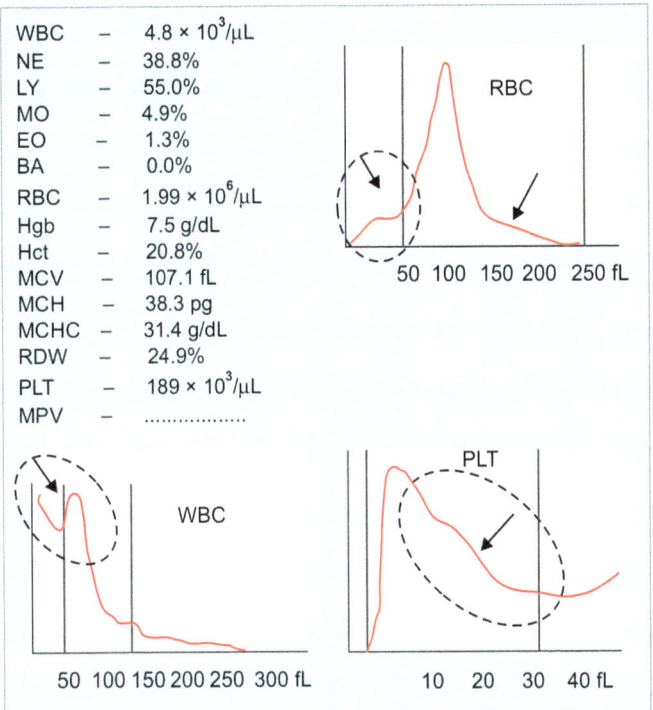

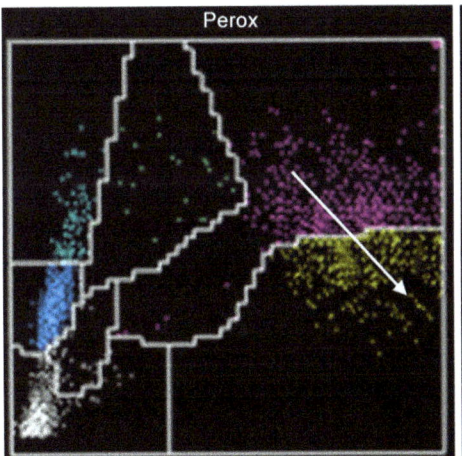

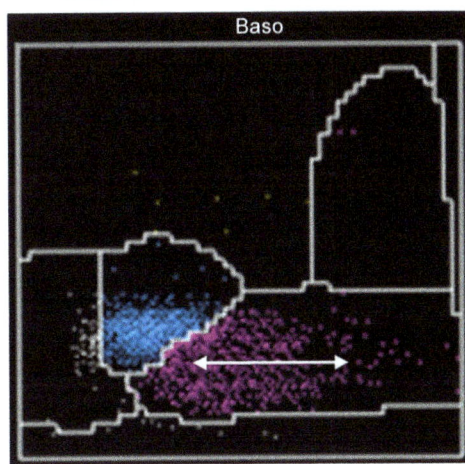

Courtesy: © Siemens Healthcare GmbH 2020

CASE NO. 25 CYTOTOXIC CHEMOTHERAPY

HISTORY
A 55-year-old female with breast malignancy receiving chemotherapy.

OBSERVATION

RBC

Normocytic (normal MCV) without any heterogeneity of cell population (Normal RDW) with reduced RBC count.

WBC

Marked leukopenia with predominant presence of lymphocytes that is also reflected in the WBC histogram.

Platelet

Marked thrombocytopenia with low MPV.
Overall picture is that of impaired production of all cell lineages.

DISCUSSION

The hypoplastic picture may be seen in:
* Aplastic (hypoplastic) anemia
* Megaloblastic anemia
* Severe sepsis
* MDS
* Drug-induced or postradiation marrow depression.

INTERPRETATION

Normocytic homogeneous red cell population (normal MCV and normal RDW) rule out the possibilities of MDS, aplastic and megaloblastic anemia.
   Marked thrombocytopenia with low MPV excludes peripheral platelet destruction.
   Marked reduction in the count is unlikely in sepsis although the condition needs clinical correlation.
This type of normocytic RBCs with hypoplastic cell count picture is suggestive of "drug-induced marrow depression or metastatic marrow replacement".

DIAGNOSIS

Drug-induced marrow depression.

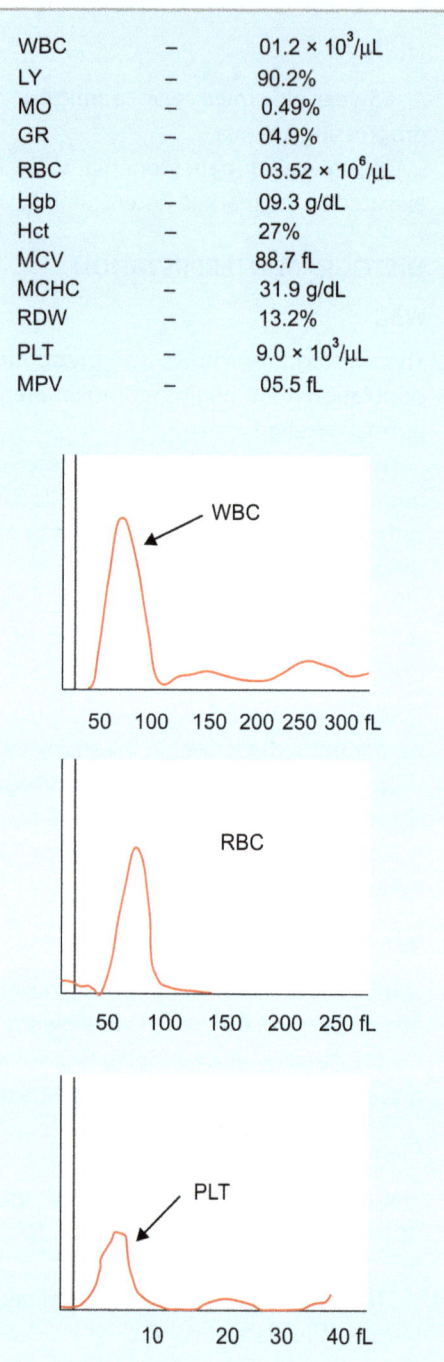

WBC	–	$01.2 \times 10^3/\mu L$
LY	–	90.2%
MO	–	0.49%
GR	–	04.9%
RBC	–	$03.52 \times 10^6/\mu L$
Hgb	–	09.3 g/dL
Hct	–	27%
MCV	–	88.7 fL
MCHC	–	31.9 g/dL
RDW	–	13.2%
PLT	–	$9.0 \times 10^3/\mu L$
MPV	–	05.5 fL

CASE NO. 26 EOSINOPHILIA

HISTORY

The case is of a 59-year-old female with a history of cardiac disease admitted for chest pain.

CBC revealed marked eosinophilia.

WBC

The histogram shows a strikingly increased mixed cell curve which peaks at 95 fL due to eosinophilia. When eosinophils are the predominant cell in the mixed cell population; they will generally peak to the right of the usual monocyte peak location (90 fL), which is on the left of mid cell population peak in a trimodal WBC curve.

Scatterogram: Increased eosinophils being exhibited in both the Baso and Perox channels.

The eosinophils will fall in the specific **Eosinophill threshold area** in the **Perox channel**.

The eosinophils will fall in the **belly of the worm** in the **Baso channel** as a result of the band form eosinophils.

RBC

Unremarkable.

Platelet

Unremarkable.

DISCUSSION

Eosinophilia is seen in various sets of situations, including:
* **Allergic disorders:** Asthma, allergic vasculitis, hay fever, eczema, serum sickness.
* **Drug allergy:** Penicillin, sulfonamides, aspirin, cephalosporin, etc.
* **Parasitic infections:** Cysticercosis, helminthiasis, filariasis, etc.
* **Malignancies:** CML, Ca. stomach, Ca. lung, Hodgkin's lymphoma, etc.
* **Hypereosinophilic syndrome:** Idiopathic and secondary.

DIAGNOSIS

Eosinophilia.

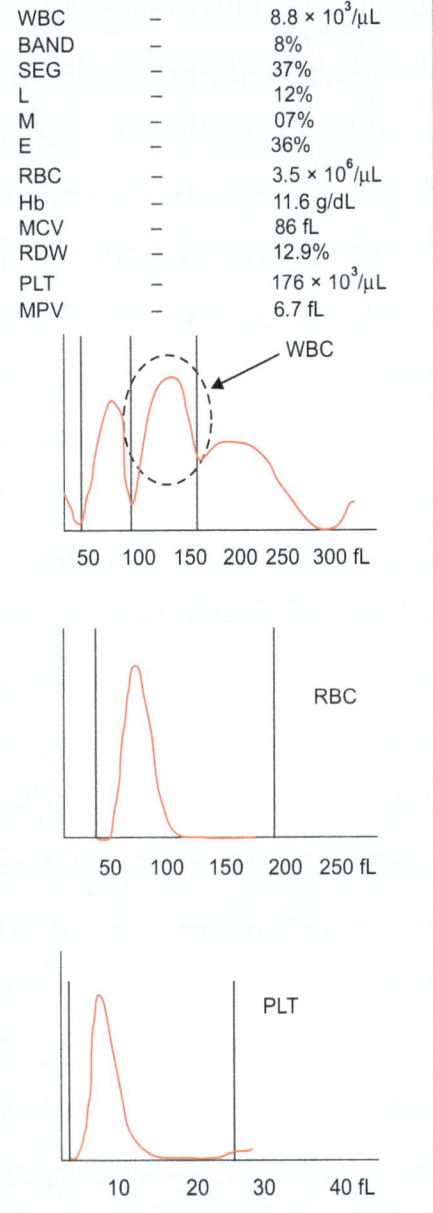

WBC	–	$8.8 \times 10^3/\mu L$
BAND	–	8%
SEG	–	37%
L	–	12%
M	–	07%
E	–	36%
RBC	–	$3.5 \times 10^6/\mu L$
Hb	–	11.6 g/dL
MCV	–	86 fL
RDW	–	12.9%
PLT	–	$176 \times 10^3/\mu L$
MPV	–	6.7 fL

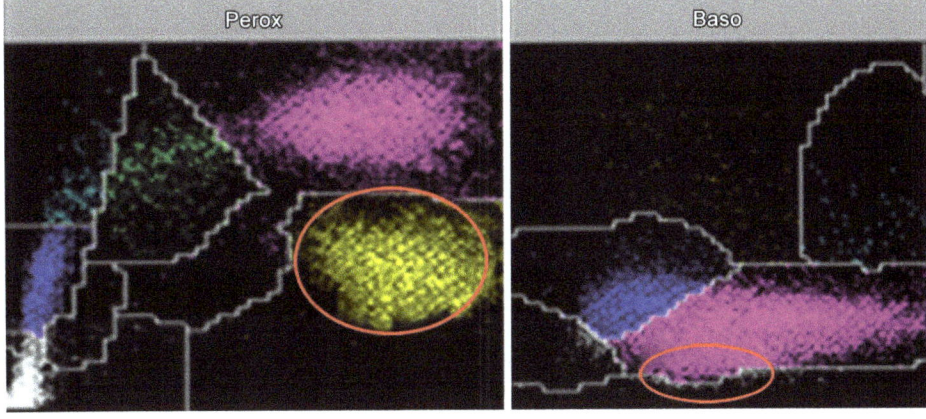

Courtesy: © Siemens Healthcare GmbH 2020

CASE NO. 27 EDTA-INDUCED PLATELET AGGLUTINATION (EIPA)

HISTORY

A 37-year-old male patient admitted with the C/O swelling of the left lower limb. Complete blood count (CBC) revealed:

WBC

The histogram and differentials are normal.

RBC

The histogram is normal.

Platelet

The count is abnormally low.

The platelet histogram patterns are consistent with platelet clumps, fragmented red cells, or ultramicrocytic red cells (black dotted circle).

Cytogram: Presence of platelet clumps in perox cytogram (red circle) and platelet scattergram.

DISCUSSION

There is an exhaustive list of causes of thrombocytopenia, if we just consider the numerical values, but the interpretation of histogram reduces the range of differential diagnosis.

The situation strongly demands a review of finger-prick peripheral smear examination.

The finger-prick direct smear showed numerous platelet clumps.

Numerically reduced platelets with adequate clumps on PS examination are indicative of: "pseudothrombocytopenia".

The causes usually include:
- EDTA-induced platelet agglutination (EIPA)
- Giant platelets
- Fragmented red cells
- Ultramicrocytic red cells.

On peripheral smear examination, there were no giant platelets, fragmented RBC, or small RBC.

DIAGNOSIS

- Pseudothrombocytopenia
- EDTA-induced platelet agglutination (EIPA)
- Confirmed by a repeat blood specimen drawn into Sodium Citrate (Na Citrate), run on an automated cell counter, revealing normal platelet count.

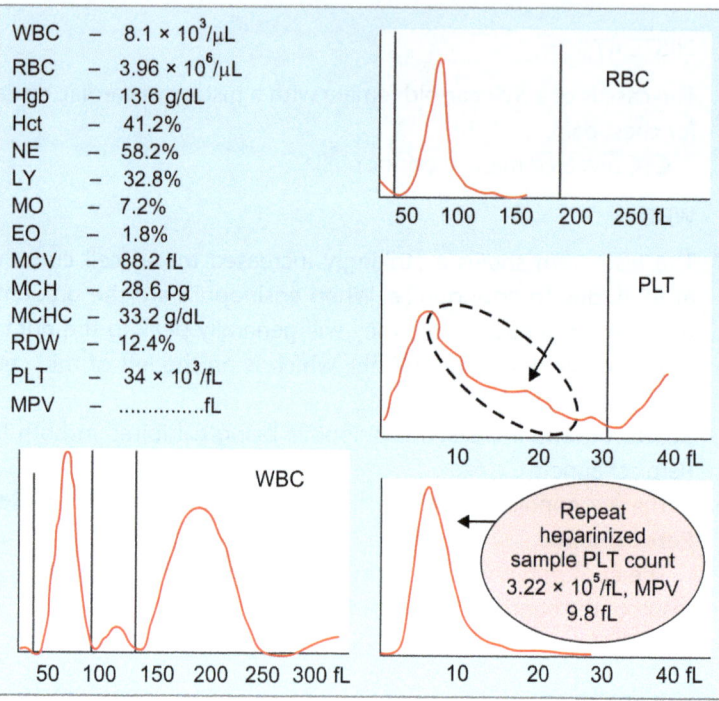

WBC	–	$8.1 \times 10^3/\mu L$
RBC	–	$3.96 \times 10^6/\mu L$
Hgb	–	13.6 g/dL
Hct	–	41.2%
NE	–	58.2%
LY	–	32.8%
MO	–	7.2%
EO	–	1.8%
MCV	–	88.2 fL
MCH	–	28.6 pg
MCHC	–	33.2 g/dL
RDW	–	12.4%
PLT	–	$34 \times 10^3/fL$
MPV	–	..............fL

Repeat heparinized sample PLT count $3.22 \times 10^5/fL$, MPV 9.8 fL

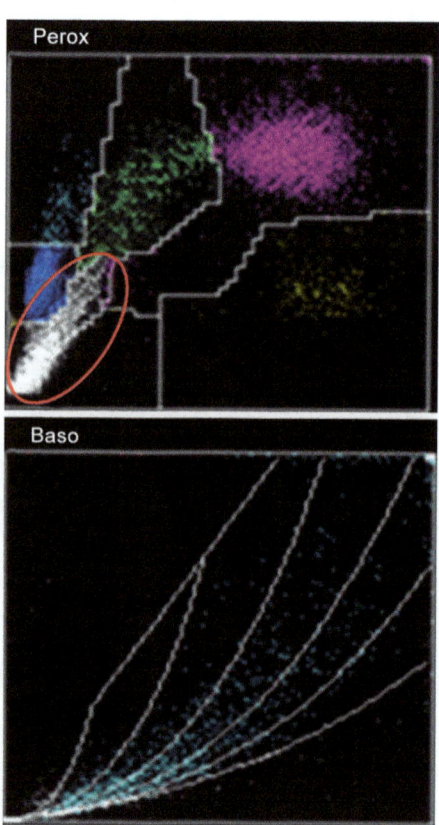

Courtesy: © Siemens Healthcare GmbH 2020

CASE NO. 28 ESSENTIAL (PRIMARY) THROMBOCYTHEMIA

HISTORY

A 37-year-old man was admitted in the trauma unit with polytrauma. A complete blood count (CBC) from the hematology analyzer revealed:

OBSERVATION

WBC

The histogram and total and differential are normal.

RBC

The histogram is normal.

Platelet

The count is remarkably high.

DISCUSSION

The causes of increased platelet counts are:
- Inflammatory disorders
- Iron deficiency anemia
- Splenectomy
- Chronic granulocytic leukemia
- Polycythemia vera
- Undetected cancer
- Essential (primary) thrombocythemia.

Since the patient had no symptoms, or any history of splenectomy, with normal WBC and RBC hemograms, the most likely diagnosis is essential (primary) thrombocythemia.

For further evaluation and confirmation of diagnosis, advice.
- Bone marrow examination (will show a significant increase in megakaryocytes and masses of platelets).
- JAK2 mutation in blood cells.

DIAGNOSIS

Essential (primary) thrombocythemia.

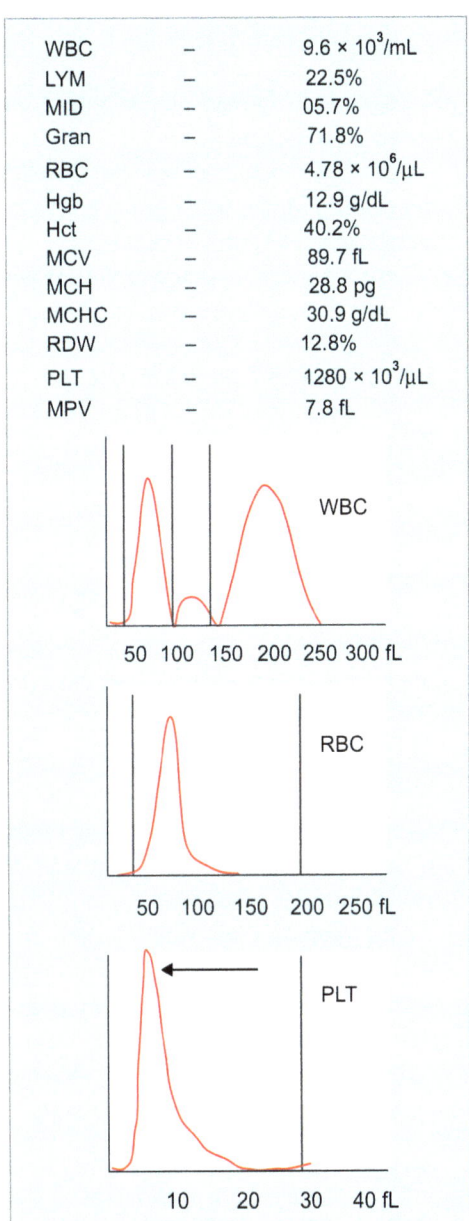

WBC	–	9.6×10^3/mL
LYM	–	22.5%
MID	–	05.7%
Gran	–	71.8%
RBC	–	4.78×10^6/µL
Hgb	–	12.9 g/dL
Hct	–	40.2%
MCV	–	89.7 fL
MCH	–	28.8 pg
MCHC	–	30.9 g/dL
RDW	–	12.8%
PLT	–	1280×10^3/µL
MPV	–	7.8 fL

CASE NO. 29 THROMBOCYTOPENIC PURPURA

HISTORY

A 60-year-old female was admitted with increased bruising. She had scattered petechiae.

CBC and other investigations revealed—thrombocytopenia, positive direct antiglobulin test, normal coagulation studies, and the presence of platelet-reactive autoantibodies.

Bone marrow biopsy and aspiration were normal except for an increased number of megakaryocytes which were morphologically unremarkable.

HISTOGRAM INTERPRETATION

WBC

Unremarkable.

RBC

Unremarkable.

Platelet

The histogram shows a broader than normal curve due to the increased size of the platelets (arrow).

DISCUSSION

Thrombocytopenia in the periphery with normal to high megakaryocytes in bone marrow indicates peripheral destruction of platelets, which is usually immune mediated.

As a general observation, when the megakaryocytes in the bone marrow are stimulated to produce platelets at a more rapid rate than normal due to peripheral destruction and challenge, as in ITP, usually the platelets produced are larger than normal.

This results in an elevated MPV. Such platelets are hemostatically more competent than normal sized platelets.

DIAGNOSIS

Idiopathic thrombocytopenic purpura.

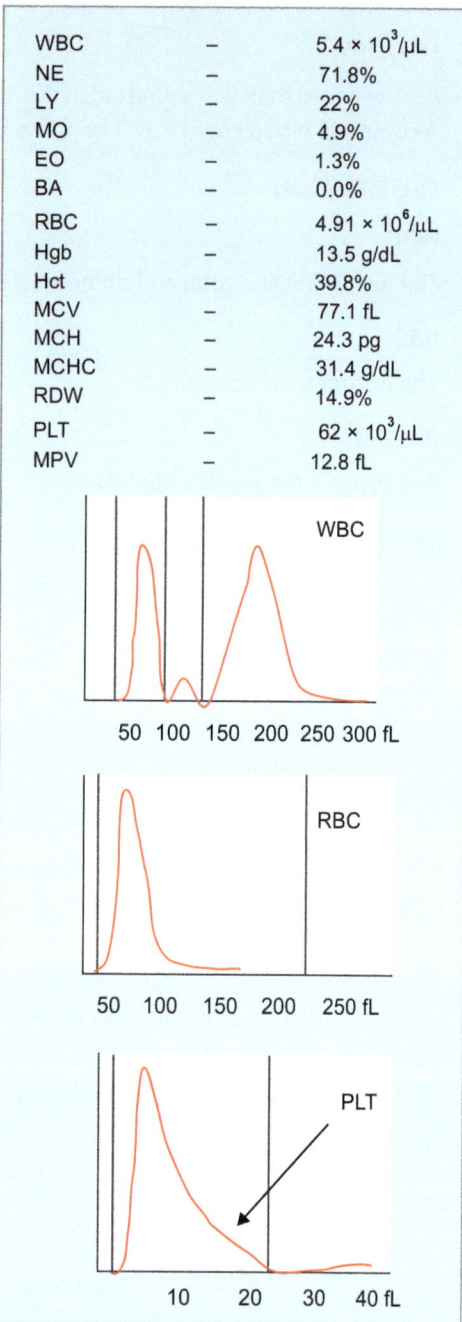

WBC	–	$5.4 \times 10^3/\mu L$
NE	–	71.8%
LY	–	22%
MO	–	4.9%
EO	–	1.3%
BA	–	0.0%
RBC	–	$4.91 \times 10^6/\mu L$
Hgb	–	13.5 g/dL
Hct	–	39.8%
MCV	–	77.1 fL
MCH	–	24.3 pg
MCHC	–	31.4 g/dL
RDW	–	14.9%
PLT	–	$62 \times 10^3/\mu L$
MPV	–	12.8 fL

CASE NO. 30 COAGULOPATHY (DIC)

HISTORY

A case of a 38-year-old female admitted for complaints of dry cough, shortness of breath, and increased bruising.

The hemogram indicated mild anemia and thrombocytopenia. After a hemostatic workup, she was diagnosed as having DIC.

WBC

The histogram shows a smaller than normal lymphocyte curve with corresponding neutrophilia.

RBC

The histogram is unremarkable but the RDW is increased which is consistent with the heterogeneity of the red cell morphology.

Platelet

The histogram is consistent with thrombocytopenia and the presence of megaplatelets evident on the descending slope of the platelet curve and raised MPV.

Extension of the descending arm of the platelet curve to the right, beyond the upper discriminator, is most likely due to the presence of red cell fragments.

DISCUSSION

Thrombocytopenia with high MPV and typical platelet histogram with ragged and extended descending arm, suggests the possibility of consumption coagulopathy.

Due to peripheral consumption of platelets and peripheral destruction, marrow was stimulated, resulting in increased production, with larger platelets.

Further investigations revealed raised D-Dimer and FDP, increased PT, and APTT.

DIAGNOSIS

Consumption coagulopathy (DIC).

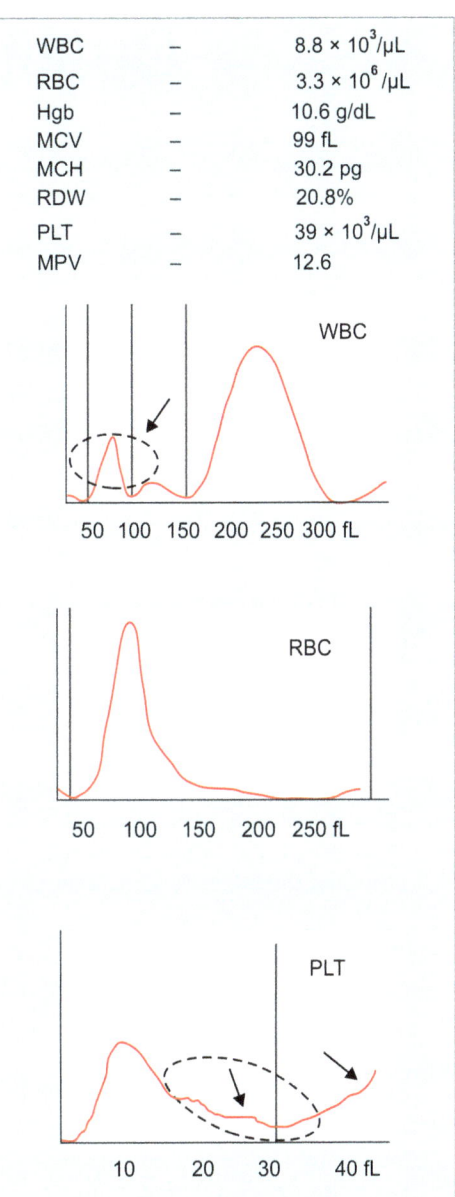

WBC	–	$8.8 \times 10^3/\mu L$
RBC	–	$3.3 \times 10^6/\mu L$
Hgb	–	10.6 g/dL
MCV	–	99 fL
MCH	–	30.2 pg
RDW	–	20.8%
PLT	–	$39 \times 10^3/\mu L$
MPV	–	12.6

CHAPTER 11

Quality Control

Courtesy: Pushpraj Singh Baghel

> Quality is not an accident, it is a product of continuous, constant commitment towards the cause —"The Quality".
> Quality implies "degree of excellence" and that of "assurance" and is the "act of giving confidence".

QUALITY ASSURANCE IN THE HEMATOLOGY LABORATORY

Quality assurance is a comprehensive and systematic process that strives to ensure reliable patient results. This process includes every level of laboratory operation. From the time a sample arrives in the laboratory until the results are reported, a rigorous quality assurance system is the key feature in ensuring quality results. Each part of the quality assurance plan or process should be analyzed, monitored, and reconfigured as necessary to emphasize excellence at every outcome.

PURPOSE OF QUALITY CONTROL (QC)

- To assure precision (a measure of reproducibility of results)
- To assure accuracy (a measure of correctness of results)
- To assure proper functionality of instrumentation
- To assure the integrity of the calibration.

Quality Control Monitoring in the Hematology Laboratory

CBC is one of the most common tests performed in the clinical laboratory. Along with clinical history, the CBC may be the first indication of a primary hematological/non-hematological abnormality, aiding the clinician with diagnosis and patient management.

With pressures for laboratories to increase productivity while decreasing costs, many are implementing auto-verification of CBC results, increasing the importance of reliable internal quality control (IQC).

Fundamental elements of any laboratory's quality management system include detailed standard operating procedures (SOPs), appropriate documentation, analyzing and monitoring QC, and external quality assessment/proficiency testing.

The analytic method in the hematology laboratory primarily includes instrumentation and reagents. For quality monitoring, both the segments are equally important and deserve attention and require a comprehensive "Quality system".

ISO defines the quality system as:
"The organizational structure, responsibilities, procedures, processes, and resources for implementing quality management".

Laboratory accreditation bodies assess the laboratories based on their quality system and accreditation is the stimulus for the quest for quality control.

Quality assurance, independent of accreditation, must be the goal of each laboratory as the test results have an important bearing on diagnostic and therapeutic decisions.

The QC program for an individual laboratory, in addition to certain essential components, also needs to take into consideration their needs, accreditation demands, and budgetary constraints.

INDIRECT QUALITY CONTROL

Indirect QC includes proper collection, identification, and labelling of the samples, hemolysis, clot or lipemia check, storage of reagents at an appropriate temperature, maintaining turnaround time, clerical error check. The various actions required for this include:

Preanalytic Variables in Quality Control

Preanalytic variables are the factors that may affect the sample before testing.

Some of the issues to be addressed are:
- Proper patient identification
- Proper phlebotomy procedure
- Proper labelling of the sample containers
- Proper anticoagulation of the sample
- Intravenous line contamination or dilution
- Timely delivery of the sample to the laboratory
- Proper mixing of the sample
- Sample tubes checked for the presence of clots
- Medications administered to the patient
- Previous blood transfusions and their influence.

Postanalytic Variables in Quality Control

Postanalytic variables refer to proceedings that ensure the integrity of the sample and precision of the final results. Some examples include:
- Delta checks
- Proper documentation of test results
- Reflex testing initiated
- Timely reporting of critical results.

Daily Start-up Procedures (Daily Maintenance)

- Daily cleaning
- Background counts
- Electronic checks
- Compare open and closed mode sampling
- Running controls.

DIRECT QUALITY CONTROL

Internal Quality Control

- This is a prospective, ongoing process on an hour to an hour and day to day basis.
- It is a continuous assessment of the performance of a particular laboratory to ensure the result's reliability.
- This involves calibration of instruments with calibrators or standards and daily monitoring with the use of controls.
- Controls should never be used for calibration of instruments.

Tools of Internal QC

Accuracy and Precision	
Accuracy	*Precision*
◆ Defined as the closeness of the result to the true (accepted) value ◆ Comparing QC terms to a target; figure illustrates that the results are accurate (in the bull's eyes) and precise (close together) ◆ Note: You cannot have accuracy without precision ◆ You can have precision without accuracy	◆ It is the agreement between repeated measurements of the same sample ◆ Defined as reproducibility of a result ◆ Comparing QC terms to a target. The figure illustrates that the results are precise (close together) but not accurate (they are not in bull's eye) ◆ It is usually expressed as standard deviation

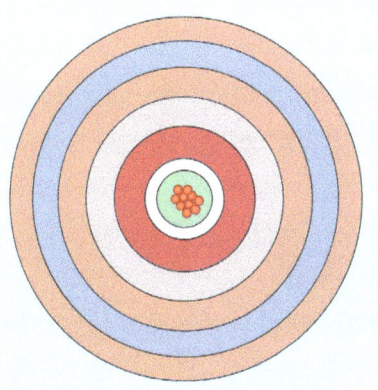
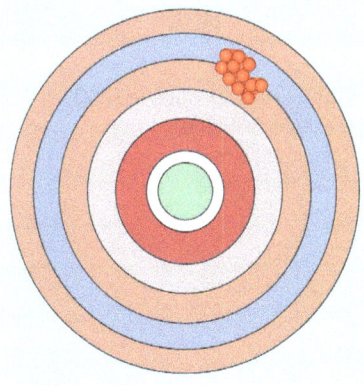

Accuracy
Refers to closeness to the true value.

Precision
Refers to reproducibility of test.

Two types of error

Systematic error (Fig. C)
- Poor accuracy
- Definite causes
- Reproducible

Random error (Fig. B)
- Poor precision
- Non-specific causes
- Not reproducible

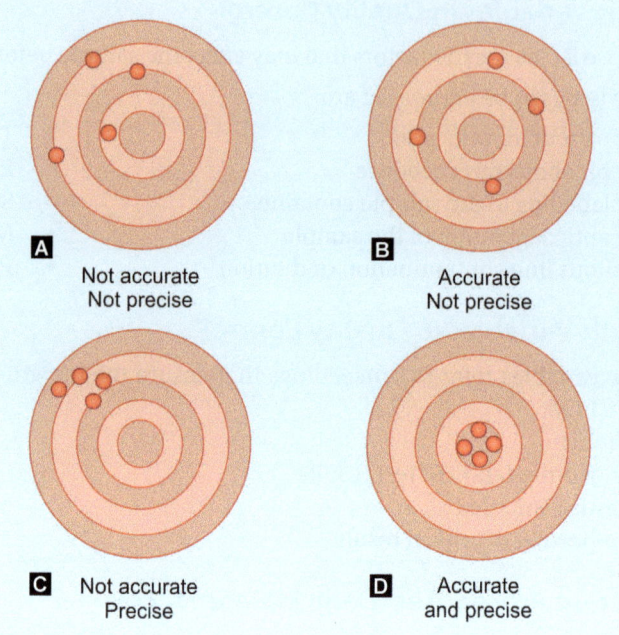

A Not accurate Not precise
B Accurate Not precise
C Not accurate Precise
D Accurate and precise

Levey Jennings Chart

- A graphical method for displaying control results and evaluating results are in-control or out-of-control
- Control values are plotted versus time
- Lines are drawn from point to point to accent any trends, shifts, or random excursions
- Ideally should have control values clustered about the mean (+/−2 SD) with little variation in the upward or downward direction
- Imprecision = large amount of scatter about the mean
- Usually caused by errors in technique
- Inaccuracy = may see as a trend or a shift, usually caused by a change in the testing process
- Random error = so pattern. Usually poor technique, malfunctioning equipment

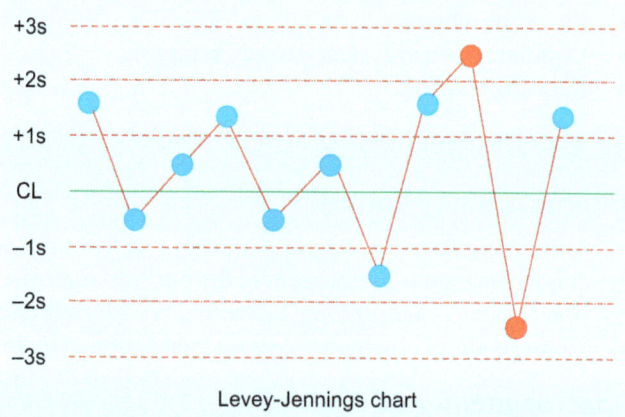

Levey-Jennings chart

Westgard Rules

- Multi-rule quality control
- Uses a combination of decision criteria or control rules
- Allows determination of whether an analytical run is "in-control" or "out-of-control"
- Commonly applied when two levels of control are used
- When a rule is violated

- Warning rule = use other rules to inspect the control points
- Rejection rule = out of control
  - Stop testing
  - Identify and correct problem
  - Repeat testing on patient samples and controls
  - Do not report patient results until the problem is solved and controls indicate proper performance

Westgard – 1_{2S} Rule

- "Warning rule"
- One of two control results fall outside ±2SD
- Alerts tech to possible problems
- Not a cause for rejecting a run
- Must then evaluate the 1_{3S} rule

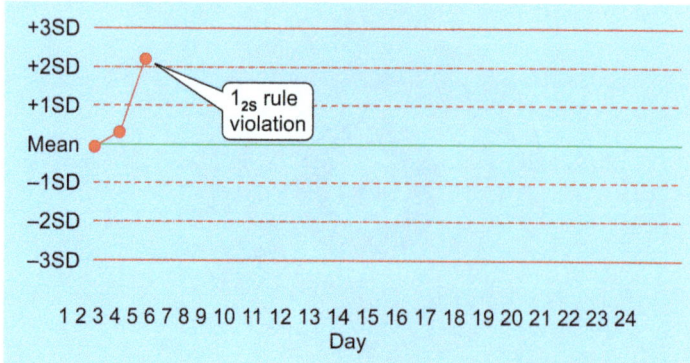

1_{2S} rule violation

Westgard – 1₃ₛ Rule

- If either of the two control results fall outside of ±3SD, rule is violated
- Run must be rejected
- If 1₃ₛ not violated, check 2₂ₛ

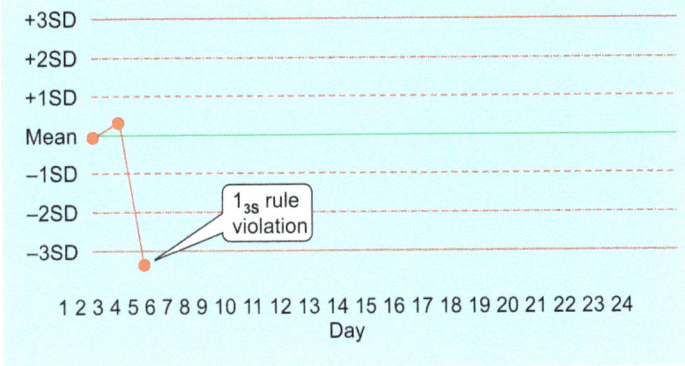

Westgard – 2₃ₛ Rule

- 2 consecutive control values for the same level fall outside of ±2SD in the same direction
- Both controls in the same run exceed ±2SD
- Patient's results cannot be reported
- Requires corrective action

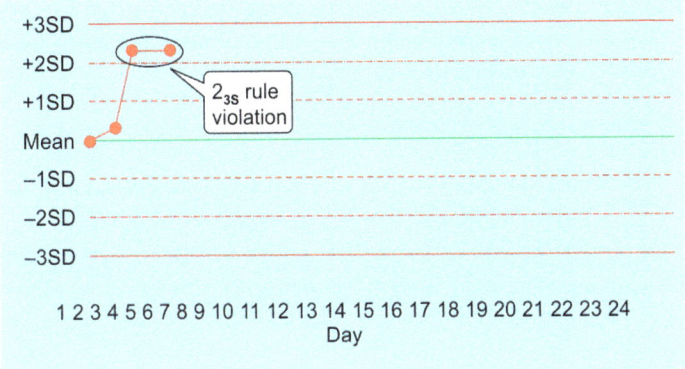

Westgard – 4₁ₛ Rule

- Requires control date from previous runs
- Four consecutive QC results for one level of control are outside ±1SD
- Both levels of control have consecutive results that are outside ±1SD

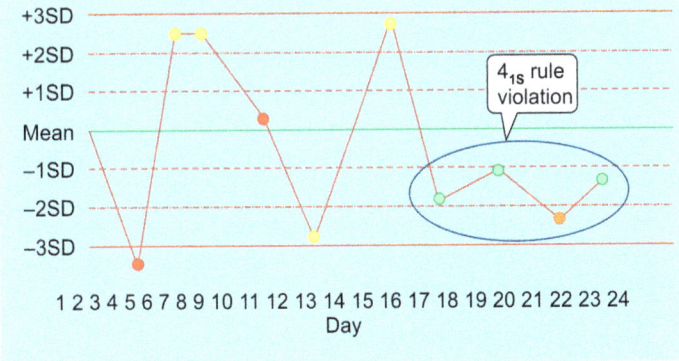

Westgard – R₄ₛ Rule

- One control exceeds the mean by –2SD and the other control exceeds the mean by +2SD
- The range between the two results will therefore exceed 4 SD
- Random error has occurred, test run must be rejected Westgard – 4₁ₛ Rule
- Requires control date from previous runs
- Four consecutive QC results for one level of control are outside ±1SD
- Both levels of control have consecutive results that are outside ±1SD

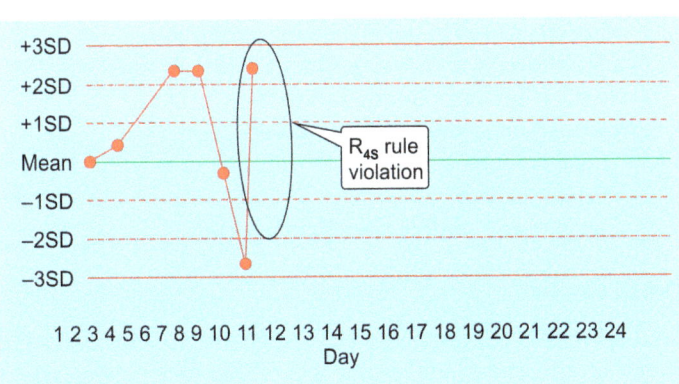

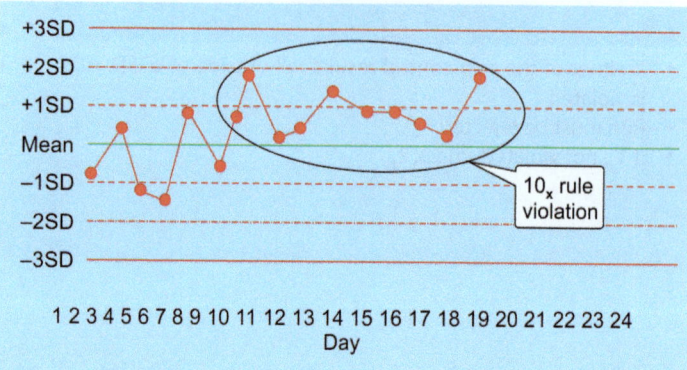

Westgard – 10_x Rule
• Requires control data from previous runs
• Ten consecutive QC results for one level of control are on one side of the mean, or
• Both levels of control have five consecutive results that are on the same side of the mean

External Quality Control

This is a retrospective process to confirm the accuracy and interlaboratory comparability.

It compares the performance of different testing sites by analyzing identical specimens allotted by an external authority. This is also termed proficiency testing.

STANDARDS OR CALIBRATORS

- Standard or calibrator are solutions having a known amount of an analyte and are used to calibrate the method.
- Standard or calibrator has one assigned or fixed, value. For example, the hemoglobin standard is 12 g/100 mL, meaning that there is exactly 12 g of hemoglobin in 100 mL of solution.
- Conversely, controls are used to monitor the performance of a method after calibration.

CONTROLS

- Controls or control materials are assayed concurrently with patient samples, and the analyze value for the controls is calculated from the calibration data in the same manner as the patient's results are calculated.
- Control materials are commercially available as stable or liquid materials that are analyzed concurrently with the unknown samples.
- The control material measured values are compared with their expected values or target range.
- Acceptance or rejection of the patient sample results is dependent on this evaluation process.
- There are three levels of control low, normal, and high.
- NABL recommendation limit: The labs must use two levels of control at least once a day.

Or

Labs working 24 × 7 will run control every 12 hours.

Quality Control Methods

- Assayed or unassayed stabilized material
  - Commercially available calibrators and control programs
  - Known values (assayed only)
  - Analyze low, normal, and high control
  - Results stored in the instrument computer
  - Monitored with Levey-Jennings charts
  - Easily illustrates trends and shifts.
- Previously analyzed patient samples
  - Easily obtained
  - Cost-effective
  - Results and samples readily available.

Delta Checks

Another method of quality control is the use of delta checks (delta means "difference") which compares a patient's values with their most previous results. If the difference between the two is greater than laboratory-set limits, the current result is immediately flagged for review. These can only be used if the instrument is interfaced with a host laboratory information system (LIS).

ANALYSIS OF QC DATA

Analysis of Control Materials
- Need data set of at least 20 points, obtained over 30 days period
- Calculate mean, standard deviation, coefficient of variation; determine target ranges
- Develop Levey-Jennings charts, plot results.

Establishing Control Ranges
- Select appropriate controls
- Assay them repeatedly over time
  - At least 20 data points
- Make sure any procedural variation is represented:
  - Different operators
  - Different times of day
- Determine the degree of variability in the data to establish an acceptable range.

Measurement of Variability
- A certain amount of variability will naturally occur when control is tested repeatedly.
- Variability is affected by operator technique, environmental conditions, and the performance characteristics of the assay method.
- The goal is to differentiate between variability due to chance from that due to error.

Measures of Central Tendency
- Data are frequently distributed about a central value or a central location
- There are several terms to describe that central location, or the 'central tendency' of a set of data
- Median = the value at the center (midpoint) of the observations
- Mode = the value which occurs with the greatest frequency
- Mean = the calculated average of the values.

Normal Distribution/Gaussian Distribution
- All values are symmetrically distributed around the mean
- Characteristic "bell-shaped" curve
- Assumed for all quality control statistics

Mean = Median = Mode

Standard deviation: It shows the dispersion of a set of values from its mean.

$$\sigma = \sqrt{\frac{\sum (x - \text{mean})^2}{n}}$$

x is a set of numbers
mean is the average of the set of numbers
n is the size of the set
σ is the standard deviation

In a normal Gaussian Curve
Out of 100 events
68 will fall in ± 1SD
95 will fall in ± 2SD
99.7 will fall in ± 3SD

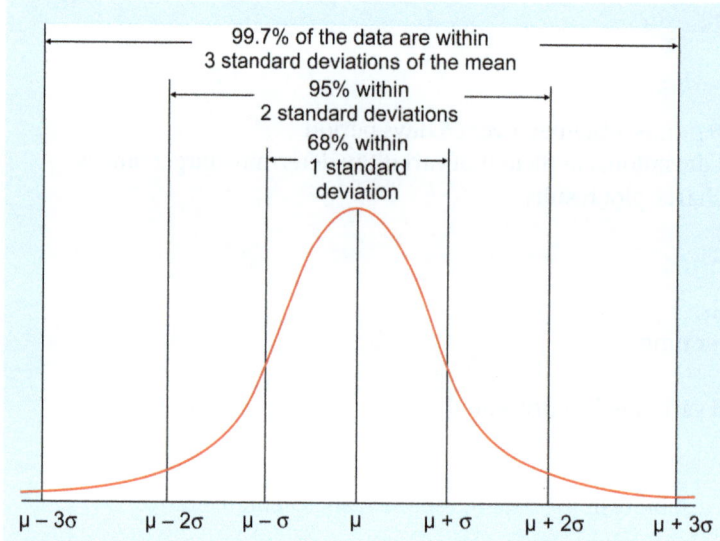

- In general, laboratories use the +/- 2 SD criteria for the limits of the acceptable range for a test
- When the QC measurement falls within that range, there is 95.5% confidence that the measurement is correct
- Only 4.5% of the time will a value fall outside of that range due to chance; more likely it will be due to error.

Coefficient of Variation

- The coefficient of variation (CV) is the standard deviation (SD) expressed as a percentage of the mean.
- Ideally should be less than 5%.

$$CV = \frac{SD}{Mean} \times 100$$

Mode to Mode

A selected specimen is run in both primary and secondary mode and results must fall within a specified limit.

In Case – "Control Out of Range"

Ensure the control

- Material was mixed properly
- Identification information, setup information, the current lot number is entered correctly
- Ensure the control material was not contaminated.

SPECIMEN-RELATED PROBLEMS

A specimen-related problem can be differentiated from an instrument problem by running a control. If the control results are acceptable, the problem is probably specimen-related. Check for:
- Clots
- Hemolysis
- Lipemia.

INSTRUMENT PROBLEMS AND TROUBLESHOOTING

- If the control shows similar problems, it indicates an instrument problem.
  - Electronic
  - Software/hardware
  - Pneumatic/hydraulic
  - Reagent.
- The subsystems are usually checked in the following order: Electronic, pneumatic/hydraulic, reagent.

Electronic Troubleshooting

- Detecting a problem in the electronic subsystem—or eliminating the electronic subsystem as the source of the problem—is simplified by indicators and electronic tests.
- Correcting electronic problems:
  - Minor problems, such as loose cables.
  - Most electronic problems require the assistance of your instrument service representative.

Pneumatic/Hydraulic Troubleshooting

- Try to identify a symptom of a malfunction, try to isolate the malfunction to the specific part of the cycle
- Then, try to isolate the malfunction to the specific components and tubing
- Next, look for one of four possible problems—Pinched tubing, plugs, leaks, or defective components.

Reagent Troubleshooting

Check the reagent containers for:
- Sufficient quantity
- Not beyond expiration date
- No precipitates, turbidity, particulate matter, or unusual color
- Proper connections between the instrument and the reagent containers.

Reagent problems can be corrected by:
- Changing the container of the reagent
- Priming the instrument with the new reagent.

Check the waste container for:
- Sufficient capacity
- Proper connections.

Flagging Signal

Parameter Errors

- Multiple flags may be generated for the entire CBC
- Usually, flags are displayed next to a specific result
- For example, an "H" indicates high results, while an "L" indicates low results
- If automated complete blood count (CBC) results present a flagging signal, operations must be performed to validate this sample. Manual methods, e.g. adding a differential count or manual slide review may be needed
- Technologists should be vigilant when hematological data are flagged because it almost always means that the sample has some abnormality
- Sometimes the histogram may show the following symbols, ***or----***, indicates that there may be sample aspiration errors or the results are exceeding the countable range
- This symbol—indicates suppressed parameter data, when histogram error codes occur. A visual analysis or manual discriminator adjustment can be done when this appears
- A manual reference method must be used in such situations for confirmation.

Critical Results

- Critical results are those results that markedly exceed or are decreased from the reference range
- These results are usually flagged by the automated instrument
- It is essential that the treating physician must be notified immediately by a member of the reporting laboratory, as many critical results involve immediate medical or patient care decisions.

SOURCES OF ERROR IN CELL COUNTS

- **Cold agglutinins may result into:**
  - Low RBC counts
  - High MCV
  - Incorrect hematocrit and MCHC
  - The right side of the red cell histogram shows an additional bump.

- **Fragmented or very microcytic red cells may result into:**
  - Decreased red cell counts
  - Flagging of the platelet count as the red cells become closer in size to the platelets and cause an abnormal platelet histogram
  - The population is visible at the left side of the red cell histogram and the right end of the platelet histogram.
- **Platelet clumps and platelet satellitisms may result into:**
  - Falsely decreased platelet counts. Platelet clumps can be seen on the right side of the platelet histogram.
- **Giant platelets may result into:**
  - The right-hand tail of the histogram remains elevated and may be seen at the left of the red cell histogram (if platelets approach or exceed the size of the red cells).
- **Nucleated red blood cells presence may result into:**
  - Interference with the WBC being counted as white cells/lymphocytes
  - WBC histogram alteration.

QUALITY CONTROL—REVIEW OF HISTOGRAMS

Variations Observed in RBC Histogram

Variations observed	Possible cause	What to do
Left of curve does not touch baseline	Schistocytes and extremely small red cells	Review smear CBC and platelet histogram
Bimodal peak	Transfused cells, therapeutic response	Review smear
Right portion of curve extended	Red cell autoagglutination	Review CBC and smear
Left shift of curve	Microcytes	Review smear and CBC
Right shift of curve	Macrocytes	Review smear and CBC

VARIATIONS OBSERVED IN WBC HISTOGRAM

Variations observed	Possible cause	What to do
Trail extending downward at extreme left, or lymph peak not starting at baseline	NRBC, pit clumping, unlyzed RBC, cryoproteins, parasites	Review smear and correct WBC for NRBC
Peak to the left of lymph peak or widening of lymph peak towards left	NRBC	Review smear and correct WBC for NRBC
Widening of lymph peak to right	Atypical lymphs, blasts, plasma cells, hairy cells, eosinophilia, basophilia	Review smear
Wider mono peak	Monocytosis, plasma cells, eosinophils, basophilia, blasts	Review smear
WBC histogram (lymph peak) does not start at baseline	Giant platelets, NRBC, pit clumping	Review smear, correct WBC for NRBC
Elevation of left portion of granulocyte	Left shift	Review smear
Elevation of right portion of granulocyte peak	Neutrophilia	Review smear

VARIATIONS OBSERVED IN PLATELET HISTOGRAM

Variations observed	Possible cause	What to do
Peak or spike at left end of histogram (2-8 ft)	Cytoplasmic fragments	Review smear
Spike towards right end of histogram	Schistocytes, microcytes, giant platelets	Review smear + CBC (↓MCV and ↑RDW) (↑MPV and ↑PDW)
Bimodal peak	Cytoplasmic fragments	Review smear

Abnormalities caused by artifacts							
Item	RBC	HB	Hct	MCV	MCH	MCHC	Artifacts appear on histogram
Red cell fragmentation	↓	↑	↓	↓	↑	↑	< 80 fL
Lymphocyte	↑	N	↑	↑	↓	↓	> 180 fL
Red cell agglutination	↑	N	↓	↑	↑	↑	150–170 fL
Hyperglycemia	N	N	↑	↑	N	↓	–
Free plasma hemoglobin	N	↑	N	N	↑	↑	–

Handling abnormal results

Platelets <40,000
- Check the integrity of the specimen (look for clots, short, etc.)
- Rule out pseudothrombocytopenia of EDTA
- Confirm count with smear review for clumps, RBC fragments, giant platelets, very small RBCs

WBC ++++
- Dilute 1:2 with isoton or further until count is within linearity (for the final result, multiply the diluted result by dilution factor)
- Do not report Hb, MCH, and MCHC as it may be erroneous. Add comment, "Unable to report Hb, MCH and MCHC due to very high WBC"
- Platelet counts are not affected by high WBC

PLT ++++
Check smear for RBC fragments or microcytes:
- If present, perform plt estimate. If they do not agree, perform manual plt count
- If not present, dilute specimen 1:2 with isoton or further until count is within linearity, multiply diluted result by dilution factor.

RBC > 7.0
- Dilute 1:2 with isoton or further until the count is within linearity, multiply the dilution result by dilution factor
- Perform spun Hct, review Hb, recalculate MCH, MCHC

MCHC> 36.5
- Decreased MCHC may be caused by swollen hyperglycemic red cell
- Perform isoton replacement or correct values using spun Hct
- Check the smear for spherocytes or lyse resistant red cells
- Check plasma for lipemia, icteremia interference If present, perform isoton replacement
- If MCHC significantly higher, check the specimen for cold agglutinin by looking for RBC clumping. If present, warm the specimen at 37°C for 5 minutes, mix well, and repeat
- If results are acceptable, report. If cold agglutinin persists, report the spun Hct and mark through, MCV, MCH, MCHC results
- Add comment, "specimen warmed before running"

Low plat, giant plat or EDTA clumps
Confirm with smear review:
- If clumps are present, recollect in blue top tube (Na citrate anticoagulant). If platelet count improves and clumps disappear (EDTA effect)
- If there are no clumps, but giant platelets are present, perform manual platelet count and smear estimate

Suggested Reading

1. ADVIA Haematology Systems: A Guide to Cytogram Interpretation by Graham Gibbs, 2014.
2. Automated Hematology Analyzer: Characteristic Patterns in Common Hematological Conditions, Lab Medicine, 2009;40:549-55.
3. Bain BJ. Blood Cells: A Practical Guide (5th Edn), Wiley Blackwell, 2015.
4. Bessman JD. Automated Blood Counts and Differentials MLAB 1315 Hematology.
5. Bessman JD, Feinstein DI. Quantitative anisocytosis as a discriminant between iron deficiency and thalassemia minor. Blood 1979;53:288-93.
6. Bessman JD, Gilmer PR, Gardner FH. Improved classification of anemias by MCV and RDW. Am J Clin Pathol. 1983;80:322-6.
7. Bessman JD, Gilmer PR, Gardner FH. Too early to put down RDW for discriminating iron deficiency and thalassemia. Am J Clin Pathol. 1986.
8. Betty Ciesla. Hematology in Practice (2nd Edn), FA Davis, 2011.
9. Cell counter User/Operation Manual of Mindray Medical International Limited, Sysmax Corporation, Abbott Laboratories, Beckman Coulter Diagnostics, Siemens Diagnostics, Merck (Medonic).
10. CLS 2523 hematology I. Automated Cell Counting and Evaluation, 2003.
11. Cornbelt J. Spurious results from automated hematology cell counters. Lab Med. 1983;14.
12. Gillian Rozenberg. Microscopic Hematology (3rd Edn), Elsevier, 2010.
13. Gottfried EL. Erythrocyte indexes with the electronic counter. N Engl J Med. 1979;300.
14. Harrison's Principles of Internal Medicine, 17th Edition, 2008.
15. Iron deficiency anemia in nonanemic subjects. JAMA. 1985;253:1021-3.
16. Johnson CS, Tegos C, Beutler E. Thalassemia minor routine erythrocyte measurements and differentiation from iron deficiency. Am J Clin Pathol. 1983;80(1):31-6.
17. MB Agarwal. Hematology Today 2007, 2008, 2009, 2010, 2011, 2012, 2013.
18. McClure S, Custer E, Bessman JD. Improved detection of early iron deficiency anemia in non-anemic subjects. JAMA 1985; 253: 1021-23.
19. Michelson A. Platelets, 3rd Edition. Elsevier, 2013.
20. Payne BA, Pierre RV, Morris MA. Use of instruments to obtain red blood cell profiles. J Med Tech. 1985;2:379-88.152.
21. Raimondi F, Ferrara, Capasso L, et al. Automated determination of neutrophil volume as a screening test for late-onset sepsis in very low birth infants.Pediatr Infect Dis J. 2010;29:288.
22. Rose MS. Epitaph for the MCHC. Br J Med. 1971;4:169.
23. Williams WJ. Examination of the blood. In: Williams WJ, Beutler E, Erslev AJ, Lichtman MA (Eds). Hematology, 3rd Edition. New York: McGraw-Hill, 1983;9-14.
24. Wintrobe MM. Principles of hematologic examination. In: Wintrobe MM (Ed). Clinical Hematology, 8th Edition. Philadelphia: Lea and Febiger, 1981.
25. Wintrobe's Clinical Hematology, 14th Edition, Wolters Kluwer, 2018.

Index

A

Abciximab 51
Abetalipoproteinemia 6, 21
ABO incompatibility 22
Acanthocytes 24
Acquired immunodeficiency syndrome 36
Acquired storage pool deficiency 53
Acridine orange 29
Acute coronary syndrome 57
Afibrinogenemia, congenital 53
African sleeping sickness 34
Aggregation defects 53
Agranulocytes 35
Alcoholism 13, 20, 53
Allergic disorders 149
Allergic reactions 36
Allergy 36
Alpha thalassemia, heterozygous 128
Alpha-granule deficiency 54
Amino acids 5
Amyloidosis, systemic 21
Anabolic metabolism 6
Androgens 5
Anemia 10, 13, 17
    advanced megaloblastic 88
    aplastic 6, 10, 13, 36, 40, 45, 51, 55, 56, 94, 136, 137, 148
    autoimmune hemolytic 14, 22
    chronic macrocytic 132
    diagnosis of 3
    dimorphic 13, 100
    drugs-induced chronic macrocytic 132
    dual deficiency 106
    dyserythropoietic 23, 25
    early megaloblastic 88
    hemolytic 3, 5, 10, 24, 38, 133
    hypochromic microcytic 14
    hypoplastic 148
    hypoproliferative 16
    macrocytic 6, 13, 14, 26
    megaloblastic 6, 10, 13, 22, 23, 25, 55, 56, 88–90, 106, 130, 131, 148
    microangiopathic hemolytic 6, 21, 22, 51
    microcytic 14
    mixed nutritional deficiency 133
    nonmegaloblastic macrocytic 13
    normocytic 13, 14
    pernicious 6, 13, 26, 130
    schistocytic hemolytic 21
    severe 26
Anisocytosis 20, 79, 141, 145
Antibiotics 53
Antibody-synthesizing lymphocytes 49
Anticonvulsants 13
Anti-inflammatory agents 53
Antimicrobials 13
Antiplatelet antibodies 53
Antitumor agents 13
Aorta, coarctation of 21
Aplasia 12
Auer bodies 41
Auer rod 41
Autoagglutination 14
Autoimmune disease 53
Automated cell counters, advantage of 70

B

Babesiosis 34
Bacterial infection 35, 38, 118
Baso channel 119
Baso cytogram 118, 120-122, 143–147
    method 118
Basophils 1, 44, 117
Bell cells 21
Bernard-Soulier
    disease 54, 55
    syndrome 52, 53
Beta thalassemia
    heterozygous 75
    major 106, 126
    minor 127
    trait 106
Bite cell 23
Bleeding
    disorders 3
    manifestation 51
    peptic ulcer 22
    severe 51
Blood
    cell 6, 66
    dyscrasias 16
    films 27, 28
        examination 33
    loss 5, 6, 12
        acute 6, 16, 53
        chronic 6
    low oxygen level in 12
    transfusion 75, 106
Bone marrow 36, 144
    aplasia 3
    aspirate 141
    failure 12, 56
    hypoplasia 51
    infiltration 51
    production defect 16
    replacement 25
    stimulation 25
    studies 16
Brugia
    malayi 33
    timori 33
Burns 21, 22, 40
    injury 38
Burr cells 22

C

Cabot rings 26
Calcium mobilization 53
Cancer, metastatic 38
Capillary blood method 33
Capillary tube method 33
Carboxyhemoglobin 7
Carcinomatosis, disseminated 21
Cardiac patch 21
Cardiac valve, abnormal 21
Cathodal proteins 26
Celiac disease 13
Cell
    counts 161
    cytogram, cell distribution of 116
    size 68
    structure density 68
    volume 68
Chagas disease 34
Chédiak-Higashi syndrome 41, 53
Chemotherapy 36, 51, 55, 56, 124
Chromatin 37, 38, 44, 46
Chronic disease, anemia of 10, 13, 20, 87, 128
Cirrhosis 10, 53
Clonal overproduction 53
Coagulopathy 153
Cobalt 5
Cold agglutinin 14, 52, 106, 135
    disease 75
Collagen
    diseases 45
    vascular disease 12, 38
Comma-shaped cytogram 96, 127
Complete blood
    cell 61
    count 1–3, 31
Composite platelet index 58
Conductivity 68, 115
Connective tissue
    diseases 26
    disorder 21
Cor pulmonale 12
Corticosteroids 38
COVID-19 49
Crohn's disease 45
Cyanmethemoglobin method 7
Cyclooxygenase deficiency 53
Cyclophosphamide 13
Cytochemistry 144, 145
Cytogram 2, 80, 101, 126, 127, 131, 133, 135, 138, 146, 150
Cytomegalovirus 25, 51
Cytoplasm 37, 38, 44–46
Cytotoxic chemotherapy 129, 148

D

Dacryocyte 21
Degmacyte 23
Dehydration 6, 12, 22
Dengue 36, 55, 57, 122
    hemorrhagic fever 12
Di Guglielmo disease 13
Diabetes mellitus 26
Diarrhea
    bloody 51
    severe 12
Disseminated intravascular coagulation 6, 21, 51, 52, 57
Döhle body 40
Dracunculus medinensis 33
Drugs 36, 53
    allergy 149
    reactions 40
Dysproteinemias 53

E

Echinocytes 22
Eclampsia 38
Electronic impedance 68
    Coulter's concept of 64
Elliptocytosis, hereditary 6, 22

Emphysema 6
Endocarditis, subacute bacterial 45
Endocrine disorders, anemia of 6
Enzyme deficiencies 6
Eosinopenia 44
Eosinophil 44, 117
Eosinophilia 44, 119, 149
Epinephrine 53
Epstein-Barr virus 51
Erythroblastosis fetalis 10
Erythroblasts, maturation of 6
Erythrocyte 5
    fragmented 56
    volume
        fraction 11
        histogram for 76
Erythroid hyperplasia 16
Erythropoiesis, ineffective 16
Erythropoietin deficiency 6, 12
Ethanol 51
Ethylenediaminetetraacetic acid 52, 61, 150
Exercise 53

F

Fanconi anemia 6
Ferritin 16
Fever 51
Fibrosis 51
    pulmonary 6, 12
Filaria 3
Filariasis 33
    subcutaneous 33
Fistula 13
Flow cytometry 80, 145
    fluorescent dyes augmentation of 67
    role of 66, 70
Fluid overload 5
Fluorescence flow cytometry 115
Fluorescent microscopy 29
    after centrifugation 29
Folate 5
    deficiency 13, 20, 36
        anemia 75, 129
        nutritional deficiencies of 12
Folic acid 3, 10
Free plasma hemoglobin 163
Fungal infection 25

G

Gametocyte 28, 29
Gastrointestinal tract lesions 6
Gaucher disease 53
Gaussian
    curve 159
    distribution 73, 159
Giant platelets 52, 162
Giemsa stain 27
Glanzmann thrombasthenia 53
Glomerulonephritis 21
Glucose-6-phosphate dehydrogenase deficiency 6, 21, 23
Glycolysis, defective 6
Golgi apparatus 47
Gram-negative bacterial infection 53
Granular lymphocyte 47
Granulocytes 35
    immature 43, 120
Granulomas 6, 51
Gray platelet syndrome 53, 54
Guinea worm 33
Gynecologic disturbances 6

H

Hairy cell leukemia 36, 45
Heart
    diseases 6, 12
    failure 6
    surgery 6
    valve prosthesis 55
Heinz bodies 23, 24
HELLP syndrome 59
Hematinic treatment 75
Hematocrit 11, 14, 64
    calculation of 2
    normal range 11
Hematological scoring system 39
    interpretation of 39
Hematology 1, 73
    automated cell analyser, basic components of 65
    automation 63
        general principles of 63
Hematopoiesis, extramedullary 25
Heme synthesis 6
Hemocytometer 62
Hemodilution 5
Hemoglobin 7, 9, 14, 64, 102
    concentration 7
    distribution width 2, 17
    measurement of 2, 8
    normal range 7
Hemoglobinopathies 3, 6, 13, 20, 21, 26
Hemolysis 12, 14, 53
Hemolytic
    disease 6, 134
    disorders 6
    uremic syndrome 21, 51
Hemoparasites 27
Hemorrhage 10, 12, 13, 38, 53
Heparin 51
Hepatitis 49, 51
Heterozygote 21
Hexokinase deficiencies 6
High fluorescence reticulocyte 10
High heparin concentration 14
High red blood cell count, causes of 6
High white blood cell counts, causes of 35
High-frequency radio wave 67
Histogram 2, 71, 73, 101, 126, 127, 139, 140
    generation, general principles of 71
    interpretation of 72
    review of 162
Hodgkin's lymphoma 36
Homozygote 21
Howell-Jolly bodies 23
Human immunodeficiency virus infection 36, 51
Hydroxyurea 13
Hyperadrenocorticism 45
Hypereosinophilic syndrome 40, 149
Hyperglycemia 105, 163
Hyperlipidemia 8
Hypersegmentation 40
Hypersensitivity reaction 38
Hypersplenism 22, 52, 53, 55
Hypertension
    malignant 21
    portal 53
Hyperthyroidism 55
Hypervolemia 6
Hypoadrenalism 13
Hypochromic cell 20, 84
Hypogonadism 13
Hypopituitarism 13
Hypoplasia 12
    megakaryocytic 55
Hyposplenia 23
Hypothyroidism 13, 20, 24
    anemia of 13
Hypoxia 10, 25

I

Idiopathic thrombocytopenic purpura 55, 152
Immature platelet fraction 2, 56, 57
    benefits of 57
Immature reticulocyte fraction 11
Immune
    hemolytic anemia 92, 93, 129
    thrombocytopenia purpura 52, 57
Impaired red blood cell production 5
Infections 6, 42, 51–53
    acute 26
    chronic 13, 26, 35
    congenital 25
    malarial 31
    mycobacterial 25
    parasitic 149
    severe 40
Inflammation 38
    chronic 6, 45
    non-infectious 53
Inflammatory disorders 151
Influenza 36
International Council for Standardization in Hematology 7
Intestinal resection 13
Iron 3, 5, 10
    deficiency 85, 86
        advanced 84
        anemia 6, 20, 22, 23, 53, 75, 106, 125, 128, 151
        early 83
        severe 21
    nutritional deficiencies of 12
    serum 16

J

Jaundice, alcoholic 26

K

Ketoacidosis 38
Kidney disease 10, 12

L

Laser
    light
        application of 66
        scatter 67
    technology 68, 80
Lead
    poisoning 24, 26
    toxicity 26
Leishman stain 34
Leishmania 3
Leishmaniasis 33
Leukemia 10, 12, 26, 36, 51
    acute
        lymphatic 145
        lymphoblastic 139
        lymphocytic 36, 121, 139
        myelogenous 121
        myeloid 36, 142, 143
    chronic
        granulocytic 53, 151
        lymphocytic 36, 53, 102, 122, 143

myelogenous 36, 56
myeloid 53
myelocytic 38
promyelocytic 121
Leukemoid reaction, causes of 42
Leukocyte
　alkaline phosphatase score 42
　maturation, stages of 36
　mononuclear 35
Leukocytosis 14, 35, 38, 118
Leukoerythroblastic reaction 21, 22, 25
Leukopenia 35, 119
Levey Jennings chart 156
Light absorption 68
Lipemia 14
Lipoxygenase deficiency 53
Lithium 38
Liver
　cirrhosis 21
　disease 13, 20–22, 25, 26, 129
　disorders 53
Low fluorescence reticulocyte 10
Low white cell counts, causes of 36
Lung diseases 6
Lupus erythematosus 12
Lymphatic filariasis 33
Lymphoblast 46
Lymphocyte 46, 47, 117, 163
　activation 49
　atypical 48
　reactive 49
Lymphocytosis 49
Lymphoma 48
　spillage 36
Lymphopenia 49
Lymphoproliferative
　disorders 51
　solid tumors, spillage of 3

M

Macrocytes 99
Macrocytic red cells 20
Macroglobulinemia 26
Malabsorption 24
Malaria 3, 6, 22, 27, 36, 51, 55
　antigen detection 31
　detection, automation based 31
　diagnosis of 27
　parasite 27
　serology-antibody detection 30
Malignancy 26, 40, 51, 53, 149
　metastatic 3
Malignant cells 36
Malnutrition 12
Manganese 5
Mansonella
　ozzardi 33
　perstans 33
　streptocerca 33
Manual reticulocyte count 9
Marrow
　aplasia 16
　depression, drugs-induced 148
Maturation disorder 16
May-Hegglin
　anomaly 51, 55
　disease 54
Mean cell hemoglobin concentration 64
Mean corpuscular
　hemoglobin 13, 14
　　concentration 13, 14

volume 13, 15, 76
　normal range 13
Mean platelet
　component 57
　mass 57
　volume 2, 52, 55, 57, 64, 113
Measles 36
Mediterranean macrothrombocytopenia, benign 52
Medium fluorescence reticulocyte 10
Megathrombocyte 52
Membrane
　filtration 33
　lipids 6
　skeleton proteins 6
Mentzer index 85
Metamyelocyte 37
Metastasis 51
Methemoglobin 7
Methotrexate 13
Microcytes 99
Microfilaria, appearance of 33
Microhematocrit tube 33
Mismatch transfusion reactions 6
Monoclonal gammopathy 141
Monoclonal proteins 14
Monocytes 117
Monocytopenia 45
Monocytosis 45
Mononuclear cells, positions of 118
Mononucleosis, infectious 45, 146
Multiple angle polarized scatter separation 66
Myeloblast 36
Myelocyte 37
Myelodysplasia 52, 55, 133, 147
Myelodysplastic syndrome 3, 6, 13, 16, 20, 24, 51, 53, 57, 120
Myelofibrosis 36, 104, 133
　idiopathic 53
Myeloid metaplasia 38
Myeloma, multiple 12, 26, 48, 141
Myelophthisic anemia 6, 13
Myelophthisis 6
Myeloproliferative disorders 16, 21, 38, 52, 53, 55
Myocardial infarction 38, 50

N

Neonatal sepsis, early diagnosis of 39
Neoplasms 13, 42
Neutropenia, causes of 39
Neutrophil 117, 120
　apparent absence of 139
　dysplasia 118
　granularity
　　index 43
　　intensity 43
　reactivity intensity 43
　volume 43
Neutrophilia 38, 45
Nonmegaloblastic macrocytosis 106
Normal red blood cells values 5
Nuclear chromatin 45
Nuclear density analysis 118
Nucleus 44
Nutritional deficiencies 3, 12

O

Onchocerca volvulus 33
Oral contraceptives 13
Organ failure 16
Ovarian tumor 124
Oxidative stress 6

P

Packed cell volume 11
Pantothenic acid 5
Pappenheimer bodies 24
Parasitemia 3, 27
Paroxysmal nocturnal hemoglobinuria 6
Pelger-Huët anomaly 41
Penicillins 51
Peripheral blood smear 141
　examination 18, 27
　preparation 18
Peripheral smear 63, 132, 143, 147
　examination 58
Perox cytogram 117, 120–122, 144, 147
　method 117
Peroxidase
　activity 118
　staining 115, 117
Phenytoin 13
Plasma
　cell 47
　protein 8
Plasmacytoid lymphocyte 48
Plasmodium
　antigens, detection of 30
　falciparum 27
　malariae 27
　ovale 27
　vivax 27
　　appearance of 28
Platelet 50, 124–153, 163
　adhesion defects 53
　agglutination 52, 150
　clumps 162
　component distribution width 58
　count 2, 50, 51, 63
　derived histograms 113
　destructions 52
　disorders of 54
　distribution
　　curves 113
　　width 56, 113
　function defects 53
　histogram 107, 113, 162
　index 113
　lineage 58
　parameters 3, 4
　production 51
　　selective marrow suppression of 51
　satellitism 52, 162
　scattergram 122
　volume histogram for 113
Pleomorphic plasma cells 141
Poikilocytosis 20
Polychromasia 25
Polychromatophilia 25
Polycythemia vera 6, 12, 36, 38, 53, 151
Polymerase chain reaction 31
Polymorphonuclear
　cells 118
　leukocytes 35
Polymorphs 38
Postradiation marrow depression 148
Post-splenectomy 13, 21, 23–25
Post-therapy megaloblastic anemia 131
Post-transfusion 22
　purpura 51
　sample 138
Pregnancy 10, 16, 58
　macrocytic anemia of 13

Prematurity, anemia of 6
Primidone 13
Progranulocyte 37
Prolymphocyte 46
Promyelocyte 37
Prosthetic
  cardiac valve 21
  valve surgery 6
Pseudoleukopenia 36
Pseudo-Pelger-Huët anomaly 41
Pseudothrombocytopenia 52, 150
Psittacosis 36
Pure red cell aplasia 6
Pyrimethamine 13
Pyruvate kinase deficiency 6, 22

Q

Quality control 154, 162
  data, analysis of 159
  direct 155
  external 158
  indirect 154
  internal 154, 155
  methods 158
  monitoring 154
  purpose of 154
Quantitative buffy coat 29
Quinine 51

R

Radiation 51
  therapy 36
Radiofrequency 1, 68, 115
Real-time polymerase chain reaction 31
Red blood cell 2, 5, 62, 124–153
  anisocytosis 79
  count 2
  cytogram 75, 80, 83, 84, 91, 92, 94, 98, 104, 125, 129, 136
  fragmentation 90, 91
  histogram 75, 82, 125, 162
    abnormal 77
  hyperchromia 80
  lineage 58
  macrocytosis 78
  maturation defect 16
  microcytosis 78
  morphology 145
    clinical importance of 19
  nucleated 25, 162
  parameters 3, 4
Red cell
  agglutination 163
  agglutinins 101
  count 63
  cytogram 88, 100, 130, 132
  distribution width 2, 15, 17
  double populations of 75
  fragmentation 91, 133, 163
Renal disease, end-stage 10
Renal failure 16, 22, 51
  acute 38
  anemia of 6
Renal insufficiency 51
Renal neoplasia 6
Reticulocyte 9
  count 10, 69
    automated 9
    normal range of 9
  hemoglobin 2
    measurement 10

production 16
proliferation index 10
Rheumatoid
  arthritis 12, 36, 53
  disease 45
Riboflavin 5
Rickettsial infections 36
Rouleaux formation 26, 141
Rubella 25
Rule of three 12

S

Sahli acid hematin method 8
Sarcoidosis 45
Schistocytes 21
Sepsis 25, 36, 55, 57, 118
  postoperative 140
  severe 148
Septicemia 140
Serum immunoglobulin electrophoresis 141
Sickle cell 25
  anemia 3, 6, 14, 55, 97, 129
Sickle crisis 129
Sideroblastic anemia 13, 20, 24, 99, 133
Siderotic granules 24
Small lymphocyte 46
Smudge cell 48, 143
Spherocytes 22
Spherocytosis 106
  causes of 22
  hereditary 6, 14, 22, 23
Spheroschistocytes 21
Spleen
  enlargement of 36
  hyperfunction 12
Splenectomy 24, 38, 53, 55, 151
Spur cell 24
Steatorrhea 13
Stem cells 6
Stomach cancer 22
Stomatocyte 23
Storage pool disease 53, 55
Stress 35, 45
  physical 35
Sulfamethoxazole 13
Sulfasalazine 13
Syphilis, congenital 25
Systemic lupus erythematosus 21, 36, 45, 51, 53

T

Tear drop cells 21
Thalassemia 3, 6, 10, 21, 25, 26
  heterozygous 96, 128
  major 21, 22
  minor 20
  trait 128
Thiamine 5
Thrombasthenia 53
Thrombocytes 50
Thrombocythemia
  essential 53, 54, 56, 57, 151
  primary 53, 54, 151
Thrombocytopenia 3, 51–53, 57, 58
  absent radii syndrome 51, 55
  amegakaryocytic 51
  causes of 51, 58
  drugs-induced 51
  gestational 59
  idiopathic 51
  infection-related 55

mild 53
severe 51
Thrombocytopenic purpura 152
Thrombocytosis 53
  reactive 57
Thrombopoiesis 56
Thrombotic thrombocytopenic purpura 21, 51, 52, 54, 57
Thromboxane
  A2 receptor deficiency 53
  synthetase deficiency 53
Thyroid hormone 5
Tissue
  damage 35
  injury 38
Toxic granulation 40, 145
Toxins 51
Transfusion therapy 24
Trauma 6
Trimethoprim 13
Trophozoite 27, 28
Trypanosoma
  brucei 34
  cruzi 34
Tuberculosis 36, 45
Tubular necrosis, acute 21
Tumors, malignant 6
Typhoid 36

U

Ulcerative colitis 45
Uremia 13, 21, 25, 53

V

Vasculitis 51
Venous blood method 33
Viral infections 35, 45, 48, 53, 122
Vitamin
  B_{12} 3, 5, 10, 13, 20, 75, 129
    deficiency 6, 130, 131
    impaired absorption of 6
  B_6, nutritional deficiencies of 12
  E deficiency 24
Volume conductivity scatter technology 115
von Willebrand disease 51, 53

W

Waldenström's macroglobulinemia 48
Water-dilution hemolysis 22
Westgard rules 156–158
White blood cell 2, 31, 35, 107, 124–153
  count 2, 35, 63
  histogram
    abnormal 108
    types of 111
  lineage 58
  parameters 3, 4
  volume histogram for 107
Wiskott-Aldrich syndrome 51, 53, 55
Wuchereria bancrofti 33

X

X-linked lymphoproliferative disease 49

Y

Y-axis 80

Z

Zidovudine 13

EU GSPR Authorised Reprsentative
Logos Europe, 9 rue Nicolas Poussin
1700, La Rochelle, France
Phone: +33 (0) 6 67 93 73 78
E-mail: contact@logoseurope.eu

www.ingramcontent.com/pod-product-compliance
Ingram Content Group UK Ltd.
Pitfield, Milton Keynes, MK11 3LW, UK
UKHW050431150426
5217IPUK00019B/1335